STRATEGIC MARKETING FOR HEALTH CARE ORGANIZATIONS

JB JOSSEY-BASS

STRATEGIC MARKETING FOR HEALTH CARE ORGANIZATIONS

Building a Customer-Driven Health System

**PHILIP KOTLER,
JOEL SHALOWITZ,
AND ROBERT J. STEVENS**

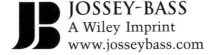

JOSSEY-BASS
A Wiley Imprint
www.josseybass.com

Published by Jossey-Bass
A Wiley Imprint
989 Market Street, San Francisco, CA 94103-1741—www.josseybass.com

Readers should be aware that Internet Web sites offered as citations and/or sources for further information may have changed or disappeared between the time this was written and when it is read.

Limit of Liability/Disclaimer of Warranty: While the publisher and author have used their best efforts in preparing this book, they make no representations or warranties with respect to the accuracy or completeness of the contents of this book and specifically disclaim any implied warranties of merchantability or fitness for a particular purpose. No warranty may be created or extended by sales representatives or written sales materials. The advice and strategies contained herein may not be suitable for your situation. You should consult with a professional where appropriate. Neither the publisher nor author shall be liable for any loss of profit or any other commercial damages, including but not limited to special, incidental, consequential, or other damages.

Jossey-Bass books and products are available through most bookstores. To contact Jossey-Bass directly call our Customer Care Department within the U.S. at 800-956-7739, outside the U.S. at 317-572-3986, or fax 317-572-4002.

Jossey-Bass also publishes its books in a variety of electronic formats. Some content that appears in print may not be available in electronic books.

Library of Congress Cataloging-in-Publication Data

Kotler, Philip.
  Strategic marketing for health care organizations: building a
customer-driven health system/Philip Kotler, Joel Shalowitz, and
Robert J. Stevens.–1st ed.
      p.; cm.
  Includes bibliographical references and index.
  ISBN 978-0-7879-8496-0 (cloth)
1. Medical care—United States—Marketing. I. Shalowitz, Joel,
1953- II. Stevens, Robert J. (Robert John), 1955- III. Title.
  [DNLM: 1. Marketing of Health Services—methods—United States.
2. Consumer Satisfaction—United States. W 74 AA1 K87s 2008]

RA410.56.K69 2008
362.1068′8—dc22

                                        2007049548

Printed in the United States of America
FIRST EDITION

HB Printing   10 9 8 7 6 5 4 3

CONTENTS

PART ONE

PART THREE

PART FOUR

TABLES, FIGURES, AND EXHIBITS

TABLES

FIGURES

EXHIBITS

To our new grandchildren, the triplets—Dante, Sapphire, and Shaina.
—Philip Kotler

To my wife, Madeleine Shalowitz, M.D., M.B.A., and children,
David, Kira, and Ilana.
—Joel Shalowitz

In memory of my late father, Jack, who inspired me to pursue a career in health
care marketing, and to Elizabeth, who has nurtured it.
—Robert J. Stevens

PREFACE

The U.S. health care system is broadly regarded as the best in the world. Affluent foreign patients needing challenging medical treatment choose to fly to our health care institutions, such as the Mayo Clinic, the Cleveland Clinic, the Massachusetts General Hospital, and Johns Hopkins Hospital.

While most U.S. health care institutions provide good-quality health care, we still have several glaring deficiencies. Consider the following six examples. First, an estimated forty-five million U.S. citizens are without health insurance. When they get ill, they cannot find the best treatment for their problem or even hope to pay the bill. Second, medical costs are highly variable and far from transparent; one finds it difficult to know in advance what a hernia operation or a knee replacement will actually cost. Third, the quality of health care varies greatly among different regions of the country and even within some counties. Fourth, the costs of care are high and rising, putting a heavy burden on average citizens as they are expected to bear more of these expenses. Fifth, Medicare and Medicaid, the two principal federal health care programs, are in financial trouble. Finally, the health system underinvests in preventive measures, such as encouraging lifestyle changes and early detection of medical problems.

Systematic health care problems are not unique to the United States. For example, in the U.K. and Canada, patients wait a long time for elective surgeries such as hip replacements. As a result of a 2001 European court decision, then-prime minister Tony Blair promised to pay for sending patients to other European countries to get more timely care. In less-developed countries, the problems are more severe: equipment, medicine, and qualified personnel are in short supply, facilities are poor, and costs of care are very high in relation to income levels.

To address these problems and identify new opportunities, we believe that health care leaders can improve their efficiency and effectiveness by taking a customer-driven view of their clients and activities. We wrote this book to serve the needs of all those who are or will be working in the health care system: physicians, nurses, medical researchers, hospital administrators, public health workers, nursing home personnel, and managers in the medical device, biotechnology, or pharmaceutical sectors. Ideally, all of these health care participants will supply products and services that enhance the health needs of citizens. To identify these needs and deliver their products and services, they will need to have marketing competencies.

Marketing is both a philosophy and a set of tools. As a philosophy, it calls for serving and satisfying the needs of customers (clients, citizens, and patients) while satisfying the practitioner's and organization's requirements. As a set of tools, marketing helps these participants learn about the market's and individual customer's needs, develop quality products and services, price them correctly, inform and communicate about their offerings, and make them accessible.

Our book is divided into four parts, following a managerial process.

- Part One (Chapters One to Four) deals with understanding the health care system and the role of marketing. We define a health care system, the providers and institutions it comprises, the determinants of health care utilization, and the role played by strategy and marketing planning.

- Part Two (Chapters Five to Eight) describes ways to analyze the users of the health care system. We explain how consumers and businesses make their health care decisions, how marketing information can be gathered, and how health care organizations can segment, target, and distinctively position their products and services within the health care marketplace.

- Part Three (Chapters Nine to Fourteen) examines the various tools of the marketing mix available to health care providers. The main tools are product and service development, branding, pricing, distribution, and communication and promotion.

- Part Four (Chapter Fifteen) explains how health care providers can organize their marketing resources, implement their marketing plans, and use control tools to reach their stated goals.

Along with this information, we provide several learning aids. For example, each chapter begins with a story that illustrates some aspect of the chapter's subject; we introduce additional stories and examples in various boxes and exhibits; and we conclude with a set of questions to stimulate further thought. Finally, we include a glossary following the last chapter.

Our hope is that this book will give you many concepts and tools that will enable you to be effective in your chosen field and make a strong contribution to the health of the nation.

March 2008

Philip Kotler
Glencoe, Illinois
Joel Shalowitz
Glencoe, Illinois
Robert J. Stevens
Durham, North Carolina

ACKNOWLEDGMENTS

We would like to acknowledge Dean Dipak Jain of the Kellogg School of Management, Northwestern University, for his support and encouragement of our project, Marge Kaffenberger for help in preparing some of the exhibits, and James Ward for help in gathering information. We would also like to acknowledge the many health care physicians, nurses, administrators, and health care company executives who were interviewed in the course of writing this book. Last but not least, we want to thank Andy Pasternack and Seth Schwartz of Jossey-Bass for their fine editorial help in guiding and producing this book.

THE AUTHORS

PHILIP KOTLER is S. C. Johnson Distinguished Professor of International Marketing at the Kellogg School of Management. He has been honored as one of the world's leading marketing thinkers. He received his M.A. degree in economics (1953) from the University of Chicago and his Ph.D. degree in economics (1956) from the Massachusetts Institute of Technology (M.I.T.). He has received honorary degrees from ten foreign universities. He is author of over one hundred articles and forty books, including *Marketing Management, Principles of Marketing, Marketing for Hospitality and Tourism, Strategic Marketing for Nonprofit Organizations, Social Marketing, Marketing Places, Museum Strategy and Marketing*, and *The Marketing of Nations*. His research covers strategic marketing, consumer marketing, business marketing, professional services marketing, and e-marketing. He has been a consultant to IBM, Merck, General Electric, AT&T, Bank of America, Motorola, Ford, and others.

JOEL SHALOWITZ is professor and director of the Health Industry Management Program at the Kellogg School of Management, Northwestern University. He is also professor of medicine and preventive medicine at Northwestern's Feinberg School of Medicine. He received his bachelor's and M.D. degrees from Brown University and completed his internal medicine residency and M.B.A. degree at Northwestern University. He currently teaches courses on the U.S. health care system as well as international health care systems. Dr. Shalowitz received a Fulbright Scholarship in 2004 to the Schulich Business School at York University in Toronto, where he is now a visiting professor. In 2007 he was a Fulbright Senior Specialist and visiting professor at Keio University Medical School in Tokyo. In addition to international health care, his current interests are health care quality and safety, health insurance, and cultural influences on health care. Honors have included election to Sigma Xi, Beta Gamma Sigma, and Fellowship in the American College of Physicians.

ROBERT J. STEVENS is president of Health Centric Marketing Services, a health care marketing research firm. He teaches health care marketing as an adjunct professor at the Kenan-Flagler Business School at the University of North Carolina–Chapel Hill, at the School of Public Health at the University of North Carolina–Chapel Hill, and at the Owen Graduate School of Management at Vanderbilt University. Stevens received a B.A. degree from Colgate University, an M.A. degree in English from

Duke University, and an M.B.A. degree from the Kellogg School of Management at Northwestern University. His background includes executive marketing positions with a health care consumer package goods company, a health care system, a publicly held physician staffing and billing company, and a publicly held physician information systems company.

PART

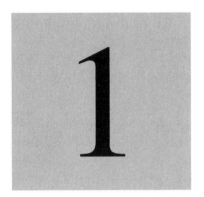

1

UNDERSTANDING THE HEALTH CARE SYSTEM AND THE ROLE OF MARKETING

CHAPTER

THE ROLE OF MARKETING IN HEALTH CARE ORGANIZATIONS

LEARNING OBJECTIVES

In this chapter, we will address the following questions:

1. What are the major areas in health care in which marketing is regularly applied and practiced?

2. What is the purpose of marketing thinking and planning in health care organizations?

3. What are the major concepts, tools, and skills in marketing?

4. How is marketing normally organized in health care organizations?

OVERVIEW: MARKETING IS PERVASIVE IN HEALTH CARE

Readers might find it strange to hear that marketing plays an important and pervasive role in the health care marketplace. They are probably aware of the marketing efforts of pharmaceutical and medical device companies to sell their branded products and services. But what about hospitals, nursing homes, hospices, physician practices, managed care organizations, rehabilitation centers, and other health care organizations?

These organizations, for the most part, didn't think about marketing until the early 1970s. But today we see a great deal of marketing taking place in health care organizations. Consider the following facts:

- Virtually every hospital places ads in newspapers and magazines to tout its facilities and services. Some hospitals run community health programs. Some hospital CEOs appear on talk shows. All of these efforts go toward building their brand.

- Managed care organizations (MCOs) develop health insurance products and use marketing tools to vie with other companies in promoting themselves to employers and their employees.

- New physicians seeking to open their own practices use marketing to help determine good locations, attractive office designs, and practice styles that will attract and retain new patients.

- The American Cancer Society, American Heart Association, and other associations turn to social marketing to encourage more people to adopt healthier life styles, like quitting smoking, cutting down on saturated fats in their diet, and increasing exercise.

These illustrations demonstrate one side of marketing, namely the use of influential advertising and selling to attract and retain customers. But marketing tasks and tools go beyond developing a stream of persuasive messages. Consider the following:

FOR EXAMPLE

Two Vignettes

A hospital is considering adding a sports medicine program to its portfolio of services. Before deciding whether to launch such a program, it plans to do market research to gauge the size of the community need, discover which competitors already offer such a program, consider how it will organize and deliver the program, understand how to price its various services, and determine how profitable the program is likely to be.

Walgreens is opening store-based clinics to provide basic health care services, such as measuring blood pressure, providing vaccinations, and treating such common conditions as sore throats, ear infections, and colds. Key marketing tasks it must perform include deciding which stores will have this service, setting prices, and, most important, determining how physician customers will view this service as possible competition.

From these examples, we recognize that many health sector participants are trying to solve their problems by relying on marketing tools and concepts. Readers who already work in the health care field may recognize some of these tasks as the realm of epidemiology; however, the discipline of marketing is much broader. The American Marketing Association offers the following definition: *Marketing is an organizational function and a set of processes for creating, communicating, and delivering value to customers and for managing customer relationships in ways that benefit the organization and its stakeholders*.

Marketing takes place when at least one party to a potential transaction thinks about the means of achieving desired responses from other parties. Thus marketing takes place when

- A physician puts out an advertisement describing his practice in the hope of attracting new patients.
- A hospital builds a state-of-the-art cancer center to attract more patients with this affliction.
- A health maintenance organization (HMO) improves the benefits of its health plan to attract more patients.
- A pharmaceutical firm hires more salespeople to gain physician acceptance and preference for a new drug.

- The American Medical Association lobbies Congress to gain support for a new bill.

- The Centers for Disease Control and Prevention (CDC) runs a campaign to get more people to get an annual flu shot.

- Health Canada develops a campaign to motivate more Canadians to exercise more and eat healthy foods.

Thus a marketer may aim to secure various responses: a purchase of a product or service; an increased awareness, interest, or preference toward an offering or supplier; a change in behavior; or a vote or expression of preference of some kind.

THE ELEMENTS OF MARKETING THOUGHT

In this section, we introduce the purpose of marketing, some important marketing concepts and skills, and how marketing is organized in health care organizations. We will discuss these topics in greater depth in the following chapters.

The Purpose of Marketing

There are two quite different opinions about marketing's purpose. One might be called the *transaction view*, which says that its aim is to get an order or make a sale. Marketing's role is, therefore, to use salesmanship and advertising to sell more "stuff."[1] The focus is on doing everything possible to stimulate a transaction.

The other opinion about marketing can be called the *customer relationship-building and satisfaction view*. Here the focus is more on the customer and less on the particular product or service. The marketer aims to serve the customer in such a way that he or she will be satisfied and come back for more services or products. In fact, the marketer hopes that the satisfaction will be sufficiently high that the customer will recommend the seller to others. For example, we know that a physician who develops an excellent service reputation will attract many new patients as a result of word-of-mouth recommendations. Also, as patients experience new medical needs and problems, they will return to the same physician for treatment and advice.

Some marketers question the use of terms such as *consumer* and *patient*. The traditional view of a consumer or patient is that of someone who is passively consuming something, but today's consumers are also producers. With respect to health care products and services, they are actively sending messages about their experiences, creating new uses, providing new findings from the Internet and other resources to their physicians, and lobbying for more and better benefits. Predicting this current environment, Peter Drucker viewed marketing as playing the role of serving as the customer's agent or representative.

In fact, more organizations are moving from the transaction view to the relationship view of marketing, in a shift from Old Marketing to New Marketing. In this environment, the New Marketer's job is to create a long-term, trusted, and valued relationship with customers, which means getting the whole organization to think about and serve customers and their interests. For instance, hospitals that have built a pervasive marketing culture will usually outperform those that see themselves simply as selling visits, tests, and services, one at a time.

Marketing Uses a Set of Concepts

The first question a health care organization must ask is, Who is potentially interested in the kind of products or services that we offer or plan to offer? Examples include young women and obstetric services, older adults and bypass surgery services, and diabetics and portable blood sugar testing devices. Very few organizations try to serve the entire market, preferring, instead, to distinguish different groups (segments) that make up a market. This distinguishing process is called *market segmentation*. The organization will then consider which market segments it can serve best in light of the segments' needs and the organization's capabilities. We call the chosen segment the *target market*. Building on this concept of a target market, we can summarize the customer-focused marketing philosophy with the acronym CCDV; the aim of marketing is to *create, communicate, and deliver value*. Value is the fundamental concept underlying modern marketing. It is not value just because the supplier believes he or she is giving value; it must be perceived by the customer. One job of the marketer is to turn invisible value into perceived value. We can extend CCDV into CCDVT, with the T standing for a *target market*. Instead of an organization generating general value, it aims to generate specific value for a well-defined target market. If a nursing home decides to serve a high-income market, it must create, communicate, and deliver the value expected by high-income families, with the price set high enough to cover the extra costs of better facilities and services.

We need to extend the expression further to CCDVTP, with the P standing for *profitably*. The marketing aim is to *create, communicate, and deliver value to a target market profitably*. Even a nonprofit organization must earn revenues in excess of expenses in order to continue its charitable mission.

To help their firms prepare a valued offering, marketers have long used a tools framework known as the 4Ps *marketing mix*: *product, price, place*, and *promotion*. The organization decides on a product (its features, benefits, styling, packaging), its price (including list price as well as rebate and discount programs), its place (namely, where it is available and its distribution strategies), and the promotion mix (such as advertising, personal selling, and direct marketing) (see Figure 1.1). It turns out that the 4Ps are already present in the CCDVT formulation. Creating value is very much about developing an excellent *product* and appropriate *price*. Communicating value involves *promotion*. Delivering value requires an understanding about *place*. Thus CCDV is a more active way to state the 4Ps. Some critics have also proposed adding more Ps (*people, passion, process*, and so on).

Marketers recognize that the 4Ps represent the set of the seller's decisions, not the buyer's decisions. Part of the transition from the Old Marketing to the New Marketing, mentioned previously, involves marketers looking at everything from the buyer's or consumer's point of view. For a consumer to be interested in an offering,

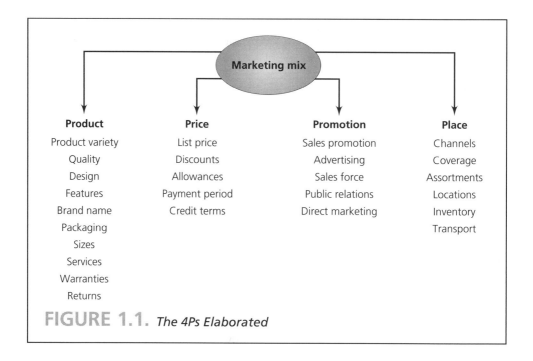

FIGURE 1.1. *The 4Ps Elaborated*

the consumer must have *awareness* of the offering and find it *acceptable*, *available* at the right time and place, and *affordable*. Professor Jagdish Sheth calls these attributes the "4As of marketing."[2]

We introduce one final concept—positioning. An organization or company positions itself to be the place of choice for its target market. Thus a hospital might position itself as having the most advanced medicine or the best patient service, or being the most efficient hospital. Good positioning requires looking at how to best implement the 4As of that target market. We refer to these steps of *segmentation*, *targeting*, and *positioning* by the acronym STP.

Combining this concept with those just described, we now have a more robust model of marketing strategy: first segment, next target position, then determine the 4As, and finally set the appropriate 4Ps.

When we say that marketing's purpose is to create value for the customer and profits (or surpluses) for the organization and its stakeholders, we don't mean that the organization should give customers everything that they want. Customer desires and needs must correspond with the mission or purpose of the organization. For example, a rehabilitation hospital does not need to open a cardiac bypass program just because some of its patients have heart disease. A further problem arises when the customer wants something that is not in his or her best interest. For example, a patient may request an antibiotic to treat a cold or ask for a narcotic for nonmedical reasons.

The Main Skills of Marketing

Marketers rely on seven traditional skills: marketing research, product design, distribution, pricing, advertising, sales promotion, and sales management.

Effective marketing must start with marketing research, which in turn consists of other skills. Suppose a hospital is planning to build a second facility in one of several neighboring communities. It clearly needs to conduct systematic marketing research to find which site is the most promising.

The marketing research will use both secondary and primary data. Secondary data comes from existing sources and yields information about such factors as the population's size, age, income, and education distribution as well as land costs and transportation resources. Primary data comes from making firsthand observations in each community by hosting focus groups to gather consumer reactions to different proposals, conducting in-depth interviews with specific community members, undertaking surveys to get a more accurate picture of customer attitudes and needs, and, finally, applying statistical techniques to draw insights from the data. By combining primary and secondary data, the hospital hopes that some neighboring community will emerge as the best target market to be served by a second facility.

Product design is the second marketing skill. Suppose a manufacturer of hospital beds wants to design a product that patients can more easily adjust on their own. It will assign a product team to design the new bed, consisting of an engineer, a designer, and a marketer. The marketer will supply some preliminary data about how patients feel about different features of a hospital bed, including functions, colors, and general design appearance. After the design is developed, the marketer might test it with a number of patients.

Although we are talking about designing a physical product, the same principles apply to a service. Many people complain about their experience in emergency rooms (ERs), including long waiting times, crowded facilities, and perfunctory service. Marketers are increasingly studying how to improve the ER experience, because hospital administrators realize that it is the place in which patients often experience their first encounter with the institution and that influences their probability of choosing it for future care.

The third traditional skill of marketers is distribution. Marketers have to choose places in which their products and services will be readily accessible and available to the customers. Marketers have learned to work with different types of wholesalers, jobbers, brokers, retailers, and transportation companies. This knowledge is very useful in activities ranging from pharmaceutical channel distribution to setting up a regional or national chain of in-store medical clinics.

Pricing is the fourth traditional skill of marketers. Marketers have gained much of their experience through setting prices and adjusting them for different markets and in different circumstances. They are guided by both internal constraints (such as their companies' production cost structure) as well as the realities of the marketplace (such as price elasticity of demand). In the realm of health insurance, the marketplace also demands flexibility to customize the product, with an attendant set of fixed and optional services and their varied prices.

The fifth traditional skill of marketers is the use of advertising. Marketers have extensive experience in working with ad agencies in designing messages, choosing media, setting budgets, and evaluating outcomes of advertising campaigns. The marketer must advise the organization about the best media mix to use, choosing among newspapers, magazines, radio, television, and billboards. Within each medium, the marketer must also make such decisions as whether to employ full-page or part-page ads, thirty-second TV spots or infomercials, and which radio stations will best reach target customers at certain times of the day.

The sixth traditional marketing skill is sales promotion: the use of incentives to stimulate trial or purchase of a product or service. Sales promotions include a wide variety of incentives. For example, community leaders might want 100 percent of citizens to get a flu vaccination; to achieve a big turnout, they may offer a discount for family members, a free booklet on staying fit, or a free coupon for a blood test.

The seventh traditional skill of marketers is management of a sales force. For example, the General Electric (GE) Medical Products division uses a well-trained sales force to sell sophisticated diagnostic imaging equipment to hospitals. This equipment is expensive, so hospitals must be convinced not only that they need this technology, but also that they should prefer to purchase it from GE. GE's professional sales force will explain the benefits of buying this equipment as justifying its high cost. Thus GE needs to hire, train, compensate, motivate, and evaluate hundreds of skilled professional salespeople.

Many suggest that, in addition to these seven skills, organizations need some newer marketing know-how, including:

- Direct marketing (mail and e-mail)
- Telemarketing
- Public relations
- Product placement
- Sponsorship
- Event management
- Internet marketing
- Blogs and podcasts

These skills, along with the more traditional marketing skills, are discussed in later chapters of this book.

How Marketing Is Organized in Health Care

Formal marketing positions (such as marketing researchers, sales managers, and advertising managers) have existed in pharmaceutical firms, medical device firms, and medical supply firms for many years, but it wasn't until 1975 that an American hospital first appointed a head of marketing. The Evanston Hospital in Evanston, Illinois (now Evanston Northwestern Healthcare), appointed Dr. John McLaren, a physician, to be its vice president of marketing.

As more hospitals began to appoint a marketing head, two variations emerged: director of marketing and vice president of marketing. The director of marketing provides and orchestrates marketing-related activities and resources. The vice president of marketing performs these activities and also sits with the other hospital officers in developing policies and strategies. The VP of marketing also brings the voice of the customer (VOC) into management and board meetings.

When hospitals first started appointing marketing heads, the public relations (PR) person on the staff often objected on the grounds that he or she was doing the marketing. The PR person's job was to generate good news about the hospital and defend it against bad news. Hospital CEOs soon realized, however, that PR and marketing have quite different roles and skills, although there is some overlap.

Public relations persons are trained in communication skills and work closely with media (editors, journalists) and occasionally with government officials, although the latter contacts are often handled by public affairs officers. Marketing people, on the other hand, are trained in economic analysis and the social sciences to understand and analyze markets and customer choice behavior. Marketers use the tools detailed earlier to provide estimates of a defined market's size and its needs, preferences, perceptions, and readiness to respond to alternative offers. Marketers develop a strategy and tactics for serving the target market in a way that will meet the organization's mission.

Today the marketing department in a large hospital may be staffed with a marketing researcher or analyst, an advertising and sales promotion manager, a sales force director, and in some cases product managers and market segment managers. Even when there are no specific positions dedicated to the functions of product development, pricing, communication, and distribution, these will be carried out by various people in the organization.

SUMMARY

Marketing plays an important role in helping participants in the health care system create, communicate, and deliver value (CCDV) to their respective target markets. Modern marketers start with the customers rather than with the products or services; they are more interested in building a lasting relationship than in securing a single transaction. Their aim is to create a high level of satisfaction so that customers come back to the same supplier.

Marketers have used many traditional skills, including marketing research, product design, distribution, pricing, advertising, sales promotion, and sales management. These skills need to be supplemented by newer ones emerging from new technologies and concepts for reaching and serving customers with messages and offers.

DISCUSSION QUESTIONS

1. You are the president of a hundred-bed hospital that has a public relations person and a development officer but no marketer. Do you need a marketer? How would this person's role differ from the others? Make an argument pro and con for hiring a marketer.

2. The governor of your state believes that more state funds need to be invested in preventing illness and accidents. He hires you as a social marketer with the mandate to raise consciousness about healthier life styles and to focus on two causes that will have the highest impact. How would you approach this assignment and what would you suggest?

3. You head the marketing department for a medical device firm whose sales department reports not to you but to a vice president of sales. Do you think that the vice president of sales and the sales force should report to you, or is it better to run marketing and sales as separate departments? What are the likely problems? What are the arguments for and against combining the departments?

4. A physician in private practice asks you, as a marketing consultant, how to attract more patients. The practice is serving about ten patients a day and cannot run profitably unless the physician sees about twenty patients a day. What questions would you ask before starting to make suggestions?

CHAPTER

2

DEFINING THE HEALTH CARE SYSTEM AND ITS TRADE-OFFS

LEARNING OBJECTIVES

In this chapter, we will address the following questions:

1. What framework can be used to understand the health care system regarding who pays, how much is paid, and where and to whom care is provided?

2. Who are the main stakeholders in the health care system?

3. What are the main trade-offs among cost, quality, and access that health care organizations must face in allocating their resources?

OPENING EXAMPLE

The State of Oregon Faces Some Hard Decisions with Respect to Allocating Medical Care   In the late 1980s, the State of Oregon faced a crisis. About 18 percent of all Oregonians and more than 20 percent of its children had no health insurance. The state wanted to provide coverage, but its Medicaid plan (mainly used to cover the state's poor) already faced high costs. To control these costs, three options were open: cut already-low payment levels to providers, raise eligibility requirements and serve fewer residents in need, or reduce benefits. Early in 1987, the state chose the third option. One benefit it removed was for organ transplants. In the fall of that year, seven-year-old Coby Howard's leukemia relapsed, requiring a bone marrow transplant. Despite private fundraising, he never received the procedure, and he died on December 2. In the outcry that followed, others needing transplants came to the public's attention. While defending the cutbacks, a spokesman for Oregon Medicaid said the money saved by denying the transplant was used to pay for other programs, including prenatal care for 1,500 women.

The ensuing debate over restoration of funds was led by Senate president John Kitzhaber (a former emergency room physician), who framed the argument in terms of making the best use of existing resources for the greatest number of people. This framing and subsequent establishment of the Oregon Health Plan (OHP) incorporated three unique characteristics. First, policy makers agreed that they had a fixed budget to spend on health care. Although most countries accept this notion, the United States has never explicitly budgeted for health care, and cost overruns are commonplace. Second, in order to gain consensus for an innovative plan, the newly formed Health Services Commission held eleven public hearings and about fifty town meetings to gauge what people in the state wanted from a health plan. These discussions included broad representation from interested stakeholders, including providers and consumer organizations representing Medicaid recipients. The result was a prioritized list of procedures and diagnoses of declining benefit/cost ratios. Given the amount of money in the budget, the state would set a cutoff in this list, below which the service would not be funded. The federal government approved the plan in March 1993 and it became operational the following February. Dr. Kitzhaber was elected governor that November.

The resultant OHP covered more people, but costs were greater than before the start of the program. Further, the economic turnaround of the 1990s enabled Oregon to offer extra services, without the same explicit analysis. When the economy worsened again after 2000, the state was once again forced to reduce benefits. Most recently, Oregon and other states have implemented co-payments for Medicaid recipients for certain services. Although these charges have led to lower state spending, many policy analysts attribute this benefit to decreased enrollment caused by the higher out-of-pocket expenses. The cycle appears to be starting anew.

Sources: http://www.oregon.gov/DHS/healthplan/index.shtml; Dranove, D. "What's Your Life Worth?" *The Oregon Plan*. Upper Saddle River, N.J.: Prentice Hall, 2003; Bodenheimer, T. "The Oregon Health Plan: Lessons for the Nation" (Part 1). *New England Journal of Medicine*, 1997, *337*, 651–655.

OVERVIEW: DEFINING A HEALTH CARE SYSTEM

In this chapter we will define the term *health care system* and show how its key components interact with and relate to each other.

There is a widespread tendency to define health in terms of the absence of disease of tangible body parts. Consider the Oxford English Dictionary (OED) definition of *disease:* "A condition of the body, or of some part or organ of the body, in which its functions are disturbed or deranged."[1] Instead, we prefer the World Health Organization (WHO) definition of *health:* "the state of complete physical, mental, and social well-being and not merely the absence of disease or infirmity."[2]

The World Health Organization also provides a comprehensive definition of a *health care system* as one that ". . . encompasses all the activities whose primary purpose is to promote, restore, or maintain health . . . and include[s] patients and their families, health care workers and caregivers within organizations and in the community, and the health policy environment in which all health related activities occur."

The way in which a nation defines its health system has significant implications for such marketing tasks as customer research, pricing, sales, advertising, and coordination of channels of distribution. The definition also has management implications for such initiatives as continuity of care programs, alignment of financial incentives, and quality assessment. Unfortunately, because the U.S. health care system is an ill-fitting mosaic, it might be defined as: *an apparently ad hoc arrangement of small units, each with its own goals and incentives, whose purpose is treatment of acute diseases of insured populations*. This "system" places the emphasis on disease management rather than overall health.

Because this system emphasizes disease management rather than overall health, there is a great need for an overall set of leading indicators to reflect major health concerns at the beginning of the twenty-first century. Some of these indicators are:

- Physical activity
- Overweight and obesity
- Tobacco use
- Substance abuse
- Responsible sexual behavior
- Mental health

- Injury and violence
- Environmental quality
- Immunization
- Access to health care

These ten indicators represent areas that can motivate action, can be measured through available data, and are important public health issues.[3]

A FRAMEWORK FOR UNDERSTANDING HEALTH CARE SYSTEMS

Deciphering any country's health care system can be a daunting and confusing task. Most approaches use economic models but fail to include such important considerations as culture, politics, and underlying national demographics. Two prominent models are those proposed by Odin Anderson[4] and Milton Roemer.[5]

Anderson's model describes a "market-minimized–market-maximized continuum." In the market-maximized version, one is "more likely . . . to favor private insurance, and, furthermore, profit-oriented insurance" (p. 27). In the market-minimized version, "one eventually subscribes to a completely state-owned, state-financed, and state-salaried health services system, paid for out of general tax revenues" (p. 27). The United States is the best example of a market-maximized system; Cuba's health care system is a market-minimized system. Most countries fall somewhere between the limits of this continuum. Roemer's model starts with the political (policy) spectrum of Anderson (ranging from laissez-faire to socialist), but adds an economic dimension (spanning affluent to poor).

Although these political and economic factors are important, one must consider a number of other, equally significant dimensions when describing a health care system. Table 2.1 illustrates these additional dimensions in a systematic way to help you understand how any nation organizes its health care. To use this framework, we present some *sample* questions and comments for each numbered cell.

Who Pays?

Cell 1. Political/Regulatory/Judicial. The first question you can ask is: Where does the power reside to make decisions about payment for health care services and products?

The answer depends on the degree of centralization or decentralization of the health care system. In the United States, except for federal programs like Medicare and Medicaid, regulatory authority for health insurance resides at the state level. Even in countries with national health laws (such as Canada), there is often a regionalization of health care payment and delivery. An extreme example of decentralization is the existence of insurance plans in small cantons in Switzerland.

Another question concerns the extent to which the public or private sector pays for health care. In the United States, private insurance companies are largely

TABLE 2.1. **Features of Health Care Systems**

Domains for Analysis	Who Pays?	How Much Is Paid (Costs/ Budgets)	Who and What Are Covered?	Where Is Care Provided?	Who Provides the Services and Products?
Political/ Regulatory/ Judicial	1.	6.	11.	16.	21.
Economic	2.	7.	12.	17.	22.
Social/Cultural	3.	8.	13.	18.	23.
Technological	4.	9.	14.	19.	24.
Demographic	5.	10.	15.	20.	25.

Source: Joel Shalowitz, 2005.

responsible for health care payments. Most of this private insurance is purchased through employer and employee contributions at the workplace. At the opposite end of the spectrum is Cuba, where the entire health care system is publicly financed. Between these two extremes there are a large number of variations. For example, in Canada, private insurance can provide coverage only for products and services that are not furnished by the provincial health insurance plans. In Chile, employees have the option to use the mandatory tax on wages to buy into either the state-sponsored health insurance plan (FONASA) or a private insurance company (ISAPRE). In yet another example, workers in Argentina (who purchase their health insurance with mandatory payroll deductions from their union) must use after-tax money if they want to enroll in a private insurance plan.

Cell 2. Economic. The state of a country's economy can also determine who pays for products and services. For example, in the 1990s, when the United States economy was rapidly expanding, many companies provided rich health care benefits for their employees. During the subsequent economic downturn, however, companies shifted more of the responsibility for payment to their workers. If the public sector has been largely responsible for financing health care, during bad economic times it may withdraw considerable support, leaving individuals to shoulder substantial financial responsibility. Extreme examples of this latter situation are rural China and parts of the former Soviet Union.

Cell 3. Social/Cultural. The social/cultural characteristics of a country will ultimately determine the mechanisms and sources of payment. In essence, these factors shape a country's health care "mission statement" (see Table 2.2 for examples from the World Health Organization, the U.K., and Canada). It is noteworthy that although many countries have crafted such statements, the United States government has not done so. For example, contrast two publicly funded programs. The U.K.'s National Health Service is funded from general taxation with a set budget, whereas the Medicare program in the United States is largely financed from employer and employee salary-based contributions and does not have an explicit cap on spending.

Cell 4. Technological. In this context, technology incorporates drugs, devices, and procedures that are used in health care settings. The key question we must ask is, How closely are safety and efficacy evaluations combined with cost considerations in determining whether a technology is approved and used? For example, in the United States, the Food and Drug Administration (FDA) will determine that a pharmaceutical is safe and efficacious. This decision is totally independent of whether or not there are many similar pharmaceuticals in the same class already available in the marketplace; if the newly approved drug is much more costly than its competitors, given equivalent benefits; or both. Contrast the FDA approval process with England's National Institute for Clinical Excellence (NICE). NICE approves pharmaceuticals based not only on safety and efficacy but also on cost-effectiveness. This disparity exists principally because, in the former case, the United States federal government does not directly pay for most pharmaceuticals, whereas the British government does have such fiscal responsibility. Even more recently, with Medicare's new system of payment for drugs, the federal government decided not to bargain directly with pharmaceutical companies.

Cell 5. Demographic. Demographic characteristics of the population will also determine who pays for products and services. For example, one of the key questions facing many countries is how they will care for their growing elderly populations. Who will pay for their care? How much will the elderly be expected to contribute themselves and how much will the public sector finance?

How Much Is Paid?

Cell 6. Political/Regulatory/Judicial. In most countries, the political process is the origin of public health care budgets and fee schedules. Even in the United States, where most care is provided by the private sector, government-set global fees for hospitals (diagnosis related groups or DRGs) and per-service fees for physicians (resource based relative value scale or RBRVS) have been adopted by the private sector as benchmarks for paying those providers. An example of judicial influence on costs comes from the debate on so-called "grey markets" for pharmaceuticals—the practice of importing drugs from lower-cost countries into higher-cost countries. This issue continues to be a contentious one in the United States (particularly with respect to reimportation of drugs from Canada) but has also been addressed by the courts in the European Union, where such practices were found to be legal.

TABLE 2.2. **Socioeconomic and Cultural Views of Health Care**

1. Universal Declaration of Human Rights. Adopted and proclaimed by General Assembly Resolution 217 A (III) of 10 December 1948.
    Article 25.(1)
    "Everyone has the right to a standard of living adequate for the health and well-being of himself and of his family, including food, clothing, housing and medical care and necessary social services, and the right to security in the event of unemployment, sickness, disability, widowhood, old age or other lack of livelihood in circumstances beyond his control."

2. According to Gordon Brown who was at the time U.K. Chancellor of the Exchequer (March 2002), taxation to fund health care is fair compared to . . .
    User charges—"It does not charge people for the misfortune of being sick."
    Private insurance—"Does not impose higher costs on those who are predisposed to illness, or who fall sick."
    Social insurance—"It does not demand that employers bear the majority burden of health costs."

3. Policy and administrative objectives for Canadian health care:
    Public administration
    Comprehensiveness
    Universality
    Portability
    Accessibility
    Efficiency, value for money
    Accountability, transparency (Canada Health Act and Commission on the Future of Health Care in Canada, 2001, Romanow Report)

4. Health System Goals According to the World Health Organization, 2000
    Maximizing population health
    Reducing inequalities in population health
    Maximizing health system responsiveness
    Reducing inequalities in responsiveness
    Ensuring health care equitably

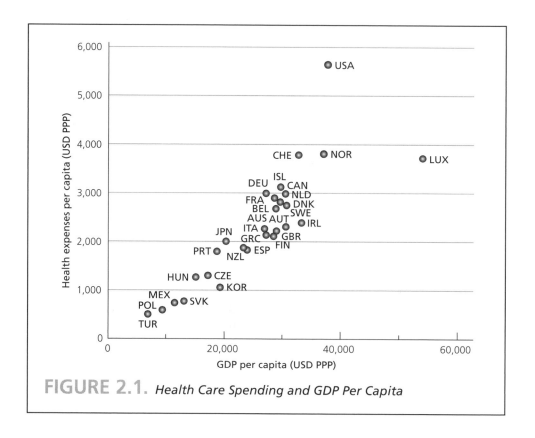

FIGURE 2.1. *Health Care Spending and GDP Per Capita*

Cell 7. Economic. Although politics determines the final amount countries will spend on public programs, overall spending is determined by the state of a country's economy. As shown in Figure 2.1, the gross domestic product (GDP) per capita is, by far, the single greatest determinant of a country's health expenditure per capita. The reason the United States is so high in per-capita health expenditures relative to its GDP is because prices are comparatively higher than in other countries.[6] Luxembourg falls below other countries mostly because of its high GDP per capita.

Cell 8. Social/Cultural. Given the political and economic determinants for health care budgets, the social and cultural characteristics of a country lay the groundwork for what is possible regarding such factors as the government's role in providing health care benefits, extent of government support, types of services covered, and relative amounts of payments. As examples, in the United States, procedures are valued relatively more than cognitive services and hence are paid at higher rates. In Sweden, the government realized a need for higher-level workers in the long-term care sector and raised salaries.

Cell 9. Technological. The effect of technology on health care costs can be found by answering the following question: How much does technology add to the cost of care as opposed to helping reduce overall expenses? The most significant factor in rising health care costs across all countries is new expenses related to technology. This new technology is, by and large, "layered on" to the old technology rather than replacing it. A good example is balloon angioplasty and stenting of coronary arteries. These relatively less invasive techniques were supposed to replace many coronary artery bypass surgeries; in fact, the overall effect was to add a large number of patients who would not have been eligible for the latter procedure. Another example is positron emission tomography (PET scanners) for cancer staging. This diagnostic test, whose cost is about $2,000, is added to computerized tomography (CT) and magnetic resonance imaging (MRI) rather than replacing either. The effect on cost has been a rapid increase in those sectors. On the other hand, the introduction of medicines to treat peptic ulcers has all but eliminated the cost of surgery for this condition.

Cell 10. Demographic. As mentioned earlier, one of the key demographic factors faced by all countries is the aging of the population. The relevant question for this category is, how much does a country want to spend on its elderly versus its younger population? The U.S. government has recently answered this question by making a substantial (though largely unfunded) commitment to adding a subsidy for noninjectable pharmaceuticals for Medicare recipients. (Non-self-administered medications, like chemotherapy, have been covered for many years.)

Who and What Are Covered?

Cell 11. Political/Regulatory/Judicial. The political process plays a significant role in determining who will be covered and what health care benefits they will receive. For example, although all Canadian citizens are covered by government-sponsored insurance, the exact benefits vary by province. In the United States, examples in this category include state laws (called *mandates*) that require health insurance companies to offer certain benefits to their members. To some, certain of these mandates, such as infertility treatment and hairpieces for chemotherapy patients, stretch the limits of what health insurance should cover.

Cell 12. Economic. In addition to determining the amount of money allocated for the health care system, the economic climate will also determine what benefits are offered. In good economic times benefits may be added, but during downturns even government benefits may be withdrawn. For example, in 2004 the Ontario government withdrew benefits for routine optometry, maintenance physical therapy, and chiropractic services under the Ontario Health Insurance Plan. In addition, increased charges were levied because of severe budget pressures.

Cell 13. Social/Cultural. These factors can have an important impact on who and what is covered by public and private systems. For example, when economic conditions required benefit cutbacks in Germany, one of the most contentious programs that was eliminated was spa care—long a staple of that country's health care system.

Cell 14. Technological. The influence of technology in terms of coverage can be assessed by answering the following questions: What technologies are lifesaving, life enhancing, or lifestyle enhancing, and how are they prioritized? An example in which this question was recently addressed is the U.S. government's consideration of coverage for erectile dysfunction drugs under its Medicare drug coverage plan. (After much debate, the government decided not to cover these medications.)

Cell 15. Demographic. Which populations require health care will also determine who or what is covered. The dilemma is, to what extent should the health care system focus on those with acute illnesses, or those with chronic disease, or those who should receive preventive services?

Where Is Care Provided?

Cell 16. Political/Regulatory/Judicial. Governments license providers and may enact portability laws to ensure that the quality of care will meet certain standards and that their populations will be treated equitably no matter where they need care. For example, with regard to portability and access to care, the European Union's courts have confirmed the rights of its citizens to obtain health care across the borders of member nations. In Canada, portability of coverage is guaranteed by the federal Canada Health Act. In the United States, the federal Emergency Medical Treatment and Active Labor Act of 1986 (EMTALA) requires that a hospital with an emergency department provide "an appropriate medical screening examination" to any patient who "comes to the emergency department" for examination or treatment. Further, the emergency department (and hospital, in general) must provide ongoing care until the patient's condition is stabilized. It is important to note that the patient's insurance coverage status is not a factor that hospitals can take into consideration in accepting the patient for treatment.

Cell 17. Economic. In countries like the United States, with both public and private health care systems, during times of economic expansion payers allow patients to receive care at and from nearly any licensed facility and provider. During more difficult economic times, payers tend to be more selective about where patients can receive their care. The example that epitomizes this concept is managed care, whereby a select group of primary care physicians will provide and coordinate services for members of such plans.

Cell 18. Social/Cultural. These considerations also have a strong influence on where care is provided. For example, many communities want a local hospital, even though regionalization would make more economic sense with respect to economies of scale. Also, for cultural reasons, some populations are much less accepting of a trade-off between cost and site of care. Particularly in the United States, health insurers recognize that providing customers with freedom of choice of providers is an extremely important feature in marketing their plans.

Cell 19. Technological. In recent years there have been two opposite major trends in technology with respect to location. The first has been consolidation to a single site for services to treat highly complex conditions. These sites have been commonly called *centers of excellence*. The contrary trend has been a move away from centralized locations to the point of care in the community. Technologies ranging from diagnostics to laser treatments have followed this pattern. In addressing the issue of where care is provided, one must also understand the extent to which technology enables care to be provided at "alternate" sites. A further trend is remote delivery of care, sometimes called *telemedicine*. Examples include consultations using audio and video conferencing over the Internet and treatments by robotic surgery.

Cell 20. Demographic. With respect to the demographic determinants of where care is provided, one must address fundamental questions about access to this care. For example, how do the physically impaired elderly get to regular physician appointments? How are rural populations served when the closest health care facility or practitioner may be hours away? What is the role of telemedicine in providing care for the homebound and geographically remote populations?

Who Provides the Services and Products?

Cell 21. Political/Regulatory/Judicial. The first question one must ask in this category is, what are the regulations and laws defining who is allowed to care for patients and to handle and prescribe such products as pharmaceuticals and medical equipment? Related to this question is the matter of the scope of such practitioners; for example, what are nurse practitioners and physician assistants allowed to do vis-à-vis the practice of physicians? The U.S. medical community makes extensive use of nurse practitioners and physician assistants, whereas these professionals are absent from the clinical scene in Japan (the exception being nurse midwives). Another related question is, who licenses these professionals? In the United States and Canada, such licensure is conducted by states and provinces, respectively. With increased globalization, such as in the European Union, there is some pressure to make such licensure transnational. Another major question in this category is, how is the supply of practitioners regulated, if at all? As an example, contrast the processes in the United States and Argentina for medical school admission. In the United States, admissions occur after a rigorous screening process; once students are admitted, however, few drop out. In Argentina, any student who can pass basic entrance requirements will be admitted to a public university, where tuition is free; however, the rigorous curriculum leads to a much higher dropout rate than in the United States. Further, the vast majority of medical school graduates in the United States go on to postgraduate residency training, whereas the number of such positions in Argentina is severely limited. A related question is, who accredits these training programs? In countries with public educational institutions, the government performs this function. In the United States, where most of these schools are in the private sector, there are a number of accrediting bodies that review the quality of training. Ultimately, the U.S. Department of Education is responsible for oversight of these accrediting organizations. Finally, what is the nature of the laws and regulations governing anticompetitive practices and fee sharing? For example, in some countries it is perfectly legal and ethical for the referring physician to receive compensation from the specialist for sending patients. In the United States, this practice is considered both illegal and unethical.

Cell 22. Economic. One could ask several questions to determine the extent economics influence who provides care. First, how are the fees for services and products determined? That is, are they set by government regulation, subject to free market factors, or a combination of the two? Within this payment structure, however it is determined, is there equity among and between practitioners? For example, are procedural specialists (surgeons) and cognitive specialists (primary care doctors) paid at equal rates for similar services based on such factors as time, risk, and skill? Also, how are nonphysicians (such as nurse practitioners and physician assistants) paid compared to physicians for performing identical services? Finally, what is the role of the marketplace in determining the overall numbers of providers and their distribution both geographically and by specialty? In the United States, the marketplace largely determines the answers to these questions. In other countries, however, the government may have a more direct influence.

Cell 23. Social/Cultural. The principal questions in this category are, how does a society determine and value who is accepted as a "legitimate" provider of care, and what are culturally valid treatments? One must look at who is allowed to provide nontraditional health care services in a country and how much of the overall care fits into the category of alternative and complementary medicine. One can also ask if these nontraditional providers and treatments are regulated or if there is any oversight by the government. For example, traditional Chinese medicine is regulated in Singapore, yet many nutritional supplements in the United States are not likewise scrutinized. Also, how does the society view the integration of traditional and nontraditional practitioners and the services they provide?

Cell 24. Technological. The primary question here is, how do decisions about technology adoption and use affect who provides care? To answer this question, it is important to know who designs the educational content for training providers and who gets to use the technology based on training, licensure, or certification. For example, in some areas, interventional radiologists perform peripheral angioplasties, while in other locations these procedures would be done by vascular surgeons. One must also know the process through which technologies are adopted, particularly when there is competition for resources. For example, is the decision made based on population needs, return on investment, or political pressure from an individual or special interest groups?

Cell 25. Demographic. The summary question one must pose here is, How do demographic characteristics of the population determine who provides the care? Answering this question requires an assessment of where the providers are located, similar to the earlier question regarding *where* the care is provided. One also must look at the demographic characteristics of those who are delivering the care. Finally, the existing and projected population demographics and disease patterns will determine the needed specialty mixes. For example, the aging population requires more practitioners who perform colonoscopies (gastroenterology), cataract removals (ophthalmology), and other geriatric services. Likewise, if diseases such as HIV/AIDS or other widespread infections occur, practitioners in that specialty will be required.

STRATEGIC CHOICE MODEL FOR ORGANIZATIONS AND HEALTH CARE SYSTEMS

As mentioned in the previous chapter, one of the most important innovations in marketing strategy in recent years is a change from the notion of *selling* existing products and services to that of *understanding* and *meeting* customer perceptions, desires, and needs.

With respect to health care, the term *customer* refers to those who purchase a product or service after determining that its characteristics meet a need or desire. By comparison, a *consumer* is the one who actually uses the product or service.

A customer may or may not be a consumer. For example, a parent would be the customer for snack food companies while the child might be the consumer. The health care setting is a bit more complicated, so we need more terms. Note the terms used in the following situation:

FOR EXAMPLE

A visiting aunt tells the mother that the mother's child looks sick and should be taken to a doctor (aunt = *influencer*). The mother decides to take the child to an emergency room (mother = *decider*). The child is treated by a physician (child = *patient*). The physician prescribes medication for the child (pharmaceutical company = *supplier*). The physician and hospital (physician and hospital = *providers*) notify the mother's health insurance company to pay for the service that was rendered (insurance company = *payer*).

Further, consider that society as a whole might be interested in this transaction if it is for treatment of an infection that may spread to the rest of the population. Given these complex relationships, we need a term that encompasses all those persons and groups who have an interest in such matters as the funding, delivery, product development, and receipt of health care services and products. We call all these interested parties *stakeholders*.

Stakeholder Identification

Following identification of its stakeholders, a health care business will inevitably confront conflicting needs and wants. For example, both payers and patients are important stakeholders for pharmaceutical companies and health care providers. Also, just as health plans may impose unreasonable constraints on the delivery of patient care, patients can express unrealistic demands for the provision of medical services and products. Balancing conflicting stakeholder requirements is therefore a constant and difficult challenge.

From country to country, stakeholders vary in such important dimensions as power and scope. For example, in Cuba, physicians are employees of the state-owned and -run system. By contrast, in Japan, the Japan Medical Association is a politically powerful organization that mainly includes private practitioners. Given these broad disparities in health system designs, a descriptive model of stakeholders must be appropriately flexible. See Figure 2.2, which divides stakeholders into three groups.

The first, central set of stakeholders is *individuals and their advocates* in the private sector. Included in this group are not only the recipients of care (the patient), but also other individuals who have an interest in these patients, such as family members, legal guardians, close friends, and community members. As well, this category includes private sector organizations that advocate on behalf of patients with similar characteristics, such as age, disease, or geographic location. For example, the Pediatric AIDS Foundation meets the first and second criteria; the second and third criteria describe the American Lung Association of Metropolitan Chicago.

The second stakeholder is the *public sector*. The feature of note here is that *public programs are differentiated from one another by who they cover for health care benefits*. Even in countries with universal coverage, separate systems of funding

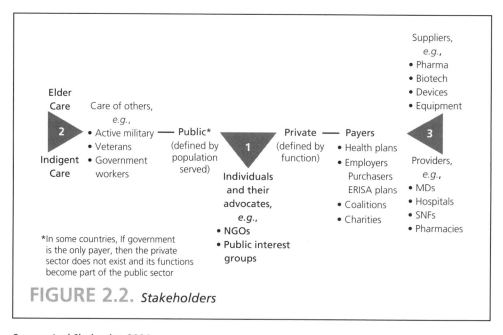

FIGURE 2.2. *Stakeholders*

Source: Joel Shalowitz, 2004.

and care may exist for subcategories of the population, usually the elderly and the poor, as well as other groups. Sometimes these categories are combined; for example, the Programa de Asistencia Medica Integral (PAMI) in Argentina covers the elderly and the poor. These categories are exemplified in the United States by Medicare, Medicaid, and government programs for those who serve it in various capacities, such as active military, veterans, and government employees.

The third group of stakeholders operate in the private sector; they define themselves by *what they do*. The traditional divisions are among *payers, providers*, and *suppliers*. Payers include not only insurance companies but also employers (who may self-fund all or part of employee health insurance), unions (the oldest form of health insurance and still the predominant method in Argentina), business associations, and charitable organizations. Pharmaceutical, biotechnology, device, medical supply, and diagnostic companies are significant suppliers of health care products. Providers comprise such categories as physicians, hospitals, nursing homes, pharmacies, and independent diagnostic facilities (such as laboratory and radiology).

Although this stakeholder model may at first glance seem clear-cut, there is much overlap and blending. Several examples illustrate this concept.

- In Canada, provincial health care is publicly funded but privately delivered.

- In almost every country where the state employs physicians to provide publicly funded care, these same practitioners also see self-paying patients in private offices apart from government facilities. An example is a number of National Health Service physicians in the U.K.

- Providers such as hospitals and physicians can be closely linked to a payer organization through exclusive arrangements or mutual ownership. An example of the former is the Kaiser-Permanente Plan in the United States.

- Some community advocate organizations have established their own health care funding and delivery systems. Group Health Cooperative of Puget Sound in Washington State was such an example.

This stakeholder framework is meant to be used as a heuristic device for thinking about the different arrangements and combinations required for successful strategic decisions in health care marketing. In other words, it is a guide to exploring themes and variations.

Developing a Strategy

Given these stakeholders, how can you formulate a strategic marketing plan to address the needs of one or more of them? In other words, how can you develop a value proposition for your health care customers and other interested stakeholders? Before exploring the answer to this question, we must consider one more key term—*strategy*—and highlight three of its important characteristics. First, although businesses are often involved in many small day-to-day decisions, strategy considers approaches to handling *major issues* with which the enterprise must deal now or in the future. Second, strategy involves setting the organizational direction for the medium to long term. These time frames are, of course, relative and vary by firm and industry. Third, useful strategies take into account that short-term decisions *do* need to be made. Strategy, therefore, provides a framework for making those decisions within the context of the organization's long-range goals.

Trade-off Analysis

Although there are a number of strategic approaches for organizational and industry analysis—such as strength/weakness/opportunity/threat (SWOT) analysis and Five Forces Analysis[7]—the one used in Figure 2.3 provides a useful framework for understanding the health care industry.

A brief explanation of this model will lay the foundation for its applicability to the health care field. The model posits that a successful company can choose to be excellent in one of the three areas, but not all three. In other words, there is a *trade-off* when a company makes its strategic business choice. To be sure, the two dimensions not chosen as the strategic focus cannot be neglected, but they have a supporting, rather than a primary function. For example, no one will buy a product just because it is cheap if it is very poorly made and does not solve a customer's needs.

The low-cost strategy is not just about pricing, but how it is achieved through operational efficiency and standardization. This approach and the customer trade-offs are best illustrated by the globally ubiquitous warehouse clubs Sam's Club and Costco. These companies are supply chain experts who buy in bulk and stock stores in a standard manner. Although they may carry fine products, the selection is based not on best of category, but on what is available at the lowest prices. Therefore a product found once at a particular store may not always be available there. To keep costs down, these stores also limit personnel. If customers want low prices, they must sacrifice a great deal of both choice and personal attention.

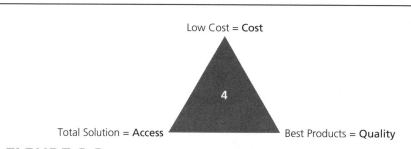

FIGURE 2.3. *Strategic Choices to Deliver Health Care Stakeholder Value*

Examples of firms that focus on "best product" strategy can range from computer chips to fashion. Chip manufacturers are always trying to improve their technology and willing to leapfrog current products for new and better versions. Fashion firms constantly try to anticipate or shape new trends, again with the willingness to abandon old styles. However, fast chips and designer clothing do not come cheap. Nor do they offer a great deal of choice. Chanel dresses and Hugo Boss suits are high quality, but they are expensive and do not come in all styles and colors.

Consulting or personal service companies provide good examples of "total solution" strategies. For example, a customer may ask consultants to provide analysis and recommendations for a health information system. The consultants will frequently recommend software and hardware as well as procedures for using them effectively and efficiently. Each product that they recommend may not be best of class, but together they will provide a compatible, integrated solution. Such custom services are also expensive.

What should be clear from these examples is that each company must make strategic *choices*. It cannot be all things to all people.

STRATEGIC IMPLICATIONS FOR HEALTH CARE

How do these concepts relate to the health care field? For many years, academicians and policy makers have recognized that choices in health care should involve trade-offs among cost, quality, and access. We use the word *should* instead of *must* because, more often than not, stakeholders are not willing to choose. They insist on having all three simultaneously, putting tremendous stress on the system and causing periodic crises.

For example, in the United States, health care is the most expensive in the world when measured by price parity, spending per capita, and percent of GDP. Technology is readily available and is not rationed by cost when, for example, the Food and Drug Administration (FDA) makes approval decisions for pharmaceuticals. What we sacrifice is access by those without health insurance. Countries with a national health system, like the U.K., spend less money than the United States on health care, not only because the service prices are lower, but because health care is budgeted along with other government programs. Also, government agencies like the National Institute for Clinical Excellence (NICE) incorporate cost into their analyses of technology approval. Although all citizens are covered by public insurance, the limited budget strains the system by constraining the supply of resources, thus causing long queues and reducing access.

If these trade-offs were that easy to explain, health care marketing, strategy, and policy would be relatively simple; but to fully appreciate these characteristics, each must be further broken down into its components. Like the three major features in the previous section, the elements that define them can also require balancing and trade-offs, thus creating a cascade of interdependent attributes.

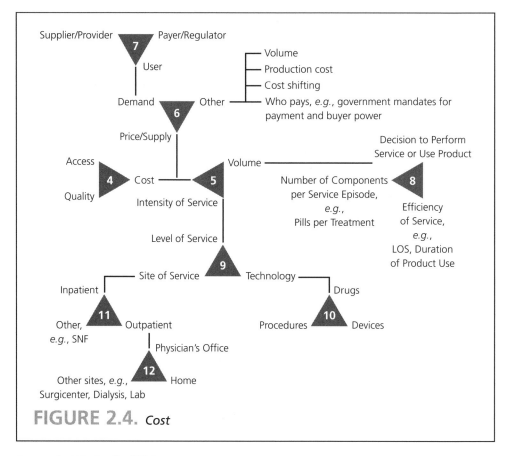

FIGURE 2.4. *Cost*

Source: Joel Shalowitz, 2004.

We will now discuss each aspect, starting with Figure 2.4, and present a unified scheme after all components have been explained. The reader should note that, for completeness, some redundancy is built into this model. For example, technology, which is presented in the cost section, could as easily be discussed under quality. Further, there is extensive overlap and interrelationships among elements of different sections, so a true representation would appear as a complex web rather than elaborations of three discrete branches.

Cost

We begin by examining cost, which we define as an *actual payment*, based on listed price or a prenegotiated rate. The total cost of products or services is governed by the following relationship (see item 5 in Figure 2.4):

$$Cost = f(P, V, I)$$

where f = function; P = price of the service or product; V = volume, or number of units; and I = intensity of service or product.

Two examples will illustrate the use of this formula:

■ Each year, national pharmaceutical expenditures are announced and increases are attributed to three categories: increase in prices of existing drugs (price), increase in use of existing medications (volume), and introduction of new products or technologies (intensity).

■ The total cost of a hospitalization for a patient can be broken down into three elements: level of care, such as intensive care unit versus a bed on a regular medical/surgical floor (intensity); number of days (volume); and price per day at different levels of care (price).

Understanding these components can lead to important insights not only for strategy but also for public policy. To check rising health care costs, one can address any or all of these fundamentals; however, the political consequences of manipulating each are significant, and addressing one without also confronting the other two is futile. For example, the federal government has been dealing with rising physician costs by lowering the fees for their services. Doctors respond by increasing volume or, more important, by increasing the technology applied to care. For example, a benign skin lesion that can be effectively removed by freezing can also be destroyed using a laser, at a significantly higher reimbursement. Also, imagine cost-control strategies that deal only with volume—that is, by rationing care—or those that address only intensity—for example, by withholding new technology. Price reduction is obviously the easiest short-term tool for cost control, but without management of the other two components, overall costs will never be adequately managed.

We can now deconstruct each of these three elements (see item 6 in Figure 2.4).

Price. Classical economics dictates that price is determined by supply and demand for a product or service. This principle is true for health care, but only to a point. With regard to *demand*, customer demand for goods can influence price, but in health care that is not the whole story. Suppliers can also manipulate customer demand by such measures as direct-to-consumer advertising and physician-requested revisits. Recall from the discussion on stakeholders that one of the unique features of health care is the presence of parties in addition to those who supply the goods and those who consume them. Payers and regulators (such as the government) can also influence demand through such direct or indirect measures as rationing services and regulating pricing, respectively. *Supply* may also influence price, but it is not always subject to free market conditions. For instance, in many countries, supply is centrally regulated. As an example, some governments regulate such items as the number of students admitted to medical school slots or advanced diagnostic imaging machines.

In addition to supply and demand, *other factors* also determine the price of health care goods and services. At least four other elements are involved in determining prices (see these to the right of item 6 in Figure 2.4).

- *Volume.* As in other fields, volume discounts are often available; however, some goods do not display the usual volume or experience (the so-called "learning curve") relationships to price that, say, calculators or computers did. For example, coronary artery bypass surgery prices have not decreased commensurate with the experience and standardization of the technology.

- *Production costs.* Prices are often linked to production costs, as an example from Medicare illustrates. The federal government determines physician reimbursements based on computing practice costs and the work that goes into providing the service. This method is the resource based relative value scale (RBRVS) introduced earlier.

- *Cost shifting.* Prices often have nothing to do with the good itself, but rather reflect the other resources consumed in the same setting. For example, one hears about a hospital charging $5 for an aspirin. Obviously, the aspirin's actual cost is nowhere near that amount, but other hospital services are often paid at below production cost. Also, some services, like maternity care, are "loss leaders." Other services (such as personnel-intensive disability evaluations) are truly underpaid, but the hospital must offer them in order to fulfill its mission of providing comprehensive care to the community. This practice of cross-subsidization is called *cost shifting*. The price of a good can therefore depend on the opportunity and need to cost shift.

- *Who pays.* This factor can greatly influence the price, regardless of supply or demand for the good or service. This category is what Porter refers to as "buyer power" and also reflects nonmarket forces. For example, Medicare has set its reimbursement for injectable pharmaceuticals at 6 percent over "average sales price (ASP)" and inpatient hospital payments based on the patient's diagnosis (diagnosis related group, or DRG).

Volume. We now turn to the *volume* determinant of cost (see 8 in Figure 2.4). Determinants of volume can be divided into three components. The first portion concerns the decision whether or not to use a product or deliver or receive a service. Although this might seem simple, there has been much debate over related issues in health care, prompting questions like these:

- Is the comprehensive annual physical really necessary for all adults?

- When is watchful waiting better than aggressive treatment? (One answer is, for certain cases of prostate cancer.)

- Are screening tests worthwhile? (The answer depends on the condition and the screening method.)

Another important consideration is that once experts agree an action is indicated (an exam must be performed, a test ordered, treatment administered), which among the options is the best choice? Obviously, choosing one may mean that the other actions are not taken. For example, assume a patient has blockages in the coronary (heart) arteries that require invasive intervention. Is the appropriate action stenting or coronary artery bypass graft surgery (CABG)? Although the answer depends on the extent of the blockages, where they occur, and how many arteries are involved, experts do not often agree on the best method for individual patients.

These examples and questions deal only with professional decisions. Patients and other stakeholders also have a role in determining whether or not actions are taken. For example, patients often pressure physicians for antibiotics for viral infections when none are needed. Public interests also may determine whether something is done or not. For instance, due to a national budget (in England), the National Health Service at one time did not pay for hemodialysis for persons over age fifty-five.

Once the decision has been made to act, two further inputs under item 8 will determine the overall volume. The first is efficiency of execution. For example, once the patient and physician agree that surgery is an appropriate option, how long is the patient to remain in the hospital and how many resources will be used for that episode of care? The second issue is the number of units of care to be applied. For example, there are various antibiotic regimens for treatment of certain bacterial infections, ranging from thirty pills (one amoxicillin pill three times a day) to one dose of medication (Zmax formulation of azithromycin).

Intensity of Service. The third determinant of cost is the *intensity of service* (see item 9 in Figure 2.4). The first component is *level of service*. For example, does a hospitalized patient require intensive care or is a regular medical/surgical bed sufficient? Once the level of care is determined, the price and then cost will follow. Another illustration of this point is choice of antibiotics. Does a patient require a short course of oral medication or prolonged intravenous treatment?

Intensity of service also comprises use of medical *technology*, which consists of drugs, devices, and procedures (see item 10 in Figure 2.4). Sometimes these modalities are used in combinations; at other times they are substitutes for one another. For instance, there are different preferred treatments for diverse heartbeat irregularities. Some are best treated by medication (amiodarone, for example); others should be cared for by devices (implantable defibrillators or pacemakers); still others require surgery (whereby the source of the rhythm disturbance is surgically ablated). Each of these different technologies carries its own cost.

Finally, the *site of service* is an important determinant of intensity and, hence, cost (see items 11 and 12 in Figure 2.4). Sites of care can be divided into institutional and noninstitutional settings. Of the former category, hospitals come to mind first. We refer to care in the acute care hospital setting as *inpatient* care. Other institutional settings consist of skilled nursing facilities (sometimes called SNFs) or long-term care settings, such as chronic ventilator facilities. We refer to care in noninstitutional sites as *outpatient* care. Common sites are the physician's office, the patient's home (with varying degrees of skilled home health care), and various other locations for diagnostic and therapeutic services. In this latter category we include same-day (ambulatory) surgery (whether at a hospital or a free-standing surgicenter), dialysis facility, diagnostic laboratory and radiology facility, and physical therapy location.

These different types of sites can be substitutes for one another or appropriate sequential choices. For example, an elderly patient should be hospitalized for repair of a hip fracture. After this treatment she may recuperate and receive physical therapy in a skilled nursing facility and then be sent home with appropriate services there. On the other hand, the majority of surgical procedures are now performed on a same-day basis, substituting for inpatient treatment. Further, diagnostic and therapeutic technologies are also moving from centralized medical centers to outpatient points of care. For example, many tests that were formerly only done in a hospital laboratory can now be performed with the same quality in physicians' offices.

Quality

Quality is still a major concern in health care; many lives are lost or harmed by problems or errors in health care delivery. More hospitals need to establish better infection control practices (especially against staphylococcal infection). More needs to be done to reduce harm from high-alert medications such as anticoagulants, sedatives, narcotics, and insulin. Surgical complications must be reduced by implementing needed changes in patient care. To address these types of problems, the Institute for Health Care Improvement has launched a Five Million Lives campaign to enlist four thousand hospitals to implement twelve interventions geared toward preventing five million "incidents of patient harm."[8]

A detailed discussion of patient safety and quality is beyond the scope of this book. For now, refer to items 13 and 14 in Figure 2.5.

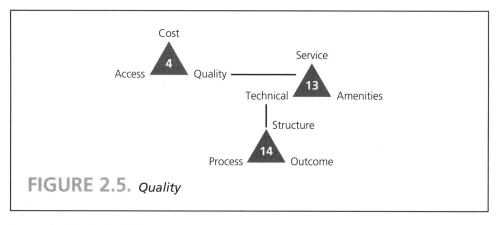

FIGURE 2.5. *Quality*

Source: Joel Shalowitz, 2004.

The dimensions of quality can be divided into the amenities, service aspects, and technical components. To illustrate and contrast these elements, consider a hospital stay:

- The *amenities* aspect may consist of the items that form a first impression about the facility; for example, the building style, landscaping, and ease and cost of parking. Although the marketing implications of these items are clear, they bear no relation to the actual desired outcome, for example, the success of a surgical procedure.

- The *service* aspect comes closer to affecting outcomes. Inpatient services may consist of meals, how quickly personnel respond to patient requests, and housekeeping. Although these functions support the actual business of delivering care and can more strongly influence opinions about the institution than the amenities, they are still not part of the core activities in delivering treatment.

- The *technical* aspect is the work that most directly affects outcomes. Examples of such activities are expertly performed surgery, choice of appropriate medication, and skillfully administered nursing care.

Because someone lacking expertise in medicine often cannot assess the quality of the technical component of care, the amenities and, to a greater extent, the services are important strategic considerations for health care marketing.

Evaluation of the technical dimension of quality is traditionally divided into structure, process, and outcome measures. Structural components are those that are either present or absent and are easily measured, such as licensure, board certification, or the presence of a critical piece of equipment. Process assessment gauges whether personnel followed acceptable procedures. Outcome, of course, measures the results of all health care inputs. As mentioned earlier, a detailed analysis of these elements is beyond the scope of this book.

Total Solution: Access

The third part of this strategic trade-off derives from the business model of providing a comprehensive, customer-intimate or total solution. In the health care realm, this concept translates as issues of access or equity (see item 15 in Figure 2.6).

Availability. The first consideration regarding access or equity is whether certain resources are available. Availability can be assessed by answering some of the questions posed earlier in Table 2.1. To expand on this inquiry, we can ask who has health insurance coverage as well as who does not. These two issues, although apparently two sides of the same coin, address different strategic purposes. As an example of the former question, a pharmaceutical company will target the insured population for sales of a new product. The latter issue raises the question, how many uninsured people can our society accept? In virtually all countries except the United States, the answer to this question is *none*.

A third aspect to this question concerns who will accept the patient's insurance. For example, in the United States, Medicaid (the joint federal-state program for

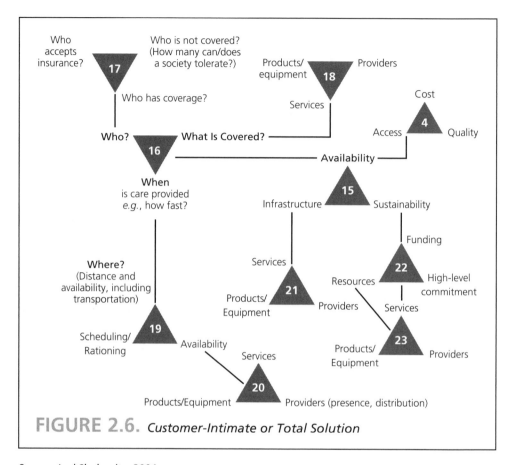

FIGURE 2.6. *Customer-Intimate or Total Solution*

Source: Joel Shalowitz, 2004.

the poor and other select populations) ensures that eligible persons have at least a modicum of health insurance coverage. Unfortunately, this program often pays physicians so little and so late (nine month in accounts receivable aging is not unusual) that there may be few who choose to see Medicaid insured patients. Also, not every commercial insurance plan will contract with every provider; patients must then seek those practitioners and institutions with whom their insurance companies contract in order to reduce the percentage of the cost for which they will be responsible.

What is covered? is the next question that defines availability. Even for the insured, not all services, products and equipment, or providers are covered or covered at the same level. For example, most insurance plans in the United States do not cover expenses related to prescription eyeglasses (they may pay for the professional exam but not the glasses themselves), and generic drugs have lower co-payments than do branded equivalents.

The third aspect of availability is *when* care can be provided. This feature depends on whether services, providers, and products exist or are close enough to patients to be helpful. For example, some developing countries may lack certain technology or personnel skilled in its use. Even if these are available, their location is extremely important. By location, we refer not only to rural locales or developing nations but also to urban centers. For instance, making free prenatal care available to inner-city women is a futile gesture unless they have a way to affordably and easily get to these services. Finally, even if health care is close and easy to reach, services that are in short supply may be explicitly or implicitly rationed. Queues in the U.K. for certain services are examples of this problem.

Infrastructure. In addition to availability, the two other dimensions of access we must consider are *infrastructure* and *sustainability*. These two topics are of particular concern for developing countries as well as rural and inner-city populations in developed nations. Although thinking about infrastructure can raise questions similar to the "where" and "availability" themes, this topic is concerned more with the supporting roles played by services, providers, and products and equipment (see item 21 in Figure 2.6) than with the primary activity or product. For example, think of a program to deliver immunizations to children in rural locations in a developing country. Assume that a pharmaceutical company donates the supplies and that health care practitioners volunteer time to administer injections. The infrastructure dimension of this program includes not only the traditional items, such as roads to get to needy populations, but also medical support services such as an information system that logs and tracks who received the shots and when recipients are due for booster immunizations.

HIV/AIDS treatment presents another example. Supplying medication is necessary but not sufficient for successful treatment programs. The infrastructure must also include health care personnel who make sure patients take the medication as prescribed and are available for support when side effects inevitably arise.

Wealthy nations also have infrastructure problems. Consider the following examples:

- A hospital advertises an innovative program, only to find it cannot accommodate the volume of phone calls or schedule the service in a timely fashion.

- Shortly after a pharmaceutical company gets approval to market a new "blockbuster" drug, its production plants cannot keep up with demand; in the meantime, a competitor releases a substitute and garners significant market share.

- A producer of unique diagnostic equipment experiences quality problems in its factory that cause a lengthy cessation of manufacturing, reduced revenue, and a plummeting stock price.

Sustainability. Contemplating the infrastructure problem naturally gives rise to considerations of *sustainability* (see items 22 and 23 in Figure 2.6). Experts often use the simile that effecting lasting change in the health care arena is more like a marathon

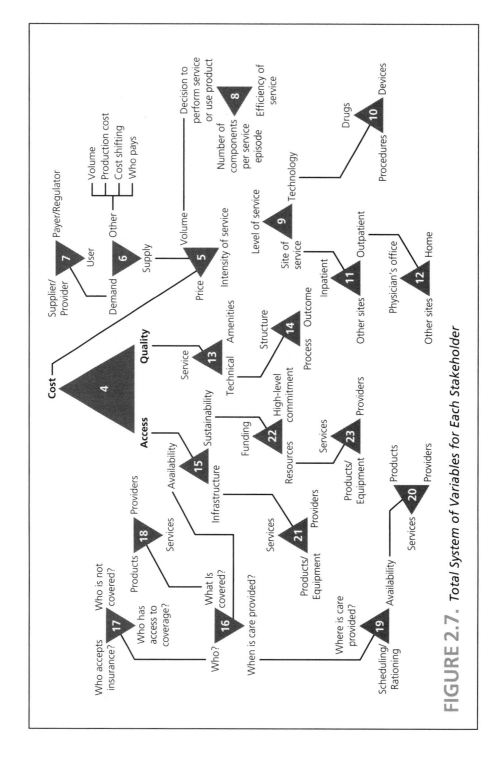

FIGURE 2.7. *Total System of Variables for Each Stakeholder*

Source: Joel Shalowitz, 2004.

than a sprint. Sustainability starts with high-level commitment by appropriately empowered authorities. (Although grassroots activities are worthwhile, their purpose is often to convince decision makers to act.) Funding is also critical. For example, hospital administrators (like university presidents) are often reluctant to accept large donations for buildings because of the anticipated (and unfunded) ongoing maintenance costs. Similarly, relevant follow-up activities must be budgeted. Finally, decision makers and funders must commit appropriate resources for the long run. These resources must not only be available for episodic interventions but also provide continuity.

We can finally put all these concepts together (see Figure 2.7).

In using this model, we must first consider that each stakeholder will have different preferences among the cost, quality, and access dimensions. When two or more stakeholders are involved in a given issue, conflicts will often arise between them regarding these choices. The initial strategic choices, therefore, require answers to these questions: Who are the important stakeholders? What are their relative preferences?

Another important consideration is that when any one element changes, it can have far-reaching effects on the entire system. As mentioned previously, Figure 2.7 really should look like a spider's web, with all points connected to all other points. For example, assume a state government lowers payment rates for physicians caring for Medicaid patients (item 6 in Figure 2.4). How will that action affect the availability of physicians willing to care for those patients (item 17 in Figure 2.6)? As another example, consider a new diagnostic technology that can be used in the physician's office at the time of a patient's visit, providing quicker results (items 10 and 12 in Figure 2.4). What are the implications of this test for volume, and hence cost (item 8 in Figure 2.4), versus patient satisfaction (item 13 in Figure 2.5).

SUMMARY

In this chapter we have presented some initial definitions and two working models that will help students and professionals understand different health care systems, the relevant stakeholders, and the effects of their strategic decisions on other elements of the health care marketplace. We encourage you to think about how you can use these models in your sector of the industry and practice using them, especially when it comes to challenging marketing decisions that are discussed in later chapters in this book.

DISCUSSION QUESTIONS

1. Your company has just received marketing approval in the European Union (EU) for an implantable orthopedic device and, you have been transferred to Frankfurt to manage the rollout. Unfortunately, you know very little about those health care systems. Pick one EU country and use the framework in this chapter to help you understand that health care system with respect to your product.

2. You are working for a U.S. senator who is very concerned about rising health care costs. To address this problem, she and her colleagues are proposing a single national fee schedule that would apply to all providers and suppliers. What do you tell her about the sustainability of this approach to reduce overall costs and trends?

3. Suppose you design a benefit plan for an insurance company that wants to provide the highest-quality services, contracting with university medical centers for complex care. Who are the customers for this product? What are the trade-offs they must be willing to make to receive this level of care?

CHAPTER

3

THE HEALTH CARE INDUSTRY AND MARKETING ENVIRONMENT

LEARNING OBJECTIVES

In this chapter, we will address the following questions:

1. What are the major characteristics and weaknesses of the U.S. health care system?

2. What are the characteristics of an ideal health care system?

3. Who are the major active participants in health care systems?

4. How is the health care system changing demographically, economically, socially, culturally, technologically, politically, and legally?

OPENING EXAMPLE

Dr. Arthur Agatston and Others Now Putting the Accent on Illness Prevention Programs Dr. Arthur Agatston, a Miami cardiologist and author of *The South Beach Diet*, does not take a conventional approach to practicing medicine. Convinced of the benefits of smoking cessation, exercise, and diet, he claims that only three of his 2,800 patients had a heart attack in 2006. Cardiologists estimate that the right preventive care can reduce heart attacks by 80 percent.

The U.S. health care system, however, has traditionally focused on treating acute illness. Doctors and hospitals are rewarded for performing expensive tests and procedures when cheaper preventive measures might actually produce better results. Consider heart care: nuclear scans and invasive procedures such as bypass surgery have high levels of reimbursement. In 2005 Medicare paid almost $15 billion, or about 5 percent of its total budget, for bypasses, stents, and other invasive cardiology, according to Jonathan Skinner of Dartmouth University. Yet the appropriateness of such measures for many patients remains unproven.

According to Dr. Gregg W. Stone, director of cardiovascular research at Columbia University, the three keys to effective disease prevention are (1) frequent patient visits to a physician, (2) a close relationship between the physician and the patient, and (3) a very committed patient. For example, Dr. Agatston's nurses give patients specific cholesterol goals to meet and also help them deal with the side effects of the drugs they are taking. A nutritionist meets with them frequently to discuss issues such as how to stick to a high-fiber, Mediterranean diet even on a cruise or a business trip. Unfortunately, while stressing this preventive approach to medicine, Dr. Agatston is actually losing money. He is able to make up for this shortfall through his best-selling book sales, but other physicians who practice prevention and who are not celebrities often suffer financially.
Source: D. Leonhardt, "What's a Pound of Prevention Really Worth?" *New York Times*, Jan. 24, 2007, pp. C1, C4.

Dr. Agatston's story may be discouraging, but there is progress in the move toward more preventive medicine. In California, Massachusetts, and other states, officials have announced plans to provide universal health insurance to residents, and this type of financial restructuring could benefit physicians who focus on preventive services. The most likely path, however, to shaking up practice patterns and payments may be through local governments and pilot programs. For example, Humana will soon begin studying six thousand high-risk patients to better understand how they can be motivated to follow a preventive approach to health. If these pilots are medically and financially successful, other payers are likely to adopt health prevention programs.

OVERVIEW: THE U.S. HEALTH CARE SYSTEM NEEDS IMPROVEMENT

Health care is one of the most extensive and complex industries found in modern economies. It touches every family and involves a considerable number of institutions and professionals. In the United States, health care accounts for about 16 percent of the gross domestic product (GDP) and that percentage is expected to continue rising, in spite of a plethora of cost-containment efforts.

What's worse, the system isn't working. Consider the following:

1. About 45 million persons lack health insurance coverage in the United States.

2. The quality and safety of health care varies greatly from local area to local area. Great geographical variation exists in the choice of procedures to address different illnesses. Access to medical facilities and services is highly uneven. In addition, there are too many medical errors occurring in the provision of health care.

3. Many patients are unhappy about the high and rising costs of health insurance and the limits placed on their choice of physicians and procedures.

4. Patients are also dissatisfied with pharmaceutical companies and what they consider to be outrageous prices for medications.

5. Physicians are angry because of falling remuneration, restrictions on their freedom to choose procedures, and the high cost of malpractice insurance in an overly litigious society.

6. Employers are unhappy because they see their medical insurance premiums rising, in some cases to almost unaffordable levels.

7. Hospitals face rising, uncompensated costs of new technology that rapidly needs to be replaced by still newer technology.

8. Health care benefits are confusing, coverage is limited, and patients' out-of-pocket expenses are increasing for professional services, products, and prescriptions.

9. Patients, physicians, employers, and health plans face substantial paperwork and bureaucratic hurdles.

10. Government, patients, physicians, and hospitals are concerned about what measures are necessary to place the Medicare and Medicaid programs on a stable financial footing.

11. All stakeholders agree that widely accessible, yet secure electronic health records are necessary, but few are willing to pay for such a system.

12. The health care system needs to spend more on prevention, early detection, and lifestyle changes that will reduce illness from conditions such as obesity, heart disease, breast cancer, prostate cancer, and HIV/AIDS.

The striking fact is that the United States devotes substantially more resources to its health care system than other advanced nations as measured by per capita and percent GDP spending. The nearly $2 trillion a year in U.S. health care expenditures is about twice what many other countries pay per capita for health care. The problem is not only the total cost but the relatively poor results. "On 37 measures of health outcome, quality, access, equity, efficiency and innovation, the United States lags behind many other industrialized nations."[1] (See Figure 3.1.)

The reasons for the disparities between the United States and other countries include the following:

1. Health care is not a declared right in the United States as it is in other countries. (For example, this right is written into the constitution of South Africa.) Because we do not have a delineation of rights, we cannot agree on common goals.

2. All countries except the United States have budgets for health care. We set benefit mandates and then try to fund them; other countries have at least implicit budgets and try to spend the money so it does the greatest good for the greatest

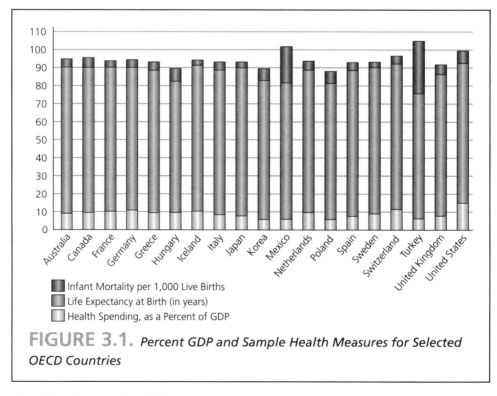

Infant Mortality per 1,000 Live Births
Life Expectancy at Birth (in years)
Health Spending, as a Percent of GDP

FIGURE 3.1. *Percent GDP and Sample Health Measures for Selected OECD Countries*

Note: Most figures are for 2003.
Source: OECD Health Data, June 5, 2005.

number. Trying to deliver on promises of coverage to all recipients without a budget is futile.

3. Unlike other countries, the United States does not have a centralized technology approval process. For example, the Food and Drug Administration (FDA) evaluates the safety and efficacy but not the cost-effectiveness of new technology. New technology is the strongest driver of higher health care costs.

Combining these three statements, one could say we don't know where we are going, and we have no budget and no control over the reasons that costs are increasing.

DEFINING A WELL-DESIGNED HEALTH CARE SYSTEM

Is the unsatisfactory performance of the U.S. health care system due to the fact that it is largely in private hands and relies on competition to create positive health outcomes? Research does not support this conclusion. For example, according to McGlynn, "Extensive research into quality of care in different countries yields no conclusive findings that one system is better or worse than others. Quality does not necessarily vary with financing mechanisms . . ."[2] Despite such findings, many still advocate replacing the current employer-based system with a single-payer system run by the federal government. Further, some still confuse universal coverage with the need to have a single payer. Many are also unaware that almost all nations operate a privately financed system along with a government-sponsored one. Critics of U.S. health care admit that public systems are not free of problems, such as long waits for elective surgery, delays in replacing aging infrastructure, and limits on the availability of new technology. Still, they believe that preventing personal financial tragedies due to health care expenses is worth the change. Further, they point to lower administrative costs of public programs, highlighting the high marketing and underwriting expenses of competing health insurers. They even point out that the Veterans Administration, run by the government, is one of the most efficient health care systems in the United States.

Others believe that the private, for-profit U.S. health care system is still superior to a single-payer system and can be further improved through such measures as controlling the price of drugs, limiting duplicative technology, holding down the premiums that health plans charge, covering the uninsured, and discouraging physicians from overtesting and overmedicating. Unfortunately, as we discussed in the previous chapter, attacking one problem at a time will trigger counterreactions in other parts of the system and may end up worsening performance.

Still others advocate that the health care system should remain private and competitive, but point out that too many of the system's participants work at cross-purposes. Michael Porter and Elizabeth Teisberg distinguish between a competitive system operating on a zero-sum model, whereby the winners gain at the expense of losers, and one operating on a positive-sum model, whereby everyone wins.[3] They assert that the private, competitive system needs to operate on a new principle, namely that *every health care practice and activity should be judged on the value that it contributes to patients' health*. Although this suggestion seems novel in the United States, it is widespread in other countries, which use cost-benefit analysis to evaluate new technologies. Health outcomes should be measured and reported for different procedures and practices and made transparent to patients, physicians, health plan providers, and employers so that excellent practices will be patronized and poorer practices avoided.

When people are asked what they desire or expect in an ideal health care system, they usually mention the following: low cost, high medical quality, and easy access to the providers they want. As explained in the previous chapter, these three features are trade-offs; however, many insured Americans are unwilling to sacrifice on one dimension to enhance or maintain the benefits of the others. This book takes the position that a health care system should be judged by the extent to which it helps its citizens maintain or improve their health over their lifetimes, given the availability and prudent use of limited resources. (See Field Note 3.1 for an expanded view of medical care outside traditional Western medicine.)

FIELD NOTE 3.1.

A Tour Through Alternative and Complementary Medicine   For years, Western medicine has adhered to the scientific method in establishing the effectiveness and safety of new drugs, treatments, and procedures. It took less notice of medical theories and practices in other parts of the world, or of non-evidence-based medical claims and nostrums. With the rise of the humanistic movement in the 1960s and the growing interest in such practices as meditation, biofeedback, and visualization, some physicians began to take a more open-minded view of these practices. The rise of interest in herbal medicine and acupuncture from China opened further doors.

The term used for many of the new medical therapies was *alternative medicine*. If a cancer patient was not being helped with Western medicine, the patient would resort to other alternatives, including herbs, hydrotherapy, therapeutic touch, incantations, and others. But some expressed concerns about alternative medicine practice, chiefly (1) the therapeutic value is not evidence-based, (2) there can be harm from relying on it, and (based in part on the first two concerns) (3) health insurers generally will not pay for it.

On the other hand, the term *complementary medicine* describes helpful practices used in conjunction with conventional medicine. Complementary and alternative medicine (CAM) describes both branches.

A still more recent term, *integrative medicine*, encompasses conventional medical treatments and those CAM treatments for which there is some high-quality scientific evidence of safety and effectiveness. Integrative medicine focuses on wellness and calls upon the physician and the patient to pay attention to all components of lifestyle, including diet, exercise, stress management, and emotional well-being.

The following are some of the most common CAM practices:

Ayurveda: This two-thousand-year-old Indian system places emphasis on restoring natural harmony between body, mind, and spirit. An Ayurvedic doctor identifies an individual's overall health profile and metabolic body type and then recommends a specific treatment plan (diet, exercise, yoga, meditation, massage, and herbal tonics) to recapture the natural harmony.

Body work and massage: This therapy involves pressing, rubbing, and manipulating muscles and other soft body tissue, causing them to relax by improving the flow of oxygen and blood to affected areas to relieve back, neck, and shoulder pain. Body work includes acupressure, chiropractic, martial arts, massage therapy, Rolfing, and shiatsu. Massage itself has over seventy-five forms, such as Swedish message, deep-tissue massage, neuromuscular massage, and manual lymph drainage. Chiropractic focuses on spinal manipulations to unblock nerve signals sent by the brain so that the body can heal itself. It is used to treat back problems, headaches, nerve inflammation, muscle spasms, and other injuries and traumas.

Diet-based therapy: This approach recommends specific diets to improve health and longevity, to control weight, and to treat specific health conditions such as high cholesterol. Examples include macrobiotic, vegetarian, low-fat, and low-carbohydrate (such as Zone and Atkins) diets.

Energy therapies: The name refers to alternative treatments that involve the use of purported energy fields. Examples include magnet therapy and therapeutic touch.

Exercise-based therapy: This treatment consists of a variety of forms of physical exercise to improve health and longevity, increase muscle mass, treat specific health conditions, and relieve stress. Examples include aerobics, Alexander technique, bodybuilding, Feldenkrais method, martial arts, Pilates, stretching, Tai Chi, and weight training.

Herbalism: This practice consists of making or prescribing herbal remedies for medical conditions.

Homeopathy: This practice uses minute doses of remedies that include plants, metals, and minerals to treat a wide variety of ailments such as seasonal allergies, asthma, influenza, headaches, and indigestion.

Hypnotherapy: Hypnotism has been used to treat symptoms, diseases, and addictions. The procedure accesses various levels of the mind to effect positive changes in a person's behavior such as losing weight, desisting from smoking, overcoming fear of flying, improving sleep, and reducing pain and stress.

Mind-body interventions: This variety of techniques is designed to enhance the mind's capacity to affect bodily function and symptoms. Examples include Alexander technique, aromatherapy, autosuggestion, Feldenkrais method, hypnotherapy, journaling, meditation, visualization, and yoga.

Traditional Chinese Medicine: This system of health care is based on the Chinese philosophy of harmony and balance within the human body as well as harmony between the body and its outside environment. Examples include acupressure, acupuncture, Chinese martial arts, Chinese pulse diagnosis, massage, and herbalism.

MAJOR PARTICIPANTS IN THE HEALTH CARE SYSTEM

We introduced the concept of stakeholders in Chapter Two; here we will explain more about them and their interaction with one another. The following are the seven major types of participants in most health systems:

1. *Care providers*, including institutions (such as hospitals, nursing homes, rehabilitation centers, surgicenters, clinics, physician offices, and in-store medical centers) and the professionals who work in them (such as physicians, nurses, dentists, pharmacists, and therapists)

2. *Payers*, including managed care organizations (MCOs) (such as health maintenance organizations [HMOs] and preferred provider organizations [PPOs]), traditional insurance companies, governments, and individuals

3. *Employers*

4. *Government organizations* (such as the Centers for Medicare and Medicaid Services, the Centers for Disease Control and Prevention, and the National Institutes of Health)

5. *Medical associations* (such as the American Medical Association, American Dental Association, and various specialty societies)

6. *Health advocacy organizations* (such as the American Cancer Society)

7. *Supply companies* (pharmaceutical, biotechnology and medical device, equipment and supply companies)

Figure 3.2 depicts where the United States spends its health care dollars.

In the following sections we describe the role played by each type of participant.

Care Providers

Care providers are organizations that provide medical services. They include hospitals, nursing homes, hospices, rehabilitation centers, surgical centers, outpatient medical clinics, individual physician offices, and in-store medical centers, among others (see Figure 3.3). They also include the professionals who work in these organizations.

Each provider type contains many variations and thus may constitute a different type of customer for the health care marketer. For example, consider hospitals, which can be classified by size (gauged by number of beds), location (urban, suburban, or rural), scope of services (general hospitals versus specialty hospitals, which may cover

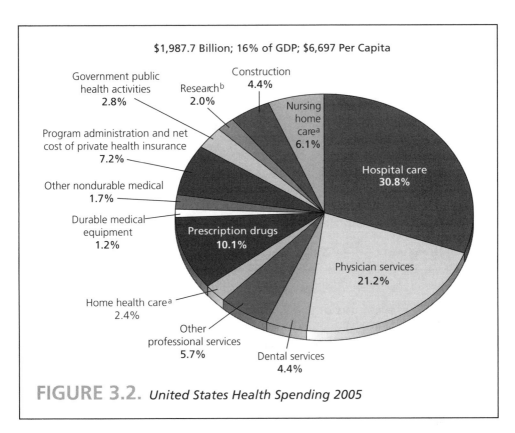

$1,987.7 Billion; 16% of GDP; $6,697 Per Capita

FIGURE 3.2. *United States Health Spending 2005*

[a]Freestanding facilities only. Additional services of this type are provided in hospital-based facilities and counted as hospital care.
[b]Research and development expenditures of drug companies and other manufacturers and providers of medical equipment and supplies are excluded from "research" expenditures and instead are included in the category in which the product falls.
Source: Centers for Medicare and Medicaid Services, Office of the Actuary, National Health Statistics Group, U.S. Dept. of Commerce, Bureau of Economic Analysis and Bureau of the Census.

only such specialties as pediatrics, psychiatry, women's health, rehabilitation, or cardiac care), sponsorship (religious, secular, or government), and for-profit status. Of the approximately 4,900 hospitals in the United States, about 60 percent are urban and about 70 percent have fewer than two hundred beds. What is especially important for health care marketers to know is that more than 80 percent of hospitals belong to a system or network and seven in ten participate in a group purchasing organization (GPO). To highlight the importance of GPOs, note that the top three (Premier Purchasing Partners, Novation, and MedAssets) account for about $60 billion per year in purchasing.

The way in which marketing and sales take place in this sector will therefore have much to do with these institutional characteristics and affiliations.

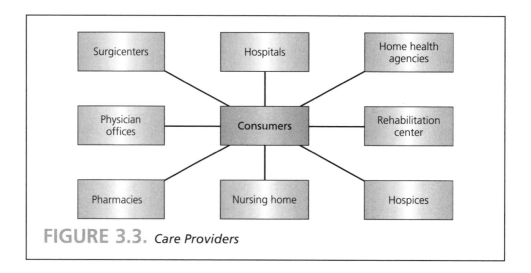

FIGURE 3.3. *Care Providers*

Residential care consists of various levels of service, ranging from independent living facilities to those providing skilled services similar to some hospital care. Nursing homes also differentiate themselves according to types of patients, income levels, and medical conditions (see Field Note 3.2).

FIELD NOTE 3.2.

Nursing Homes: Are They the Best Solution? Many communities have set up nursing homes to serve elderly, poor, or disabled patients who have no alternative place to go for care. For example, San Francisco has the massive Laguna Honda nursing home in which hundreds of residents live in regimented wards of up to twenty-eight beds each. It was founded back in 1866 and combined two functions, serving as both a long-term home for the poor and elderly and a public hospital. It represents one view of nursing homes as places that warehouse the elderly and frail before they die.

The city has decided to erect a large modern replacement building—which will feature suites of rooms, internet access, and flat-screen televisions—to offer more humane treatment for the residents. Opposition has arisen, however, to the idea of a large-scale impersonal nursing home. Opponents prefer to see the Medicaid money spent on providing home care or smaller assisted-living facilities sprinkled throughout the community. They supply studies showing that average Medicaid costs for home care may be almost a third less than for nursing homes—$34,400 versus $46,612 per year. They argue that not only is the cost less but also the patients feel more stimulated and better served in home care or in small assisted living facilities.

Those who favor large nursing homes argue that these facilities are needed as a safety net when sufficient alternatives don't exist. They further argue that large nursing homes can provide better medical and hospital care for residents who have serious medical conditions. And finally, these nursing homes can be modernized and made more pleasant and stimulating.

This debate on how to serve the indigent, elderly, and disabled will undoubtedly continue, and cost will be one of the prime factors determining the outcome.

Source: "Battle on Home Front: San Francisco's Massive New Nursing Facility Draws Criticism as Institutions Lose Favor," *New York Times*, May 7, 2007, pp. A1, A12.

The professionals who work in these settings are of diverse types as well. For example, physician specialties range from surgical subspecialties (such as neurosurgery and cardiovascular surgery) to general primary care (family practice). Currently, there are more than 885,000 physicians in this country.

Payers

Most insured people in the United States receive their coverage through their employer. If small employers provide such coverage, they usually purchase it from an insurance company; most large employers, however, self-insure and have other firms manage the benefit on their behalf. Regardless of who bears the financial risk, the vast majority of these plans are considered managed care organizations (MCOs) (see Figure 3.4). We define managed care as follows: "A process to maximize the health gain of a community within limited resources, by ensuring that an appropriate range and level of services are provided, and by monitoring on a case-by-case basis to ensure that they are continuously improved to meet national targets for health and individual health needs."[4] What differentiates managed care from fee-for-service care is financial and clinical accountability aided by enhanced coordination of services.

MCOs consist mainly of three types of plans: health maintenance organizations (HMOs), preferred provider organizations (PPOs), and a hybrid called a point of service (POS) product. To effectively market to these types of plans or work within this sector, the health care marketing specialist must understand how they differ.

Health Maintenance Organizations. *An HMO is a health care plan that delivers comprehensive, coordinated medical service to voluntarily enrolled members on a prepaid basis.* Several parts of this definition require a more detailed explanation. First is the key word *comprehensive*. With regard to scope of services, many traditional, non-HMO plans cover acute care but not routine preventive services. A founding precept of a health *maintenance* organization is the provision of care that prevents illness and maintains health. In fact, for all the bad press these plans have received, the research indicates that HMOs do provide more preventive care than other forms of

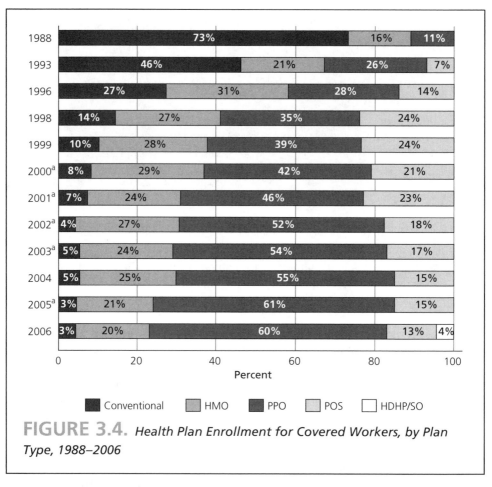

FIGURE 3.4. *Health Plan Enrollment for Covered Workers, by Plan Type, 1988–2006*

[a]Distribution is statistically different from distribution for the previous year shown at p <.05. No statistical tests are conducted for years prior to 1999. No statistical tests are conducted between 2005 and 2006 due to the addition of HDHP/SO as a new plan type.
Source: Kaiser/HRET Survey of Employer-Sponsored Health Benefits, 1999–2005; KPMG Survey of Employer-Sponsored Health Benefits, 1993, 1996, 1998; The Health Insurance Association of America (HIAA), 1988.

insurance coverage.[5] Another part of the comprehensiveness is financial coverage. For example, many insurance products have lifetime limits on expenses, usually ranging from one to five million dollars. HMOs do not have such caps.

The next key concept is *coordinated medical service*. This term implies that someone is directing the care to ensure that it is delivered in a high-quality, cost-effective manner. Although the term *gatekeeper* is often applied to this function, it is more appropriate to say that it is the responsibility of a *primary care physician*. We define the latter term as follows:

Primary care is the provision of integrated, accessible health care services by clinicians who are accountable for addressing a large majority of personal health care needs, developing a sustained partnership with patients, and practicing in the context of family and community. The term integrated is used to denote the provision of comprehensive, coordinated, and continuous services that provide a seamless process of care.[6]

Note the essential features in this definition: these physicians must be capable of caring for a majority of common conditions (such as diabetes, asthma, high blood pressure, and arthritis) and can treat patients on a long-term basis in whatever setting they need care. The specialties that fit this definition, therefore, are family medicine, internal medicine, and pediatrics. The HMO requires that patients coordinate care through their primary care physicians; except in nonemergency situations, the HMO will generally pay only for services that the primary care physician authorizes. Because this process restricts freedom of the patients to self-refer to specialists of their choice, this practice has become a source of member dissatisfaction with this type of plan. Other health care arrangements (such as PPOs) may not require these referrals, accounting in part for their popularity and growth vis-à-vis HMOs.

The final key term is *prepaid*. This term means that the physicians receive a set monthly fee (capitation) in advance of providing services. The amount is based on the total number of patients assigned to that practitioner (or group), usually adjusted by age and sex. The amount paid on behalf of an individual patient is usually called the *per member per month* (PMPM) payment. This method of payment is intended not only to provide physicians with a financial incentive to keep patients healthy, but also to remove a barrier for patients who would otherwise delay care because of out-of-pocket costs.

HMOs perform better than other types of plans in containing cost because they are designed to change physician behavior, which accounts for about 75 percent of health care expenses. One reason some countries fail to achieve successful cost containment strategies is that they usually address only the *amount* of payment to providers and suppliers rather than the *method* of payment that will result in a change in physician behavior. Capitation is the hallmark of HMOs. If a plan does not involve capitation, it is not truly an HMO, no matter what it calls itself. Because a capitated plan means the services are prepaid, the physician does not increase revenue by doing more. *Capitation, therefore, addresses the financial incentives of provider-induced demand that occur in a fee-for-service setting.*

The concern with capitation, of course, is that the physician will be tempted to withhold services. In addressing this issue, however, Berwick noted: "If anything, the data suggest hazards and ethical problems in the overuse of services in fee-for-service settings, rather than its underuse in capitated care."[7]

Because there are several types of HMOs, an important point to remember is that the type of plan is defined by how the physicians are organized and their relationship to the insurance component. Appreciating these organizational structures and relationships are critical for marketers who must understand and identify decision makers in a managed care setting.

The first type of plan is a *staff model*. In this arrangement, physicians are employees of the plan and receive salaries as well as performance bonuses based on such measures as number of patients seen, compliance with cost-control measures, and meeting of quality goals. Although physicians are not capitated under this scheme, their employment status, supervision, and reward structure make this model a true HMO. Because these physicians are employees of the health plan, they see only patients who belong to that HMO. Also, because they are employees, their management decision-making abilities may be restricted. The real decision makers are the plan executives. Common examples of this arrangement are employer- and union-sponsored plans, which hire full-time physicians to care for all employee and family health care needs.

The second type of plan is the *group model*. In this arrangement, physicians belong to a medical group that has a mutually exclusive relationship with a health plan: the plan's patients see only the group's physicians and the group sees only patients enrolled in the plan. The group is capitated, and physicians within the group determine the distribution of funds among themselves. The decision-making authority in this model is split between the plan and the group. For example, pharmaceutical companies may convince the plan (or its designated pharmaceutical benefit manager) to offer its products to members. These companies then need to convince the group's leadership and, often, individual physicians to actually use these medications. The prototype of a group model is the relationship between Kaiser and the Permanente Medical Group.

The third model is called an *individual practice association* or IPA, which itself has organizational variations. In the first type of this arrangement, the health plan contracts with each individual physician. In another version, physicians organize into virtual medical groups for purposes of contracting with health plans. Under this arrangement, the organizing entity can be a hospital (a so-called *hospital-based IPA*), medical society, or freestanding company. The plan then contracts with and pays capitation to the IPA, which in turn pays member physicians on a fee or capitation basis. Unlike group and staff model physicians, those who belong to an IPA can see fee-for-service patients and contract with multiple plans. The decision makers are even more decentralized in this setting. They consist of the plan executives, IPA administrators, and individual physicians.

The fourth type of HMO plan is the *network model*, an organizational hybrid of the group and IPA models. In the network model, plans contract with established medical groups to provide care to enrolled members. It has thus been called an *IPA of groups*. Unlike IPAs, though, these groups are actual legal entities in which physicians share practice revenues and expenses. As is the case with IPAs, physicians in network models also see non-HMO patients and can contract with multiple plans.

The decision makers here are the plan executives, group leadership, and individual physicians. Because physicians are organized in groups, reaching them is logistically easier than with the first type of IPA model. Because they offer patients a wider network of providers and have lower capital costs for the insurer than group or staff models, the IPA and network models are the predominant types of HMOs in the United States.

Preferred Provider Organizations. The second major type of MCO is the *preferred provider organization* (PPO). PPOs emerged as an alternative to HMOs because they give patients more freedom of choice of providers. According to the American Association of PPOs (APPO): "PPOs, while difficult to define, have a number of common operational elements . . ." These elements operate as follows:

- Insurer or third parties contract with a panel of providers.

  Often the provider network is larger than a comparable HMO network; however, in view of continuing cost escalations, many of these networks are becoming more select.

- They negotiate a fee schedule with these providers.

  Instead of capitation, these providers are paid on a discounted fee-for-service basis. The rates are usually based on a percentage of the local Medicare payment rates (above or below them).

- The providers agree to abide by a utilization review process.

  Because the health plan is paying claims, the utilization review can be more administratively complex than in an HMO setting. For example, in HMOs physicians are financially as well as clinically responsible for care and tend to self-monitor utilization. Because a PPO is essentially a fee-for-service payment mechanism, more preauthorization procedures are in place to curb perceived overutilization.

- Patients are not "locked in"; that is, if they obtain care outside the panel of contracted providers, they will retain some coverage, though it will not be as comprehensive as if they had stayed within the network.

As mentioned previously, in an HMO, except for emergencies, all care must be approved and referred by the patient's primary care physician. If a patient seeks such care without a referral, the patient will be fully responsible for the bill. In a PPO, if the patient sees a contracted doctor, the plan pays that doctor according to the fee schedule. If the patient sees a noncontracted provider, the plan requires the patient to pay more of the bill, but may still pay something. In recent years, the out-of-pocket share has risen significantly for patients who obtain elective services from providers who are not contracted with the plan.

Although PPOs proliferated during the managed care backlash of the 1990s, rising health care costs have forced these plans to increasingly behave like HMOs: provider networks are narrowing, fee schedules are more "aggressive," utilization review is stricter (using more disease management programs), and financial penalties are increasing for patients who go to noncontracted providers or use nonpreferred pharmaceuticals. These changes, along with HMOs' adoption of some open features, have caused some convergence in the design of these two very different types of insurance.

We offer an important caution for providers and suppliers dealing with PPOs. Some of these companies contract with other plans to use their negotiated rates and networks without the knowledge of the providers and suppliers; they are essentially selling their contractual relationships to a third party. These arrangements are called *silent PPOs*, because those delivering the services or providing products are unaware of these secondary contracts. When payments are due, it can be difficult to identify the responsible party. Contracts must, therefore, specify the companies responsible for payment and prohibit such behavior.

Point of Service Plans (POS). POS plans are a hybrid of HMOs and PPOs and may incorporate any number of the features of each. For example, some plans have HMO benefits if the patient stays with his or her assigned primary care physician, but switch to PPO-like fees if the patient prefers to see another contracted physician. Because of the large number of variations, no one definition or lists of characteristics adequately define this type of plan.

KEY MANAGED CARE TRENDS

To meet current and future concerns about health care costs, MCOs have introduced changes in the way they do business. These measures include increasing patients' out-of-pocket expenses (in the form of higher deductibles, co-payments, and coinsurance), giving customers the opportunity to customize their health insurance (by combining desired cost structure and benefits), and establishing health savings accounts (HSAs), whereby individuals are at increased "first dollar" financial risk for their health care. The rationale for this latter measure is to make consumers of health care more prudent purchasers.

Role of the Federal Government as a Payer

Because the federal government is a single entity and has legislative powers, it wields more market power than any private payer. The populations covered by federal payments include government employees (through the Federal Employee Health Benefit Program, or FEHBP), military veterans (through the Veterans Administration, or VA), active military and their families (through a program called Tricare), and, most important, Medicare and Medicaid. We will briefly discuss these last two programs.

Medicare covered about forty-two million Americans in 2005. Eligibility for this insurance comes from two groups. The first group (35.4 million) comprises those sixty-five years of age or older, provided they or their spouse made payroll tax contributions for at least ten years and are eligible for Social Security payments. The other group consists of those less than sixty-five years old who have been permanently and continuously disabled for a twenty-four-month period and are eligible to receive Social Security Disability payments (6.3 million).

Although most payers traditionally compensate providers on some type of negotiated fee schedule, Medicare has developed innovative alternative methods, some of which have been adopted by private payers. We summarize these payment methods in Table 3.1. Although the details of each method are beyond the scope of this chapter, we encourage marketing managers who deal with each category of customer to investigate them further. Knowledge of how customers are paid is essential to delivering value to them.

Medicaid is a joint federal and state program, with the former contributing at least half of the funds. Despite federal parameters for participation, the degree of coverage for specific services varies dramatically from state to state, making generalizations unfeasible. In contrast with Medicare, whose eligibility is straightforward, the criteria for Medicaid are much more complicated, but usually include financial criteria tied to annual income as a percentage over the Federal Poverty Line (FPL). Further, individuals need to apply for benefits rather than qualifying automatically, as is the case with Medicare. Because of this latter feature, the exact number of Medicaid *eligibles* is impossible to determine. Also, because individuals and families go on and off the Medicaid rolls, the exact number of beneficiaries nationwide is constantly changing. In the past few years, the numbers of enrolled persons have been estimated to be between thirty-seven and fifty-two million. Current estimates are in the middle portion of this range.

Employers

Most large employers offer their employees two or more types of health insurance, often from the same insurance company. The marketing task for health plans is to get the employer to choose their company to provide or administer these benefits. If chosen, the plan must also market itself to the employees.

The continuing marketing challenge for these plans is to keep employer and employee satisfied while holding down costs (see Field Note 3.3). For example, employees want their medical claims paid in a prompt fashion; employers, who want satisfied employees, also desire the plans to make sure payments are made only for covered benefits and for correct amounts. Often a health plan will agree to full payment for a noncovered or nonreferred service so as to not lose the employer customer.

TABLE 3.1. **Medicare Payment Methods**

Provider	Payment Method
Inpatient Hospital	International Classification of Disease (ICD)-9CM coding that determines a diagnosis related group (DRG). Global amount paid per hospital stay.
Outpatient Hospital	Ambulatory Payment Category (APC)—Outpatient Prospective Payment System (OPPS) based on Current Procedural Terminology (CPT)-4 and Healthcare Common Procedural Coding System (HCPCS). Global amount paid per type of care; for example, emergency room visit or chemotherapy visit. May have more than one APC per encounter.
Ambulatory Surgicenter (not hospital affiliated)	Nine payment categories. After 2008, new rates will be phased in linked to the APC methodology.
Skilled Nursing Facility	Resource Utilization Group (RUG-III)—Health Insurance Prospective Payment Systems (HIPPS). Pays on per diem basis.
Physicians	CPT-4 or HCPCS codes that determine resource based relative value scale (RBRVS) per service payment.
Pharmacies	Contracted rates with either a Medicare MCO (under Part C) or Part D payer. Also, Medicare beneficiaries who do not sign up for Part C or D pay out-of-pocket charges.
Hospice	Daily rates (per diems) based on level of service: routine home care, continuous attendance at home, inpatient respite care, and general inpatient care (for palliative treatment).
Home Health Care	Outcome and Assessment Information Set (OASIS)—Home Health Resource Groups (HHRG). Pays global amount for each sixty-day episode of care (adjusted downward for increments less than sixty days).

FIELD NOTE 3.3.

Companies Struggle to Reduce Their Health Costs   In 2007, the average employee paid $2,904 a year for a family in premiums and out-of-pocket health expenses. And companies are laying out nearly $9,000 per employee. This situation will only get worse.

The new corporate imperative is to contain health care expenses. Aside from the 39 percent of companies that offer no medical benefits, the 61 percent who do are undertaking various initiatives to reduce their costs, including:

- Adopting higher-deductible plans.

- Pressing for higher co-payments to discourage going to the doctor for minor ailments.

- Instituting higher coinsurance payments by employees.

- Adding surcharges to cover spouses and partners who could otherwise get coverage from *their* employer, and audit more carefully which dependents are entitled to coverage.

The result is that employees are feeling the pain of higher medical costs.

Companies are also being more careful who they hire. Job applicants with poor medical backgrounds or likelihood of medical problems encounter discrimination, although this is never the reason given.

Companies are also exhorting their employees to live healthier lifestyles. Several companies have instituted wellness programs including smoking cessation and health-club discounts. Other companies have gone further by establishing wellness facilities on their premises, including running tracks, treadmills, and exercise equipment. Scotts Miracle-Gro in Marysville, Ohio, audits and consults on the health of each employee.

Sources: Kathleen Kingsbury, "Pressure on Your Health Benefits," *Time*, Nov. 6, 2006, pp. 53–54; "Get Healthy–or Else: Inside One Company's All-Out Attack on Medical Costs," *Business Week*, Feb. 26, 2007.

Supply Organizations

According to the U.S. Bureau of Labor Statistics, "the pharmaceutical and medicine manufacturing industry consists of about 2,500 places of employment, located throughout the country." In 2004, this sector provided jobs for about 291,000 persons and is expected to grow about 26 percent by 2014 (compared with 14 percent for all industries combined). We will furnish examples of companies in each category, but the reader should understand that there is much overlap due to diversified firms and joint ventures. For example, Johnson & Johnson comprises many divisions engaged in several sectors: pharmaceuticals (Janssen), biotechnology (Centocor), and devices (Cordis and DePuy), to name a few.

Every health system includes two types of for-profit supply organizations: (1) pharmaceutical and biotechnology companies, and (2) medical device and supply companies.

Pharmaceutical and Biotechnology Companies

The United States accounts for almost half of the $604 billion market value of the global pharmaceutical and biotechnology sector. On a sales basis, this country is the largest single market, with a 44 percent share of over $216 billion. Although biotechnology products are being rapidly developed, pharmaceuticals still dominate this field with more than an 80 percent share.[8] A detailed account of the supply chain in this sector is beyond the scope of this chapter, but is summarized in Figure 3.5 and Table 3.2. Here we will review key features of drug manufacturers, wholesalers, pharmacies, and pharmaceutical benefit management companies (PBMs).

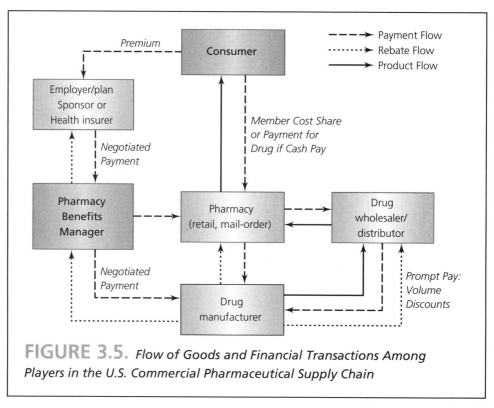

FIGURE 3.5. *Flow of Goods and Financial Transactions Among Players in the U.S. Commercial Pharmaceutical Supply Chain*

Source: The Health Strategies Consultancy LLC. This information was reprinted with permission from the Henry J. Kaiser Family Foundation.

TABLE 3.2. Channel Distribution by U.S. Sales

Rank	Channel Distribution	2006 Total Dollars (U.S. $Billions)[a] [Scripts In Millions]
1	Chain Stores	$96.1 [1,946.4]
2	Mail Service	$42.2 [232.3]
3	Independent Pharmacies	$35.5 [765.3]
4	Clinics	$30.1
5	Nonfederal Hospitals	$26.8
6	Food Stores	$22.2 [475.5]
7	Long-Term Care	$13.0 [287.0]
8	Federal Facilities	$3.7
9	Home Health Care	$2.4
10	HMO	$1.5
11	Miscellaneous	$0.9
	All	$274.8 [3,706.7]

[a]Represents prescription pharmaceutical purchases including insulin at wholesale prices by retail, food stores and chains, mass merchandisers, independent pharmacies, mail services, nonfederal and federal hospitals, clinics, closed-wall HMOs, long-term care pharmacies, home health care, and prisons/universities. Excludes co-marketing agreements. Joint ventures assigned to product owner. Data run by custom redesign to include completed mergers and acquisitions. *Source*: IMS Health, IMS National Sales Perspectives™, 3/2007.

Drug Manufacturers. Globally, the industry is still fragmented; the top six firms (led by Pfizer, Sanofi-Aventis, and Glaxo SmithKlein) account for only about 30 percent of the industry's value. Companies are frequently differentiated from one another by the types of products they produce. Some companies, such as the ones just mentioned, produce innovative pharmaceuticals that are patented and sold under trade names (branded pharmaceuticals). Other companies sell medications whose patent has expired and promote the drug using a different brand name, but stress its chemical content (generic pharmaceuticals). For example, Motrin (ibuprofen) was originally sold exclusively under its brand name; now ibuprofen is available without a prescription under a variety of names (including Motrin). Companies that manufacture generics range from U.S. firms Mylan and Barr, to Israel's Teva, to India's Ranbaxy and Dr. Redy. According to Visiongain: "In sharp contrast to the branded pharmaceutical market, which has stalled in recent years, the generics market is enjoying a period of unprecedented success. In 2005 the world generics market was worth $45 billion, a growth of 14 percent on the previous year . . ."[9] A third category of manufacturers makes complex organic molecules known as biologicals. These medications are most often administered by injection. Prominent companies in this sector are Amgen and Genentech.

According to the Kaiser Family Foundation, "Most promotional spending (86 percent) in 2004 . . . was devoted to promoting drugs directly to physicians through sampling (57 percent), detailing (26 percent), and professional journals (2 percent), with the remaining 14 percent directed at consumers. DTC [direct-to-consumer] advertising experienced the highest average annual increase (22 percent) from 1996 to 2004, compared with 15 percent for the retail value of sampling, 12 percent for detailing, and 1 percent in professional journal advertising"[10] (see Figure 3.6). Worldwide, Consumers International (a British consumer advocacy group) estimates promotional spending is about $60 billion.[11] Such spending can be divided into the following categories:

- *Detailing.* Sales representatives from pharmaceutical companies call on physicians to educate them about the company's products, often comparing them with ones offered by competitors on such dimensions as cost, drug-drug interactions, side-effect profiles, and effectiveness. Recently, revised professional codes of ethics, legislation, and voluntary efforts have limited the monetary value of gifts that can be offered during sales calls and increased the scrutiny of promotional activities. For example, the American Medical Association recommends that no single gift exceed $100; as part of enforcement of a 2004 law, the state of West Virginia has debated requiring drug companies to disclose the costs of detailing physicians;[12] and many medical students are refusing to attend lunches sponsored by pharmaceutical companies or to accept small gifts, such as pens with corporate logos and drug names.[13]

- *Sampling.* Drug companies supply physicians (and sometimes patients directly) with free samples. These samples provide the opportunity for the doctor either

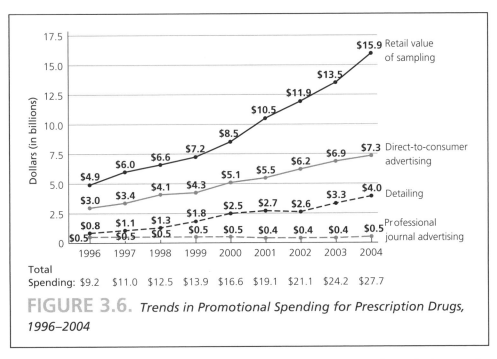

FIGURE 3.6. *Trends in Promotional Spending for Prescription Drugs, 1996–2004*

Notes: Numbers may not total due to rounding. *Sampling* is the value of samples left at sales visits to office-based physicians. The samples are valued at the prices at which they would be sold in retail pharmacies. *Detailing* is expenses for the sales activities of pharmaceutical company representatives directed to office-based and hospital-based physicians and hospital directors of pharmacies; approximately 85 percent of detailing is for office-based sales visits. *Direct-to-Consumer Advertising* is expenses for advertising to consumers through television, magazines and newspapers, radio, and outdoors. *Professional Journal Advertising* is expenses for advertising appearing in medical journals.
Source: IMS Health Web site [http://www.imshealth.com] and Kaiser Family Foundation Publication 7031.

to use a new medication or to see if a patient will respond to the medication before a long-term prescription is issued. Because of the different methods used to determine pharmaceutical costs (wholesale, retail, and marginal manufacturing costs, to name a few), the exact value of these samples cannot be accurately assessed. The 2003 retail figure used by the Pharmaceutical Research and Manufacturers of America (the industry trade group often referred to as PhRMA) was $16 billion.

■ *Direct-to-consumer (DTC) advertising.* This includes all advertisements geared to consumers, as opposed to professionals who would prescribe medications. All media have been used for this technique, including print, television, radio, and the Internet. Again, according to the Kaiser Family Foundation: ". . . for every 10% increase in DTC advertising, drug sales within the classes studied increased on average by 1%. No evidence was found that changes in DTC advertising affected the market share of individual drugs within the classes . . . This means that each additional dollar spent on DTC advertising in 2000 yielded $4.20 in additional pharmaceutical sales in that year." [14] Because DTC advertising has been in general media outlets, messages often reach many persons who are not candidates for the treatments being promoted. To further refine their advertising strategies, drug companies are adopting target marketing strategies. One of the fastest-growing methods is internet use. "As marketers shift from consumer mass marketing to more targeted opportunities on the Internet, eMarketer projects pharmaceutical companies' Internet spending will increase nearly 25% this year, to $780 million." [15] It is important to note that DTC advertising of pharmaceuticals is illegal in most of the rest of the world (New Zealand being the prominent exception).

■ *Medical journal advertising.* This cost is the value of the advertisements drug companies purchase in publications geared to prescribing physicians.

Another important marketing technique is sponsorship of educational meetings and other events for physicians and health care professionals such as nurses and pharmacists. The cost of these activities for physicians has been estimated at about $2.1 billion. [16]

A perennial question arises about drug company profit margins and often frames the public relations part of marketing this sector. This discussion begins with the cost of bringing a drug to market, which manufacturers would like to recoup at a profit over the course of its patent life. The actual out-of-pocket expense for drug development has been estimated to be $403 million (in 2000 dollars). The problem with using this figure is that it often takes more than ten years to bring a drug from discovery to market; therefore, this cash flow must include a discount rate. At 11 percent, the present value is $802 million. [17] Other estimates are higher: "Declining R&D productivity, rising costs of commercialization, increasing payer influence and shorter exclusivity have driven up the average cost per successful launch to $1.7 billion and reduced expected returns on new investment to the unsustainable level of 5%" [18] (see Table 3.3).

Wholesalers. In 2004, this sector booked $212 billion in U.S. sales. Three firms dominate 88 percent of the market: McKesson, Cardinal Health, and sourceBergen. [19] They profit from the spread between the volume discounts they get from the manufacturers and what they charge their pharmacy, hospital, long-term care facility, and physician clients.

Pharmacies. Pharmacies are the providers who deliver most of the pharmaceuticals directly to patients in the United States. (Physicians may administer certain specialty drugs, like chemotherapy.) Pharmacies may be independently owned and operated or may be part of large chains, the three largest being Walgreens, CVS Caremark, and

TABLE 3.3. Pharmaceutical Industry: Top Ten Companies in R&D Spending and Financial Performance

R&D Spending in $ Billion		R&D Spending/ Total Sales		Gross Margins (Sales-Cost of Goods Sold)		EBITDA/Sales	
1. Pfizer	$7.6	1. Biogen Idec	26.8%	1. Biogen Idec	88.9%	1. Biogen Idec	68.5%
2. GlaxoSmithKline	$6.5	2. Amgen	24.2%	2. Genentech	87.1%	2. Merck	47.4%
3. Sanofi-Aventis	$5.8	3. Merck	21.1%	3. Amgen	85.3%	3. Amgen	44.2%
4. Novartis	$5.5	4. Lilly	19.9%	4. Pfizer	84.1%	4. Genentech	42.2%
5. Johnson & Johnson	$5.0	5. Genentech	19.1%	5. GlaxoSmithKline	78.0%	5. Pfizer	42.2%
6. Merck	$4.8	6. Bristol-Myers Squibb	17.1%	6. AstraZeneca	77.8%	6. GlaxoSmithKline	38.3%
7. AstraZeneca	$3.9	7. Pfizer	15.7%	7. Lilly	77.1%	7. AstraZeneca	36.1%
8. Amgen	$3.4	8. Sanofi-Aventis	15.6%	8. Forest	76.7%	8. Forest	33.3%
9. Lilly	$3.1	9. GlaxoSmithKline	15.2%	9. Merck	73.5%	9. Wyeth	32.3%
10. Bristol-Myers Squibb	$3.1	10. Novartis	15.2%	10. Sanofi-Aventis	73.4%	10. Johnson & Johnson	29.8%
Average		Average	16.2%	Average	75.4%	Average	34.1%

Rite Aid. Regardless of ownership, one can fill a prescription in person at a local outlet or by mail from a distant warehouse (see PBMs in a later section). Additionally, some pharmacies specialize by the type of product they furnish or the customers they service. For example, Omnicare differentiates itself as "The nation's leading provider of pharmaceutical care for seniors." Although traditional pharmacies make their money on volume sales for frequently occurring conditions (such as respiratory infections) or chronic diseases (such as diabetes), the companies that supply high-cost drugs, such as biologicals, profit from low-frequency, high-cost medications. These firms are called "specialty pharmacies," and industry estimates project they will grow to a $75 billion segment in the next few years. Leading companies in this specialty sector include Accredo Health, CVS Caremark, and Priority Health Care. This niche also includes hospital pharmacies, PBMs, and independent pharmacies. Patients can traditionally buy medications in pharmacies one of two ways: using a physician's prescription to obtain drugs from the pharmacist or directly off the shelves in the store (so-called "over-the-counter," or OTC). Other countries have a third mechanism called "behind-the-counter" (BTC), which does not require the consumer to have a physician's prescription but does require consultation with the pharmacist before obtaining the drug. In the United States, the BTC method was instituted for Plan B, a "morning after" contraceptive, but is rare for other items.

Pharmaceutical Benefit Management Companies (PBMs). Employers who self-insure, and many insurance companies, contract with outside firms to provide pharmaceutical benefits for insured members. According to the Employee Benefit Research Institute (EBRI), PBMs provide pharmaceutical benefits for almost three out of four insured persons in the United States.[20] About two-thirds of total market share (in terms of prescriptions filled per year) is concentrated among the top four firms: CVS Caremark, Medco Health Solutions, Express Scripts, and ACS State Health Care.[21] PBMs may perform one or more of a variety of services for their clients:

- Pharmacy network establishment
- Mail-order pharmacy capability
- Formulary establishment and maintenance
- Beneficiary eligibility tracking
- Claims processing
- Negotiation of rebates from manufacturers
- Utilization review of prescription patterns
- Generic drug and therapeutic substitution protocols
- Disease management

These companies make their money by

■ Contracting for some or all of the administrative services mentioned above

■ Accepting risk for performance criteria for these activities

■ Retaining some of the rebates they negotiate with manufacturers

Medical Device and Supply Companies

These companies can be divided into the following categories:

■ *Diagnostics.* At one end of this category are companies such as GE, Siemens, and Toshiba that manufacture complex, expensive devices such as CT and MRI scanners and nuclear imaging equipment. At the other end are companies such as Bayer, which manufactures urine dipsticks. Along the spectrum are firms like Beckman Coulter, which produce machines to analyze blood samples. Other firms supply *products* used in diagnostic procedures; for example, Berlex furnishes contrast dye for x-rays, and Boston Scientific and Medtronic make catheters used to study the heart and other organs. Electronics and data companies, such as Hewlett Packard, have significant positions in such medical diagnostic devices as intensive care unit monitors.

■ *Therapeutics.* As with diagnostics, the therapeutics category spans products ranging from complex to simple. In the former category are such items as cardiac pacemakers and implantable defibrillators (made by such companies as Boston Scientific, Medtronic, and St. Jude Medical). In the latter group are items such as urinary catheters, manufactured by firms such as C.R. Bard, Inc. Sometimes the therapeutic device category overlaps with the pharmaceutical industry, such as in the case of drug-coated coronary artery stents.

■ *Durable medical equipment (DME).* Included in this category are such items as wheelchairs (made by companies like Invacare and Everest & Jennings), hospital beds (produced by firms like Hill-Rom and Stryker), and walkers.

■ *Prosthetics.* These items help individuals restore appearance and/or function after loss from accident or disease. Simple prosthetics include wigs for persons who lose their hair from chemotherapy. More complex items include artificial joints (made by such companies as Johnson & Johnson's DePuy Orthopedics, Zimmer Holdings, and Smith & Nephew), limbs, and heart valves.

■ *Disposables.* This category comprises many over-the-counter items, such as bandages and latex gloves. Some products in this category overlap with diagnostics and therapeutics, such as diabetic test strips and syringes (both of which, for example, are manufactured by Becton Dickenson). Many of these companies are publicly traded (such as Johnson & Johnson), but some are large privately held firms (such as Medline Industries, Inc.).

■ *Information systems.* Suppliers to this sector include not only the well-known hardware manufacturers, but also many specialty software companies. Microsoft and GE are household names; other prominent health care software companies include Epic, Cerner, Mysys, and McKesson. The products these companies provide range from electronic medical records to billing to medication dispensing and may comprise comprehensive, enterprise-wide systems.

For all of these categories one should also recognize the consulting and support services that make them function. For example, facilities need proper architectural design to maximize efficiency and comply with safety and building code requirements; supply chain experts help manage inventory; and health care consulting companies' expertise ranges from information technology to sales force management.

Medical and Trade Associations

Persons and organizations join professional and trade groups for a variety of reasons, such as professional development and recognition as well as achieving economies of scale in industry-wide research, product recognition, and lobbying. A few examples by sector are described here:

■ *Providers.* The most widely recognized organization is the American Medical Association (AMA), whose membership comprises the most diverse group of physicians; however, the AMA represents only about a third of U.S. physicians. Its divisions address issues of public health, publish respected medical journals, and lobby for legislation important to physicians. There are also a number of medical specialty societies. Some represent broad categories, such as the American College of Physicians (recently merged with the American Society of Internal Medicine) and the American College of Surgeons. Others are more specialized within a specialty; for example, The American Association for Hand Surgery, to which members of the American Academy of Orthopedic Surgeons may belong.

Other providers have their own associations based on their professional roles. Nurses have the American Nursing Association, but also subspecialty groups such as the American Association of Nurse Anesthetists. Additional groups represent such providers as respiratory therapists, radiology technicians, and others.

Specialty societies are not limited to the clinical realm. Organizations such as the American College of Physician Executives and American Organization of Nurse Executives serve clinicians who have administrative roles.

■ *Payers.* The most widely know association in this and any other category is the Blue Cross Blue Shield Association. This organization administers the franchise of its trademark, coordinates local plans that collectively serve national accounts, and provides national research. Another important group is America's Health Insurance Plans (AHIP), which represents most of the other major insurance companies.

- *Hospitals.* Two main organizations represent this sector. The American Hospital Association represents the political and economic interests of its members, while the American College of Health Care Executives fulfills a professional education and academic mission.

- *Suppliers.* Many associations exist to serve this sector. For example, the Pharmaceutical Research and Manufacturing Association (PhRMA) represents the major pharmaceutical companies. The Biotechnology Industry Organization (BIO) focuses on members in both established and emerging companies in that sector. Devices are represented by the Medical Device Manufacturers Association (MDMA) and the Advanced Medical Technology Association (AdvaMed).

- *Functional.* Other associations represent members in diverse organizations who share common functional roles. Examples include the Health Care Financial Management Association (HFMA), Healthcare Information and Management Systems Society (HIMSS), and the Medical Marketing Association (MMA).

Health Advocacy Organizations

Health advocacy organizations are mostly nonprofit groups that seek to contribute to and improve health care in the nation. Prominent examples include the American Cancer Society, American Heart Association, and American Lung Association. Their missions include increasing public awareness about health and disease, providing information and support to people with certain conditions, raising money to support research to treat specific diseases, and advocating for public support for their members. For example, the American Heart Association uses information and education channels to educate physicians and encourage people to exercise more and eat more healthily.

All of these organizations have staffs who engage in social marketing to create programs to fulfill their missions. The term *social marketing* describes the kind of activities practiced by many health cause organizations to encourage such practices as safer driving, smoking cessation, hard drug avoidance, life-long exercise, and other causes.

Organization of the Federal Government's Health Care Activities

Through the executive branch, the federal government is actively involved in health care as an insurance payer provider of health care services, regulator, health researcher, and funder of health programs and investigations. Both the legislative and judicial branches are responsible for oversight of many health care activities. The principal responsibility for health care at the national level resides in the Department of Health and Human Services (see Figure 3.7 for an organizational chart of this department). A detailed explanation of each section of this department is beyond the scope of this chapter; however, health care marketers must be aware which branch is involved in their business. For example, for vaccine manufacturers, the FDA approves the safety and efficacy, the CDC issues

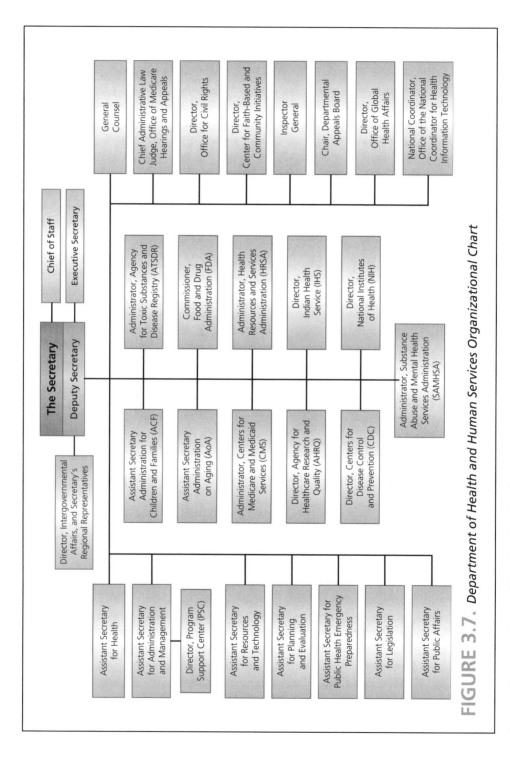

FIGURE 3.7. *Department of Health and Human Services Organizational Chart*

Source: http://www.dhhs.gov/about/orgchart.html.

recommendations for use, and the CMS determines whether the federal government will pay for it.

State and local governments differ in their organization of responsibilities for health care, including professional licensure, insurance regulation, administration of state-specific Medicaid programs, public health programs, and granting certificates of need (CONs) to organizations who wish to build new facilities that may increase the local cost of care. States such as California, Illinois, and Massachusetts have departed from traditional federal guidelines to introduce innovative health measures to provide better coverage to the uninsured and to improve access to health care.

DYNAMIC RELATIONS AMONG HEALTH CARE STAKEHOLDERS

Depending on the situation, any two or more stakeholders in the health care system may cooperate or compete with one another. One actor may value the others' contributions but at the same time object to some features of the others' behavior. Although the cooperative situations may be obvious, the potential competition and resulting conflicts may not be as clear. We present some examples of the latter type of relationship in Figure 3.8 and further highlight three of them in this section. These explanations should serve as a way for managers to consider competing and cooperative arrangements across the field.

Although all stakeholders may interact alone or in any combination with patients, for sake of clarity the patient is placed at the center of Figure 3.8, and you should infer the links that indicate these relationships.

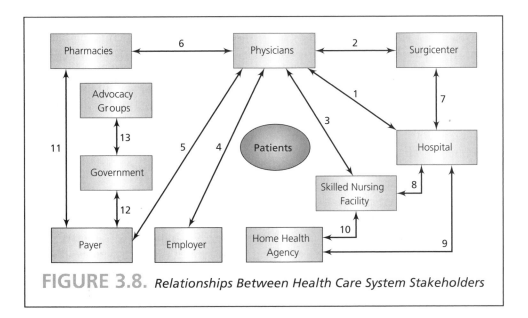

FIGURE 3.8. *Relationships Between Health Care System Stakeholders*

We will examine three relationships here and describe several others elsewhere in this book.

Physicians and Hospitals

Although hospitals credential physicians who practice on their staffs, once approved, these doctors act relatively independently, calling on the institution's resources as they see fit to provide patient care. Sources of conflict arise in these situations:

- Physicians' care is wasteful; for example, when they order unnecessary tests or needlessly prolong a patient's stay in the hospital. This situation causes financial losses to hospitals that are paid a fixed amount per patient stay or per day.

- Physicians set up businesses that compete with hospitals, such as freestanding diagnostic facilities or ambulatory surgery centers.

- Hospitals hire physicians who compete directly with independent practitioners.

Cooperation between physicians and hospitals has been hampered by federal fraud and abuse laws (so-called "Stark Laws," named after California democratic Congressman Fortney Hillman "Pete" Stark Jr.). These laws prohibit hospitals from offering physicians anything of value because of the possible illegal inducements to send patients to that particular facility. Of note is that this legal obstacle was relaxed in 2006 to facilitate cooperation in the development of information systems. Since laws frequently change, we advise the marketer to obtain legal counsel before launching new programs in this area.

Hospitals and Skilled Nursing Facilities

Hospitals and skilled nursing facilities (SNFs) most often engage in cooperative arrangements when a patient is ready to be discharged but cannot go home because of special needs. However, the line between these two institutions is increasingly becoming blurred. Many hospitals have established "step down" facilities within their walls that function as short-stay SNFs until the patient is ready to go home. In fact, rural hospitals may even use the same beds for both inpatients and SNF patients, changing the designation as the level of care changes (these are called *swing beds*). SNFs, on the other hand, are providing services that were formerly the sole province of hospitals, such as chronic ventilator care. A special designation of *subacute care facility* applies to SNFs that furnish this higher technical level of care.

Physicians and Pharmacies

Although this relationship seems straightforward, diversification by both parties has made the situation less clear. In 2006, Walgreens, CVS (now CVS Caremark), and Wal-Mart all announced that they were opening in-store clinics. This action, although not a challenge to surgeons or subspecialists, has direct consequences for primary care physicians. The companies hope that the convenient hours offered by these walk-in centers will increase store traffic and enhance same-store sales, including sales of medications. In reaction to this move, many physicians have more seriously considered implementing in-office medication dispensing, aided by management services from such firms as Allscripts.

THE CHANGING HEALTH CARE ENVIRONMENT

Health care organizations and marketers need to frequently assess the major trends in the health care environment to develop a competitive strategy that will help them achieve their objectives.

Marketers find many opportunities by identifying trends in the macro environment. A trend is a direction or sequence of events that has some momentum and durability. In contrast, a fad is unpredictable, short-lived, and without social, economic, and political significance.

For example, one trend is seen in the steady rise over the years in the percentage of people who value physical fitness and well-being. Marketers of health foods and exercise equipment cater to this trend with appropriate products and communications.

Deducing a new market opportunity from a trend does not guarantee success, even if it is technically feasible; therefore market research is necessary to determine an opportunity's profit potential. For example, some hospitals market a surgical procedure to reduce acid reflux because the incidence of this condition is growing; however, there may not be a sufficient number of people interested in having the procedure or willing to pay the required price if they can make do with inexpensive over-the-counter antacids.

Within the rapidly changing global picture, six major forces represent "uncontrollables" that health care organizations must monitor and to which they must respond: demographic, economic, social-cultural, natural, technological, and political-legal. Marketers must also pay attention to interactions among these forces to identify and take advantage of new opportunities and threats; for example, population growth (demographic), which leads to more resource depletion, and pollution (natural), which leads to more ailments, which in turn lead consumers to call for more regulations and laws (political-legal). The restrictions stimulate new technological solutions and offerings (technological). If the offerings are affordable (economic), they may actually change attitudes and behavior (social-cultural).

Demographic Environment

The main demographic force that marketers monitor is population, particularly the size and growth rate of population in cities, regions, and nations; age distribution and ethnic mix; educational levels; household patterns; and regional characteristics and movements.

Worldwide Population Growth. The world population is undergoing explosive growth, standing at over 6.3 billion and expected to exceed 7.9 billion by the year 2025.[22] Population growth is a source of concern for two reasons. First, resources needed to support this much human life (food, fuel, land) are limited and may be depleted at some point. Second, population growth is highest in areas that can least afford it. The less developed regions of the world currently account for 76 percent of the world population and are growing at 2 percent per year; the population in the more developed countries is growing at only 0.6 percent per year. In the developing countries, the death rate has been falling as a result of modern medicine, but the birthrate has remained fairly stable or is declining.

Although worldwide population growth has major implications for business, it does not mean growing markets unless they have sufficient purchasing power. Nonetheless, organizations that carefully analyze their markets can find major opportunities. With the growth of senior markets, for example, there is greater demand for long-term care and nursing home services.

Population Age Mix. National populations vary in their age mix, although there is a global trend toward an aging population.[23] At one extreme is Mexico, a country with a very young population and rapid population growth. At the other extreme is Japan, a country with one of the world's oldest populations. Childhood vaccines, baby vitamins, and pediatric services would be important offerings in Mexico. Japan's population consumes many more adult medical products.

A population can be subdivided into six age groups: preschool, school-age children, teens, young adults age twenty-five to forty, middle-aged adults age forty to sixty-five, and older adults age sixty-five and up. The most populous age groups shape the marketing environment. In the United States, the seventy-eight million baby boomers born between 1946 and 1964 are a powerful force shaping the health care marketplace. Boomers are becoming more involved with health care decisions not only for themselves, but also for their aging parents who require long-term care services. Americans over the age of sixty-five represent 12.5 percent of the population and grew from thirty-one million to thirty-four million from 1990 to 2000. The number of those aged eighty-five and over grew from three million to four million. Parents of the boomers are living longer and have increased demand for adult day care services, Alzheimer's clinics and homes, and assisted living centers, among other services. The number of skilled nursing facilities has exploded, from 5,200 in 1980 to over 17,000 currently, while the number of nursing home beds has increased 21 percent.[24] More impressive is that, according to J. Walter Thompson, "households over 50 spend more than $1.7 trillion on goods and services annually, they own 65% of the total net worth among all U.S. households, they control 50% of all discretionary income, and they are responsible for 60% of all health care spending."[25]

Ethnic Markets. Countries also vary in ethnic and racial makeup. The United States was originally called a melting pot, but people now call it a "salad bowl" society, with groups maintaining their ethnic differences, neighborhoods, and cultures. According to the 2000 census, the U.S. population of 276.2 million was 72 percent white, 13 percent African American, 11 percent Latino, and 3.8 Asian American. Moreover, of these, nearly twenty-five million—more than 9 percent of the population—were born in another country.

Each group has specific needs, wants, and buying habits that marketers need to understand. After PacifiCare Health Systems (now part of United Health Group) learned that 20 percent of its three million insurance customers are Latino, it set up a new unit, Latino Health Solutions, to market its products in Spanish and refer customers to Spanish-speaking doctors.[26] Yet marketers must be careful not to over-generalize about ethnic groups. Within each ethnic group are consumers who are quite different from each other.

Educational Groups. The population of any society falls into five educational groups: illiterates, high school dropouts, high school graduates, college graduates, and professional and post–graduate degree holders. The differences even among developed countries can be significant. In Japan, 99 percent of the population is literate; in the United States up to 15 percent of the population may be functionally illiterate. This illiteracy problem "has profound implications . . . more than 200 studies have consistently found the level of most health materials and medical documents—appointment slips, consent forms, prescriptions—to be written well beyond the functional literacy of the average reader. Yet, few findings from those studies have circulated beyond the adult literacy and health education professional communities."[27] Coexisting with this illiterate segment of the population are the approximately 36 percent of Americans who are college-educated, one of the world's highest percentages. This latter education level fuels demand for health care information from such sources as books, magazines, and the Internet.

Household Patterns. "Typical" 1950s families consisting of opposite sex, married parents and their children are no longer the norm; they account for only 25 percent of U.S. households.[28] Paradoxically, the majority of families are termed diverse or nontraditional; these designations include single live-alones, unmarried adults of one or both sexes who live together, single-parent families, childless married couples, and empty-nesters. More people than ever before are divorcing or separating, choosing not to marry, marrying later, or marrying without the intention to have children. Each group has a distinctive set of health care needs and buying habits. For example, because widows in the SSWD group (single, separated, widowed, divorced) live alone, they may need (1) help getting to and from health care appointments, (2) modifications to their homes (ramps, first-floor accommodations) if they cannot use stairs due to accidents or illnesses, and (3) emergency communications devices if they become incapacitated and are unable to call for medical assistance.

As another example, compared to the average American, respondents who classify themselves as gay are over ten times more likely to be in professional jobs, almost twice as likely to own a vacation home, eight times more likely to own a laptop computer, and twice as likely to own individual stocks.[29] Organizations such as the King County (Washington) Public Health Department have developed offerings for this population and the nontraditional household market as a whole.

Geographical Shifts in Population. This era is a time of great migratory movements between and within countries. Within countries, population movement also occurs as people migrate from rural to urban areas and then to suburban areas. Although the United States experienced a rural rebound in the 1990s as nonmetropolitan counties attracted large numbers of urban refugees, urban markets are now growing more rapidly again due to a higher birth rate, a lower death rate, and rapid growth from foreign immigration.[30]

Location makes a difference in goods and service preferences. For example, nearly half of all those over the age of five (120 million) moved at least once between 1995 and 2000. Many moved to the Sun Belt states and away from the Midwest and Northeast.[31] As a result, the demand for health care services is decreasing in the Midwest and Northeast and increasing in the Sun Belt. Also, with more of the population living in areas with greater sun exposure, there is higher incidence of sun-related skin cancers and aging conditions. These conditions, in turn, generate more demand for dermatologists and plastic surgeons. There are also regional differences that relate to health choices: people in Seattle buy more toothbrushes per capita than people in any other U.S. city, people in Salt Lake City eat more candy bars, and people in Miami drink more prune juice.

Economic Environment

Markets, as well as people, require purchasing power. The available purchasing power in an economy depends on current income, prices, savings, debt, and credit availability. Marketers must pay careful attention to trends affecting purchasing power because they can have a strong impact on business, especially for companies whose products are geared to high-income and price-sensitive consumers. For example, people with lower incomes are not good prospects for high-deductible consumer-driven health insurance plans.

Income Distribution. Nations vary greatly in level and distribution of income and industrial structure. The four types of industrial structures are *subsistence economies* (few opportunities for marketers); *raw-material exporting economies*, such as Zaire (copper) and Saudi Arabia (oil); *industrializing economies*, such as India, Egypt, and the Philippines; and *industrial economies* that are rich markets for all sorts of goods and services.

Marketers often distinguish among countries according to five different income-distribution patterns:

1. Very low incomes
2. Mostly low incomes
3. Very low and very high incomes
4. Low, medium, and high incomes
5. Mostly medium incomes

The market would be very small in countries with type (1) or (2) income patterns. Further, income distribution patterns differ across time and between countries. For example, ". . . over their 1990s business cycles, the entire distribution of after-tax household size-adjusted income moved to the right in the United States and Great Britain while inequality declined. In contrast, Germany and Japan had less income growth, a rise in inequality and a decline in the middle mass of their distributions that spread mostly to the right, much like the United States experienced over its 1980s business cycle. In the United States and Japan, younger persons fared relatively better than older persons while the opposite was the case in Great Britain and Germany."[32]

The correlation between income and health insurance coverage is strong. The likelihood that an individual has health insurance increases with income, but some individuals in relatively high-income families do not have health insurance, as shown in Table 3.4. The probability that a person with $50,000 or more in family income is uninsured is growing slightly faster than it is for lower-income individuals. Between 1999 and 2003, the likelihood of being uninsured for persons in a family with income below $25,000 increased 1 percent, while it increased 3.4 percent for persons in families with income of between $50,000 and $74,999, and 2.7 percent for persons with family income of $75,000 or more. This situation is due in part to the fact that persons in low-income families are often eligible for publicly funded programs such as Medicaid and the State Children's Health Insurance Program (S-CHIP).[33]

Health Care Costs. In 2005, U.S. health care spending increased 6.9 percent to almost $2.0 trillion, or $6,697 per person. This increase was the slowest rate since 1999, when spending rose 6.2 percent. The health care portion of gross domestic product (GDP) was 16.0 percent, slightly higher than the 15.9 percent share in 2004. Although spending on health care rose at twice the rate of general inflation in 2005, this increase was the third consecutive year of slower health spending growth.[34]

This slower growth was driven by a reduction in prescription drug expenditures, largely due to the increasing use of lower-cost generics. Spending on prescription drugs increased 5.8 percent, to $200.7 billion, well down from the peak increase of 18.2 percent noted in 1999.

Hospital spending was again the largest piece of the health spending pie, accounting for 31 percent of all money spent, and continued to be the main factor in spending growth. Inpatient and outpatient costs resulted in a nearly 8 percent annual increase. Spending for hospital and physician and clinical services grew at rates similar to those in 2004. Health insurance premium rates rose by 6.6 percent in 2005, continuing a moderating trend seen in the preceding couple of years and well below the double-digit increases seen in the late 1990s and early 2000s. Employers continued to shift some of those costs to workers through offering so-called consumer-driven plans that increased deductibles, added co-payments, or eliminated coverage for specific treatments or certain drugs.[35]

Savings, Debt, and Credit Availability. Consumer expenditures are affected by savings, debt, and credit availability. U.S. consumers have a high debt-to-income

TABLE 3.4. Nonelderly Population with Selected Sources of Health Insurance, by Family Income, 2005

| Family Income | Total | Employment-Based Coverage | | | | Public | | Uninsured |
		Total	Own Name	Dependent	Individually Purchased	Total	Medicaid	
Total	100.0%	62.7%	32.0%	30.7%	7.0%	17.7%	13.5%	17.2%
Under $10,000	100.0	12.2	6.4	5.9	10.7	46.9	42.4	34.3
$10,000–$19,999	100.0	22.8	15.5	7.4	9.0	39.7	34.6	33.4
$20,000–$29,999	100.0	41.1	26.8	14.3	8.3	26.5	21.6	29.4
$30,000–$39,999	100.0	55.9	33.9	22.0	7.9	19.3	15.1	22.1
$40,000–$49,999	100.0	66.1	36.9	29.1	7.5	15.1	10.3	17.0
$50,000–$74,000	100.0	76.2	38.0	38.2	5.9	10.3	6.3	12.2
$75,000 and over	100.0	85.8	39.1	46.7	5.3	6.2	2.6	6.5

Note: Details may not add to totals because individuals may receive coverage from more than one source.
Source: Employee Benefit Research Institute estimates of the Current Population Survey, March 2006 Supplement.

ratio, which slows down further expenditures on housing and large-ticket items. Credit is very available in the United States but at fairly high interest rates, especially to lower-income borrowers. Here the Internet is helping consumers connect with many financial services firms vying for their business.

Physicians and hospitals are now working with financial services companies to market credit cards to patients. The purpose of these joint ventures is to help physicians and hospitals reduce their mounting collection efforts, which are due to patients' bearing more responsibility for out-of-pocket spending on health care.

According to the results of a recent national survey by Access Project, a nonprofit medical consumer advocacy group associated with Brandeis University, and Demos, a public-policy research organization, about one-fifth of low- and middle-income households with credit card balances cited significant medical expenses as a reason for their debt.

Tenet Health Care, a large, publicly traded national hospital chain, is attempting to deal with its employees' escalating medical debts by offering them a line of credit. Under this innovative pilot program, employees' co-payments for doctor visits and other health care services are paid through automatic payroll deductions. The program is being offered in partnership with UnitedHealth Group, which markets health savings accounts.[36]

Social-Cultural Environment

Society shapes our beliefs, values, and norms. Almost unconsciously, people absorb a worldview that defines their relationships to themselves, others, organizations, society, nature, and the universe. Other cultural characteristics of interest to marketers include the persistence of core cultural values, the existence of subcultures, and shifts of values through time. For a given product or service, marketers should determine which of the following views are most important to the stakeholder:

- *Views of themselves.* People vary in the relative emphasis they place on self-gratification. Today, U.S. consumers are more conservative in their behaviors and ambitions. Marketers must recognize that there are many different groups with different views of themselves.

- *Views of others.* People are concerned about the homeless, crime and victims, and other social problems. At the same time they hunger for long-lasting relationships with others. These trends portend a growing market for offerings that promote direct relations among human beings, such as health clubs, and for offerings that allow people who are alone to feel that they are not.

- *Views of organizations.* People vary in their attitudes toward corporations, government agencies, trade unions, and other organizations. There has been an overall decline in organizational loyalty in U.S. society due to such occurrences as downsizings and scandals such as at Enron and HealthSouth.[37] Even in cultures with traditional long-term employer loyalty, such as Japan, workers are becoming more mobile. As a result, organizations need to find new ways to win back consumer and employee confidence.

■ *Views of society.* People have varying attitudes toward society. Some defend it, some run it, some take what they can from it, some want to change it, some are looking for something deeper, and some want to leave it.[38] Consumption patterns often reflect social attitudes; those who place high importance on exercise and diet may believe that societal health problems can be helped more by individual initiative and not as much by government intervention.

■ *Views of nature.* People vary in their attitudes toward nature. A long-term trend has been humankind's growing mastery of nature through technology. Recently, however, people have awakened to nature's fragility and finite resources. Business has responded to increased interest in camping, hiking, boating, and fishing with appropriate goods and services.

■ *Views of the universe.* People vary in their beliefs about the origin of the universe and their place in it. Most Americans are monotheistic, although religious conviction and practice have been waning through the years.

High Persistence of Core Values. People living in a particular society hold many *core beliefs and values* that tend to persist. Core beliefs and values are passed on from parents to children and are reinforced by major social institutions—schools, religious institutions, businesses, and governments. *Secondary beliefs and values* are more open to change. Marketers have some chance of changing secondary values but little chance of changing core values. For instance, the nonprofit organization Mothers Against Drunk Drivers (MADD) does not try to stop the sale of alcohol, but it does promote the idea of appointing a designated driver who will not drink; it also lobbies to raise the legal drinking age.

Existence of Subcultures. Each society contains *subcultures*—groups with shared values emerging from their special life experiences or circumstances. Members share common beliefs, preferences, and behaviors that may differ in subtle ways from the mainstream culture. For instance, health food stores seek to market their specialty products to certain populations who believe they cannot satisfy their needs in traditional grocery outlets.

Natural Environment

The deterioration of the natural environment is a major global concern. In many world cities, air and water pollution have reached dangerous levels and have triggered or exacerbated such health ailments as asthma and certain types of cancer.

In Western Europe, "green" parties have vigorously pressed for public action to reduce industrial pollution. In the United States, experts have documented the ecological damage and the global warming phenomenon. Watchdog groups such as the Sierra Club and Friends of the Earth carry these concerns into the political and social arena, calling for new regulations and investments. These groups use marketing tools to influence public opinion and initiate legislative action to stop the tide of deterioration. As a result, heavy industry and public utilities have had to invest billions of dollars in pollution-control equipment and more environmentally friendly fuels. The auto industry has had to introduce expensive emission controls in cars. The soap industry has had to increase its products' biodegradability.

Great opportunities await companies and marketers who can create solutions that reconcile company profitability with environmental protection. Companies will be rewarded for developing new materials that can be recycled and for reducing energy costs in the lighting, cooling, and heating of homes and in the use of automobiles. With better air and water quality, people will be less afflicted by environmental conditions that harm their health.

Technological Environment

One of the most dramatic forces shaping people's lives is technology. "New" technology has led to such breakthroughs as penicillin, open-heart surgery, and the birth control pill, but it is also a force for "creative destruction." Transistors hurt the vacuum-tube industry, xerography hurt the carbon paper business, and the Web hurt the magazine business. These innovations are what Christensen, Bohmer, and Kenagy have called "disruptive technologies."[39] Instead of moving into the new technologies, many industries fought or ignored them, and their businesses declined. Yet it is the essence of market capitalism to be dynamic and tolerate the creative destructiveness of technology as the price of progress.

New health care technology also creates major long-term social consequences that are not always foreseeable. The contraceptive pill, for example, led to smaller families, more working wives, and larger discretionary incomes—resulting in higher expenditures on vacation travel, durable goods, and luxury items. Marketers should monitor such technology trends as the pace of change, the opportunities for innovation, varying R&D budgets, and increased regulation.

Accelerating Pace of Change. Many common products, such as MRI scanners, were not available decades ago. The Human Genome Project promises to usher in the Biological Century as biotech workers create new medical cures, new foods, and new materials. The lead time between new ideas and their successful implementation is shortening, as is the time between introduction and peak production. Ninety percent of all the scientists who ever lived are alive today, and technology feeds upon itself.

Unlimited Opportunities for Innovation. Scientists today are working on a startling range of new technologies (such as biotechnology and medical robotics) that will revolutionize products and production processes. Researchers are working on cures and vaccines for AIDS, more potent and less addicting painkillers, safer contraceptives, and tasty nonfattening foods. They are designing robots for heart surgery and home nursing. The challenge in innovation is not only technical but also commercial—to develop affordable versions of new products.

Varying R&D Budgets. Although the United States leads the world in annual basic research and development expenditures, a growing portion is going into the development side. This strategy raises concerns about whether the United States can maintain its lead in basic science. Many organizations are content to put their money into copying competitors' products and making minor feature and style improvements. Even basic-research companies such as DuPont and Pfizer are proceeding cautiously. Increasingly, research directed toward major breakthroughs is being conducted by consortiums rather than by single companies.

Increased Regulation of Technological Change. As products become more complex, the public needs to be reassured about their safety. Consequently, government agencies' powers to investigate and ban potentially unsafe products have been expanded. In the United States, the Federal Food and Drug Administration must approve all drugs before they can be sold. Safety and health regulations have also increased in the areas of food, automobiles, clothing, electrical appliances, and construction. Marketers must be aware of these regulations when proposing, developing, and launching new products. In addition, drug companies have a moral as well as a legal obligation to monitor drug use after approval. The controversy concerning the deaths resulting from the use of the painkiller Vioxx led Merck to withdraw the drug from the market. According to the Associated Press, by March of 2007 the company faced about 28,000 law suits as well as 265 potential class action suits due to adverse cardiovascular events associated with Vioxx and the inadequacy of Merck's warnings. As a result of this instance and other concerns, new federal legislation in 2007 gave the FDA greater powers to oversee pharmaceutical and medical device companies' post-marketing surveillance. The persistent dilemma, however, is balancing the potential benefit of quick approval and introduction of technology against possible unanticipated complications.

Political-Legal Environment

Marketing decisions are strongly affected by developments in the political and legal environment. This environment comprises laws, government agencies, and pressure groups that influence and limit various organizations and individuals. Sometimes these laws also create new opportunities for business. For example, regulations related to the licensing and training of emergency medical technicians (EMTs) and paramedics have created dozens of new companies dedicated to meeting the increased demand for mandatory training. Two major trends in this environment deal with the increase of business legislation and the growth of special-interest groups.

Increase of Business Legislation. Business legislation has three main purposes: to protect companies from unfair competition, to protect consumers from unfair business practices, and to protect the interests of society from unfair business behavior. A major purpose of business legislation and enforcement is to charge businesses with the social costs created by their products or production processes.

A central concern about business legislation is, at what point do the costs of regulation exceed the benefits? The laws are not always administered fairly, and regulators and enforcers may be lax or overzealous. Although each new law may have a legitimate rationale, it may have the unintended effect of sapping initiative and retarding economic growth. For example, state certificate of need (CON) regulations control new construction or remodeling of hospital facilities. These CON laws are designed to control supply of what could be unneeded health services and hence extra costs to the system. An alternative approach would be to let market forces influence changes in capacity to make hospitals accountable and at risk for their initiatives so as to protect taxpayers.

Over the years, legislation affecting business has steadily increased. The European Union has enacted laws that cover competitive behavior, product standards, product liability, and commercial transactions. The United States has laws covering such issues as competition, product safety and liability, fair trade and credit practices, and packaging and labeling.[40] Marketers need a good working knowledge of relevant business legislation, legal review procedures, major laws protecting competition, consumers, and society, and ethical standards.

Growth of Special-Interest Groups. The number and power of special-interest groups have increased over the past three decades. Political action committees (PACs) lobby government officials and pressure businesses to pay more attention to the rights of consumers, women, senior citizens, minorities, the disabled, and gays. An important force affecting business is consumerism—an effort of citizens and government to strengthen the rights and powers of buyers in relation to sellers. Recently, consumer advocates have made inroads in the health care arena, including knowing the true cost of a medical procedure and the quality of care a provider is likely to provide. Yet new laws and growing pressure from special-interest groups continue to add more restraints on marketers, moving many private marketing transactions into the public domain. Many marketing managers in the pharmaceutical sector feel particularly constrained by their legal departments, which are concerned about fraud and abuse laws as well as accuracy of advertising claims.

SUMMARY

The U.S. health care system needs improvement, given that it spends so much more on health care than other nations and does not derive commensurate benefit. Too many parties are working at cross purposes, rather than operating in unison to achieve the main objective, namely healthy citizens. Further, the health system should invest more in wellness rather than principally in curing illness. Achievement of these goals, however, starts with providing health insurance for the entire population.

Marketers can play an important role in achieving a better health care system. Opportunities to help start with identifying and monitoring trends in six major environmental forces: demographic, economic, social-cultural, natural, technological, and political-legal.

In the demographic environment, marketers must be aware of worldwide population growth; changing mixes of age, ethnic composition, and educational levels; the rise of nontraditional families; large geographic shifts in population; and the move to micromarketing and away from mass marketing.

In the social-cultural arena, marketers must understand people's views of themselves, others, organizations, society, nature, and the universe. They must market products that correspond to society's core and secondary values, and they must address the needs of different subcultures within a society.

In the natural environment, marketers need to be aware of raw materials shortages, increased energy costs and pollution levels, and the changing role of governments in environmental protection.

In the technological arena, marketers should take account of the accelerating pace of technological change, opportunities for innovation, varying R&D budgets, and the increased governmental regulation brought about by technological change.

In the political-legal environment, marketers must work in concert with the many laws regulating business practices, ethical considerations, and various special-interest groups.

All these considerations must also be grounded in an understanding of stakeholders' preferences among cost, quality, and access.

DISCUSSION QUESTIONS

1. You are in charge of marketing your company's laboratory services to managed care plans in your region. Contrast approaches to promoting these products to a PPO and to a staff model HMO.

2. Your pharmaceutical company has just come out with a new, second-in-class pill to treat high blood pressure. As manager for institutional and government contracts, you want to make sure your hospital (inpatient and outpatient), nursing home, home health care, Medicare, and Medicaid customers will use the product. To understand their willingness to pay for it, contrast how buying your drug affects each of these client's costs.

CHAPTER

DETERMINANTS OF THE UTILIZATION OF HEALTH CARE SERVICES

LEARNING OBJECTIVES

In this chapter, we will address the following questions:

1. What are the main factors driving people to seek health care?

2. How are people influenced by their personal characteristics (such as age, gender, race, income and education) in seeking health care?

3. What are the main factors and forces that reduce the demand for health care?

4. What are the main factors that tend to increase the demand for health care?

5. How do health care coverage and incidence vary geographically?

OPENING EXAMPLE

"Just one more thing..." Mr. Ramirez had just spent twenty minutes of his follow-up doctor's appointment talking about how difficult it was to stay on his prescribed diabetic diet. After his physician came up with an alternate diet and exercise plan, and made some medication adjustments, Mr. Ramirez said, "I think I can live with that," and got up to leave the exam room. With one foot out the door, he paused and said, "By the way doc, can I talk to you about another problem?" His physician was running behind schedule and asked if it was urgent or could wait until the next appointment in a month.

"Never mind," the patient said, and he left.

Mr. Ramirez wanted to talk to his physician about erectile dysfunction, a common problem in diabetics. Although the subject is difficult for any male to bring up, in the Hispanic culture it is a particularly sensitive issue. Rather than seek proven medical treatment, many men in this situation try unproven herbal remedies, which can cause side effects with prescribed medication, or order from internet sites, which carries a risk of receiving inactive counterfeits, outdated medication, or a mislabeled drug.

As we discuss in this chapter, people seek medical care for a variety of reasons, and physicians respond to those reasons in ways that are also very individual. We hope that the insights we provide will help the reader appreciate F. W. Peabody's statement: "The essence of the practice of medicine is that it is an intensely personal matter . . . The significance of the intimate personal relationship between physician and patient cannot be too strongly emphasized . . . One of the essential qualities of the clinician is interest in humanity, for the secret of the care of the patient is caring for the patient." [1]

OVERVIEW: WHY PEOPLE SEEK HEALTH CARE

The first obvious reason to seek care is for a known illness (either acute or chronic), accident, or injury. All of the stakeholders in Table 4.1 have an interest in this reason. Those closest to the patient—family and friends—provide a strong influence to seek care. An employer also wants the patient to return to work as soon as possible and reduce health care costs.

The government's interest is represented by such federal agencies as the Food and Drug Administration (FDA), the Centers for Disease Control and Prevention (CDC), the Occupational Safety and Health Administration (OSHA), and the Environmental Protection Agency (EPA), as well as state and local public health departments. These agencies and departments are charged with the oversight and preservation of public health and safety and can request or require that an individual seek care. An example of government requiring someone to get medical attention is the case of a communicable infection such as tuberculosis or a sexually transmitted disease (STD).

TABLE 4.1. Reasons for Seeking Care and Relevant Stakeholders

	Stakeholder						
Reason	Patient	Family or Partner	Friends	Employer	Public Health and Safety	Insurance Company	Suppliers
Illness/ Accident/ Injury	X	X	X	X	X	X	X
Symptom	X	X	X	X	X		X
Prevention/ Checkup	X	X	X	X	X	X	X
Second opinion	X	X	X	X		X	
Legal	X	X	X	X	X	X	X
Administrative	X			X	X	X	X
Discretionary	X	X	X				X

Source: Joel Shalowitz.

Insurance companies have a significant financial stake in patients' seeking of health care services, ranging from preventing unnecessary visits to making sure timely and appropriate care is provided. In this category, we include not only commercial insurance plans, such as Blue Cross/Blue Shield, but also those with government sponsorship, such as Medicare and Medicaid. For example, insurance companies are now reminding patients to seek care more often to control such conditions as diabetes and high blood pressure.

Finally, suppliers, particularly pharmaceutical companies, encourage patients to seek care for a variety of known diseases and symptoms. This encouragement may occur through such measures as public service announcements, sponsorship of health fairs, or direct-to-consumer (DTC) advertising.

For the reasons "Symptom" and "Prevention/Checkup," the stakeholder interests are the same as those for acute conditions, except that insurance companies usually do not frequently encourage individuals to seek care for specific *symptoms*. As an example of government intervention in this category, the CDC may encourage patients with a high fever and cough to seek medical care during influenza season. Also, suppliers, such as those offering diagnostic tests, and pharmaceutical companies who manufacture vaccines are particularly interested in encouraging preventive services.

As far as second opinions are concerned, patients and those in their support network often want additional viewpoints about diagnoses and treatment recommendations. Further, insurance companies may request or require that a patient receive a confirmatory exam to avoid unnecessary care, such as surgery. Also, employers often require employees to obtain second opinions regarding the nature and treatment of work-related injuries, and for the timing of return-to-work clearance and functional expectations.

Legal reasons for seeking care can involve all stakeholders. Patients and those who are interested in them may believe they were physically or mentally harmed in some negligent fashion and initiate an encounter to verify or confirm this impression. Employers, government agencies, and insurance companies may request exams to determine disability payments. On the other side of the liability issue—that is, the defendant's side—stakeholders such as pharmaceutical companies may require exams to assess legal responsibility for damages.

Other stakeholders may require patients to obtain services for administrative reasons—such as preemployment physicals and documentation of immunizations or treatment—and assessment of eligibility for life and disability insurance. Note, however, that due to large group contracts, persons who work for big companies are almost always exempt from physicals to determine health insurance eligibility. Suppliers such as pharmaceutical companies may compel certain patients to have specialist exams or tests to determine eligibility to receive certain medications, such as those involving experimental protocols.

The Discretionary category listed in Table 4.1 includes services that, strictly speaking, have little to do with health as we defined it in Chapter One; for example, procedures such as cosmetic surgery. Products that may fall into this class are the so-called lifestyle medications (such as those for erectile dysfunction and baldness). From an international perspective, a given country's culture will determine what is included in this category. For example, as mentioned previously, until recently spa care was covered by the sickness funds in Germany; such a benefit is unlikely to become standard in the United States. Individuals and concerned parties are obviously interested in these discretionary services, particularly when they have disposable income. Suppliers are eager to sell these nonessential products or services by aggressively promoting their use via DTC advertising.

The strategic marketing lesson from applying this approach is to identify *what type of service is involved*, *the reason the patient is seeking care* (for example, self-motivated or required by a third party), and *the relevant stakeholders for the encounters*.

We must next consider the *personal* characteristics that influence the likelihood that an individual will seek care:

- Age
- Gender/Sex
- Race
- Income and socioeconomic status
- Education
- Availability of care (including insurance and pricing for services)
- Culture and patients' beliefs

Age

With respect to age, "children, child-bearing-age women, and the elderly use health care services the most."[2] Although this finding is from a Brazilian study, it represents the pattern in most developed countries. In the childhood category, the greatest utilization is in the first two years of life; it then declines rapidly until females reach the child-bearing years. This overall relationship in the U.S. population is displayed in Figure 4.1.

Age is also a factor for utilization of specific services (see Figure 4.2). For example, "significant age-related disparities appear to exist for both evidence-based and non-evidence-based cancer-screening interventions."[3]

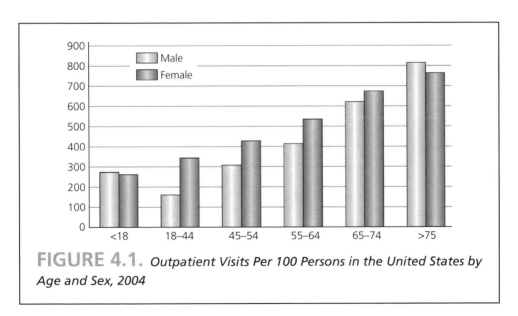

FIGURE 4.1. *Outpatient Visits Per 100 Persons in the United States by Age and Sex, 2004*

Source: National Center for Health Statistics. *Health, United States, 2006: With Chartbook on Trends in the Health of Americans, With Special Feature on Pain.* Hyattsville, Md.: U.S. Government Printing Office (DHHS Pub No. 2006–1232), 2006.

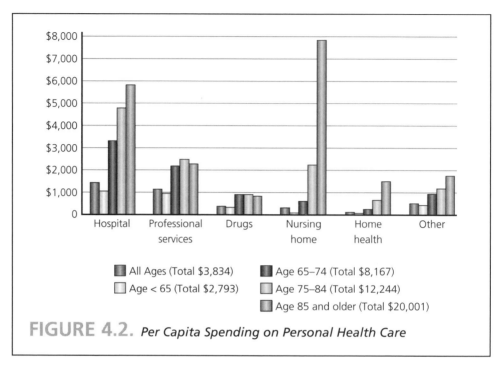

FIGURE 4.2. *Per Capita Spending on Personal Health Care*

Note: Complete data on personal health care spending by age are not readily available. The estimates in this [figure] are based on administrative data for Medicare and Medicaid, household survey data from the Agency for Health Care Research and Quality, and various provider surveys. Estimates are for 1999 and are the most current available.
Source: http://www.globalaging.org/health/us/2007/spending.pdf.

Gender/Sex

The difference between men and women regarding utilization of health care is also displayed in Figure 4.1. Note that in every age category except childhood, women use health care services and products more than men. Not only do men and women differ in their health-seeking behaviors, but providers order services at different rates for the sexes (even when reproductive services for women are excluded). These differentials can be either beneficial or harmful, depending on whether the intervention represents appropriate care versus over- or underutilization.

One very important factor that cannot be inferred from these statistics is the central role of women as the health care decision makers, not only for themselves but also for their families. This responsibility has critical marketing implications—from making sure mothers in developing countries know which products to use to treat childhood diarrhea (a leading cause of death) to persuading women in developed nations to direct their family's health care needs to a particular hospital or request a brand of medication.

Race

When considering differences due to race, one must be aware of several caveats. First, race is a difficult category to define. Often people of mixed backgrounds identify with only one race, thus confounding studies that rely on self reporting. Second, many findings associated with racial differences can be explained on the basis of socioeconomics or education (two other, independent determinants of health care usage). For example, a study of adult preventive dental care showed that racial disparities among whites, African Americans, and Mexican Americans were "no longer significant when enabling resource variables are included in the model (income level, insurance, census region, and metropolitan statistical area)."[4] Likewise, disparities in treatment outcomes may or may not be related primarily to race. An illustration of this principle is the finding that "socioeconomic factors and lack of access to health care do not entirely explain the worse prognosis" of African Americans with respect to colon cancer.[5] Further, as is the case with men and women, providers deliver care of diverse types and frequencies to people of different racial backgrounds. For example, compared to Caucasian patients, minorities are less likely to receive adequate cancer pain management, and African Americans are less likely to have access to kidney transplants.[6]

Finally, one should not assume uniformity within any racial or ethnic group. For example, variations are found among adolescents of different Latino origins with respect to frequency of and reasons for obtaining routine physical examinations. Cuban-origin adolescents in a single-parent household were *more* likely to get such an exam, whereas for those of Central or South American or Dominican background, the likelihood depended on higher income and having insurance.[7] These findings highlight the need to research the appropriate market segments for a product or service.

Income and Socioeconomic Status

Income obviously affects use of health care products and services by giving the affluent certain opportunities, but *which* services are used varies by income as well. For instance, those from higher economic strata use specialist services more than those at lower levels, when other factors, such as health status and insurance, are factored out. An additional area of investigation has been the effect of social status on health outcomes. As Fitzpatrick has noted: ". . . accumulating evidence suggests that . . . social status itself, regardless of associated material and economic advantages, may confer health benefits."[8] Here are a few international examples of the effect of income and socioeconomic status on health care utilization:

- "Socioeconomic differences in utilization were present for all services [in The Netherlands] after we controlled for age, sex, and marital status."[9]
- "Although financial barriers may not directly impede access to health care services in Canada, differential use of physician services with respect to socioeconomic status persists."[10]

■ "Lower socio-economic groups [in Belgium] make more often use of the general practitioner and nursing care at home and are more often admitted to hospital than persons with a high socio-economic status. There is, however, no socio-economic gradient when the health status is taken into account. On the opposite, persons with higher socio-economic status report more often a visit to a specialist, a physiotherapist or a dentist."[11]

■ "Women [in Britain] whose households were in the lowest income category were more likely to report back pain than those in the highest income group."[12]

Education

Education, apart from health care knowledge, is also an independent determinant of health care use. A few examples follow; note also that parental education can influence utilization for children.

■ In a cross sectional survey of 5,556 patients from fifteen European countries, "[p]atients with higher education had lower global coronary risk, than those with lower education."[13]

■ In Israel, "those with high school educations were 1.18 times more likely to be hospitalized while those with elementary school educations experienced a risk of 1.32 . . . Lower education was found to be a significant risk factor for hospitalization in most diagnostic categories."[14]

■ In Eastern Turkey, childhood "vaccination rates increased in parallel with maternal education level . . . There was no difference in vaccination rates with respect to gender, paternal education level, number of siblings and socio-economic status."[15]

■ In a survey of households in England, Wales, and Scotland, "women with no formal education qualification were more likely to report back pain than women who had a qualification. These associations were not explained by smoking, obesity, and co-existent depressive symptoms."[16]

■ In Germany, education was "independently associated with severe current back pain . . ."[17]

Availability of Care

Availability of care, including insurance status, has probably the most obvious influence on use of health care services (see Table 4.2); however, this effect is not limited to the status of the insured individual. For example, it is interesting to note that insured, low-income children with an uninsured parent are less likely to experience provider visits and well-child exams than if the parents are insured.[18] Further, with respect to availability, Paine and Wright posed the question: "With free health services, why does the Brazilian working class delay in seeing the doctor?" They found that: "The most common reason for delay in seeking medical attention was

TABLE 4.2. **Percent of Adults with Chronic Conditions Who Lack a Usual Source of Health Care, by Insurance Status**

For adults with:	Percent Without a Usual Source of Care[a]		
	All Adults	Uninsured[b]	Insured
Any chronic condition[c]	11%	38%	5%
By race/ethnicity			
White	9%	36%	5%
Black	11%	33%	5%
Hispanic	20%	46%	6%
Other	12%	34%	6%
Hypertension (2+ visits)	7%	30%	3%
High cholesterol (ever)	7%	29%	5%
Heart disease (ever)[d]	8%	37%	4%
Asthma (current)	10%	36%	5%
Diabetes (ever)	5%	25%	2%
Arthritis-related conditions (ever)[e]	7%	30%	4%

[a]Usual source of care excludes emergency room.
[b]Difference between uninsured and insured is significant at p<0.05.
[c]Hypertension, high cholesterol, heart disease, asthma, diabetes, arthritis-related conditions, anxiety/depression, severe headache/migraine, cancer, chronic bronchitis, liver condition, stroke, and emphysema.
[d]Coronary heart disease, angina, heart attack, and any other kind of heart condition or disease.
[e]Arthritis, rheumatoid arthritis, gout, lupus, or fibromyalgia.

Source: Urban Institute Tabulations of 2003 National Health Interview Survey. Used with permission from the Robert Wood Johnson Foundation in Princeton, New Jersey. Copyright 2007, Robert Wood Johnson Foundation.

the inconvenience involved in making the initial contact with a doctor; this either involved waiting too long in line to be seen at an outpatient clinic or it was too much trouble to be seen by a doctor." [19]

Culture and Patients' Beliefs

Finally, culture and patients' beliefs about the health care system have powerful effects on use of health care resources. Because the word *culture* has a number of connotations, we provide here some useful examples of how it can be defined (our emphases added to the original texts):

- *Culture* is defined "as the collective programming of the mind that distinguishes members of one group or category of people from another. . . . Culture is to a human collectivity what personality is to an individual . . ." [20]

- ". . . anthropologists do agree on three characteristics of *culture*: *it is not innate, but learned*; the various facets of culture are interrelated—you touch a culture in one place and everything else is affected; *it is shared and in effect defines the boundaries of different group* . . . there is not one aspect of human life that is not touched and altered by culture. This means personality, how people express themselves (including shows of emotion), the way they think, how they move, how problems are solved, how their cities are planned and laid out, how transportation systems functioned and are organized, as well as how economic and government systems are put together and function." [21]

- "The *culture* of a group can . . . be defined as a pattern of shared basic assumptions that the group learned as it solved its problems of external adaptation and internal integration, that has worked well enough to be considered valid and, therefore, to be taught to new members as the correct way to perceive, think, and feel in relation to those problems." [22]

The following are examples of the effects of culture and beliefs on health care utilization:

- The perception that cancer treatment had advanced in Tunisia was positively associated with use of screening in that country. [23]

- The primary reason Swedes who needed health care refrained from visiting a physician was lack of confidence in the health care system. [24]

- In a population of U.S. Chinese immigrants, one quarter of those surveyed believed cancer is contagious and many believed it is caused by immoral behavior. [25]

- "Intercultural differences in perceiving or reporting back pain can be hypothesized as the most likely explanation of the markedly different prevalence rates of the disorder in the United Kingdom and East and West Germany [more frequent in Germany]." [26]

- With regard to households from Tamil Nadu and Uttar Pradesh ". . . the status of women, and their exposure to and interaction with the outside world and control over decision making at home, explained the differences between the two groups," with the former being healthier than the latter.[27]

- "African-American women who had used religion/spirituality in the past year for health reasons . . . were more likely to have seen a medical doctor during the year prior to the interview, compared to their counterparts."[28]

MULTIPLE FACTORS INFLUENCE HEALTH-SEEKING BEHAVIOR

Figuring out why people use health care services is not as simple as identifying *the single driver* for behavior. Clearly there are multiple factors that influence these activities. One of the key tasks of the effective health care marketing strategist is to identify the relative importance of these reasons and realize that this analysis may not be generalizable to other conditions or uses of products or services. The following are examples of multifactor influences:

- With respect to asthma care, ". . . age, gender, education level, and employment status all had a significant relationship to medical utilization."[29]

- Delay in seeking care for cough in urban Lukasa, Zambia ". . . was associated with older age, severe underlying illness, poor perception of the health services, distance from the clinic and prior attendance at a private clinic. There was no relationship between delay and knowledge about tuberculosis, nor with education, socio-economic level or gender."[30]

- Focusing on developing countries, Pakistan in particular, the authors concluded that ". . . the utilization of a health care system, public or private, formal or non-formal, may depend on socio-demographic factors, social structures, level of education, cultural beliefs and practices, gender discrimination, status of women, economic and political systems, environmental conditions, and the disease pattern and health care system itself. Policy makers need to understand the drivers of health seeking behaviour of the population in an increasingly pluralistic health care system."[31]

Reducing Demand: Consumer Factors

Many health care marketing analysts stop at this point and become expert at understanding all the reasons why people may tend to use *more* health care services or products. Enhancing demand is, of course, the traditional role of the health care marketer; however, many stakeholders may wish to *reduce* demand. Consider these stakeholders who may want to lessen utilization of health care products and services: public or private insurance payers who are at financial risk for paying for health care services and products; medical groups who assume financial risk for certain services by accepting advance payments (capitation); and pharmaceutical benefit management companies (PBMs) or pharmacy companies who share with managed care companies some financial risk for overutilization of drugs. The profitability strategy in these instances changes from traditional revenue maximization to expense minimization. The following are stakeholder strategies to reduce customer demand:

- Increase out-of-pocket expenses

- Disease prevention

- Elimination or reduction of risky behaviors

- Self-management and education

- End-of-life issues

- Promotion of healthier lifestyle

As there is an extensive literature on each topic, we will discuss each category only briefly.

Increase Out-of-Pocket Expenses. The current approach to reducing health care costs is aimed at making customers more prudent about the types and amounts of health care they purchase—so-called "consumer-driven health care." The proponents of this strategy recite the mantra that a more informed and price-sensitive consumer will make "better" choices. Whether or not they make better choices regarding the quality of care under this scheme, the main outcome has been a further shifting of the cost of this care from the insurance company (or employer who pays for the premium) to consumers. A 2005 study by the consulting firm Hewitt Associates found that employees contributed 65 percent more to health care costs compared to 2002. From a quality and public policy perspective, one must ask whether increasing out-of-pocket expenses reduces utilization and, if so, whether there is a point after which such expenses are so great that consumers skimp on medically necessary services.

These questions have been asked for a number of years, but informed answers started with the groundbreaking RAND Health Insurance Experiment (HIE). (See Field Note 4.1.) The RAND experiment participants who had out-of-pocket requirements received $1,000, which was the maximum they were required to spend; if they did not spend this money, they could keep it. The "free care" group, of course, had no out-of-pocket liability, so they did not receive any funds. (See Field Note 4.1. for details of the experimental design and results. See the source document for a full explanation of the study design and critique.) The experiment results indicated that increasing out-of-pocket expenses reduces utilization. Another part of the study showed that *overall* there were no significant, deleterious effects on health status for those who received fewer services. We must, however, apply caution to unqualified acceptance of these findings. For instance, it is well known that the uninsured receive fewer medically necessary services than do the insured. Further, harmful effects of reduced utilization may not have appeared because chronic conditions, such as high

FIELD NOTE 4.1.

RAND Health Insurance Experiment (HIE) The RAND HIE randomized families to health insurance plans that varied their cost sharing from none ("free care") to a catastrophic plan that approximated a large family deductible with a stop-loss limit of $1,000 (in late-1970s dollars), which was scaled down for the low-income population. If one uses the rate of increase in per capita medical spending to convert late-1970s dollars into 2004 dollars, a $1,000 deductible then would be more than a $6,000 deductible is today. The HIE participants in the large-deductible (95 percent coinsurance) plan used 25–30 percent fewer services than those in the free-care plan; on average, they had just under two fewer face-to-face physician visits per person per year and were 23 percent less likely to be hospitalized in a year (Exhibit 1). Substantial reductions in use were found among all income groups (data not shown).

EXHIBIT 1. Use and Spending per Person in the RAND Health Insurance Experiment

Coinsurance (percent)	Visit Rates		Admission Rates		Spending (2003$)	
	Number	SE	Number	SE	Amount	SE
0 (free care)	4.55	0.17	0.128	0.0070	1,377	58
25	3.33	0.19	0.105	0.0070	1,116	51
50	3.03	0.22	0.092	0.0166	1,032	58
95 (high deductible)	2.73	0.18	0.099	0.0078	946	47

Source: Newhouse, J. P. "Consumer-Directed Health Plans and the RAND Health Insurance Experiment." *Health Affairs,* 2004, 23, 107–113.
Notes: The spending values shown are predicted from a multipart model; raw means are similar except that the spending figure for the 50 percent coinsurance plan is considerably higher because of one outlier that accounted for one-sixth of all spending on that plan. All plans with coinsurance had a $1,000 stop-loss feature, which was scaled down for lower income families. SE is standard error.

blood pressure, may take many years to manifest. With the growth in consumer-driven health plans, this study becomes even more important. The pricing lesson we can learn here is that we need to know *how much* insurance plans, the government, or employers will require the public to pay out of pocket before we can gauge the effect on use of essential services. This issue is also important for pharmaceutical pricing, as many expensive new drugs require significant out-of-pocket payments by patients.

Prevention. Because of public health concerns, governments are obviously interested in reducing illness by using preventive measures such as promoting or requiring immunizations. Pharmaceutical companies have responded to this need by developing new immunizations and combining existing ones to reduce the number of injections. Such preventive interventions are often cost-saving, as indicated by the following examples:

- "Vaccination of the 23 million elderly people unvaccinated in 1993 would have gained about 78000 years of healthy life and saved $194 million."[32]

- "A routine, universal rotavirus immunization program would prevent 1.08 million cases of diarrhea, avoiding 34000 hospitalizations, 95000 emergency department visits, and 227000 physician visits in the first 5 years of life. . . The program would provide a net savings of $296 million to society."[33]

- "The model was used to compare costs and benefits of a combined vaccination programme (CVP) including tetanus, diphtheria, and acellular pertussis (dTacp) administered at age 12, compared to current practice. . . . From the societal perspective, the CVP would be cost saving [Canadian] $858,106 at 10 years for the cohort."[34]

- If hepatitis A prevalence is 53% in patients with chronic liver disease, then immunizing this select group against this infection will save over $11,000 per 100 patients.[35]

Despite the potential future savings, these measures may add current costs to the health care and social welfare systems. With fixed budgets, many governments face the problem of prioritizing these measures to determine which delivers the best results at the lowest cost; evaluations of this type are often called cost-benefit analysis or cost-effectiveness analysis.

Elimination and Reduction of Risky Behaviors. This category includes cessation of smoking, wearing of seatbelts, use of car seats for young children, and reduction of unprotected sex. Unfortunately, sometimes attempts to legislate these behaviors run into personal freedom issues. Examples of successes in this area have been seatbelt laws and smoking bans in public places. A typical example of failure is attempts in some states to pass laws requiring helmet use for motorcyclists.

Instead of legislating behavioral changes, change agents can use *social marketing*, which we define as: ". . . the use of marketing principles and techniques to influence a target market to voluntarily accept, reject, modify, or abandon a behavior for the benefit of individuals, groups, or society as a whole."[36] Social marketing, as a discipline, has made enormous strides and has had a profound positive impact on social issues in the area of public health, safety, the environment, and community involvement. Fundamental principles at the core of this practice have been employed to encourage such behaviors as reducing tobacco use, wearing bicycle helmets, and decreasing littering. The main point is that social marketers use

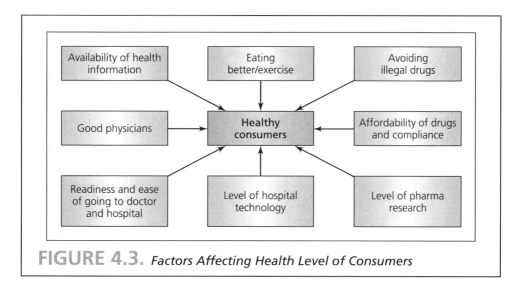

FIGURE 4.3. *Factors Affecting Health Level of Consumers*

noncoercive education, persuasion, and incentives to convince people that a change is in their self-interest or at least in the public's interest.

Prevention can be aided by listing and addressing key factors that affect the health level of consumers (see Figure 4.3 for examples).

Self-Management and Education. With the advent of consumerism, an expectation that patients will be self-empowered and learn more about their conditions and health status has arisen. To meet the needs of patients and reduce health care service costs, many insurance companies and associations have implemented programs to help patients better understand and be more involved in their care. For example, many insurance plans now educate asthmatics about initial steps they can take in the event of disease exacerbations; these programs are often called "asthma action plans." Such self-management programs are also prevalent for diabetics and sufferers of congestive heart failure. Further, patients and their families are increasingly using the Internet to find the latest treatments and most experienced providers. In this regard, while health care marketers are undoubtedly aware of the potential of the Internet, they should also be aware of the less reputable sites that compete for customer attention.

End-of-Life Issues. One often hears the complaint that a significant reason for soaring health care costs is the needless expenses of end-of-life care. This issue is a contentious one, fraught with conflicting data. Medicare statistics indicate decedents in their last year of life cost about six times as much as those who receive care but do not die. Even establishment of a Medicare-funded hospice program in 1983 (with a tripling of enrollees in the 1990s), changes in payment methods for skilled nursing homes and home care services, and the dramatic increase in use of advanced directives (so-called Do Not Resuscitate or DNR orders) have not slowed the rate of increase in these costs. Although *total* costs have been rapidly rising, the *percentage* of Medicare costs for this population has been stable for the past two decades.[37] In fact, these patients cost about the same as those with similar illnesses who are treated for cure rather than palliation. The reasons for this finding are complex, but can be best summarized by Emanuel and Emanuel: "Even when patients refuse life-sustaining interventions, they do not necessarily require less medical care, just a different kind of care."[38]

Despite these conclusions, we need to make two further distinctions regarding this topic. First, we differentiate between rationing and the provision of futile care. "Rationing refers to the withholding of efficacious treatments which cannot be afforded. Futility refers to ineffective treatments."[39] Second, we point out that the statistics cited are *averages* across all patients and sites. There are opportunities for savings in this category through identifying best practices and reducing nonhelpful variations in care. For example, Wennberg and others found that: "(s)triking variation exists in the utilisation of end of life care among US medical centres with strong national reputations for clinical care."[40]

Promotion of Healthier Lifestyle. These activities, though distinct, may be seen as complementing the elimination of risky behaviors. They include such behaviors as eating a proper diet and exercising regularly. For example, in March 2004 the Centers for Disease Control and Prevention released a study that found 400,000 deaths in the United States are linked to poor diet and lack of physical activity, representing an increase of 33 percent since 1990. This area is another example in which social marketers are active in promoting positive health behaviors.

Demand: Provider Factors

Although consumers usually initiate contact with the health care system, understanding their behavior is only half the story. For decades, economists have been studying a phenomenon called *provider-induced demand* (PID); that is, providers stimulating use of their services or products, presumably for financial gain. Not surprisingly, physicians have been the subjects most studied. The ongoing debate among academicians has been over whether this practice actually exists and if so, to what extent.

In interpreting the data, one must be aware of the following differences in research studies:

- Variation in analytical methodology
- Environmental conditions that could cause PID, such as increased density of physicians in a particular geographic area or a change in payment amount or method
- Cultural influences

With regard to *methodology*, Dranove and Wehner "proved" the thesis of their article "Physician-Induced Demand for Childbirths."[41] The point of this research was to discredit a methodology (two-stage least-squares regression) by confirming an obviously absurd notion. *Environmental events* might include a change in the number of practicing physicians in a given specialty within a defined geographic area (physician density) or a shift from fee-for-service payment to capitation or salary. The following examples highlight the effect of *cultural influences*: in France, when physician density increased, Delattre and Dormant found an increase in the number of services per visit;[42] under similar conditions in Norway, Sørensen and Grytten did not find this behavior.[43]

One must also realize that, although financial incentives have a powerful effect on physician behavior, they are only one of a number of influences on such conduct. As Eisenberg pointed out:

> . . . the factors that influence physicians' use of medical services are complex. They include personal considerations of the physician, such as the aspiration for income, the enjoyment of a satisfying practice, and the desire for approval from peers. Characteristics of the patient and the clinical encounter are also influential, such as consideration of the patient's economic well-being, maintenance or improvement of the patient's health, and the understanding of the patient's perceived values and desires.[44]

Other reasons for physician behavior include factors influencing local area variations in practice patterns, organizational cultural norms (which may be separate from peer approval issues), and professional aversion to uncertainty—particularly in the context of malpractice fears. Although we focus here on the behavioral implications of financial incentives, one should recognize that these other issues are also important for changing physician conduct. As Eisenberg further notes, "Education, feedback, participation, administrative rules, incentives and penalties may each address different factors that govern medical decision making. Any one by itself is less likely to be successful than an orchestrated combination." The following examples help to illustrate the possibilities.

Provider-Induced Demand: U.S. Examples

- ". . . larger fee differentials between caesarian and normal childbirth for the Medicaid program leads to higher caesarian delivery rates."[45]

- "Other things equal, a 10 percent increase in the surgeon/population ratio results in about a 3 percent increase in per capita utilization. Moreover, differences in supply seem to have a perverse effect on fees, raising them when the surgeon/population ratio increases."[46]

- "A 10 percent increase in surgeons per capita . . . results in a 0.9 percent increase in overall surgery per capita and 1.3 percent increase in elective surgery. The positive surgeon-availability elasticity, due primarily to elective surgery, supports the hypothesis that more discretionary surgical procedures are performed in areas of high surgeon concentration." [47]

■ In an investor-owned ambulatory care center, changing compensation from an hourly salary to an hourly minimum plus bonus based on monthly gross charges resulted in increases in the following areas: laboratory tests per patient (+23 percent), number of X-ray films per visit (+16 percent), total charges per month (+20 percent), and average number of patient visits per month (+12 percent). The authors also noted that "all physicians in this study, including those who never received a bonus, increased the intensity of their practices after the bonus system was instituted." [48]

Provider-Induced Demand: International Examples

■ In France, where fees are fixed, when physician/population ratios increase, both general practitioners and specialists "counterbalance the fall of the number of encounters by an increase of the volume of care delivered in each encounter." [49]

■ "After controlling for a patient's detailed characteristics, we found that increases in the relative numbers of" Japanese hospital and physician services are "significantly related to physician-initiated expenditures and the effect is higher for high-tech treatments." [50]

■ After 1961, most Danish physicians were paid a mix of half capitation and half fee-for-service. Doctors in Copenhagen were paid primarily capitation until 1987, when they were able to bill patients for their services. Observing utilization patterns before and after the change and comparing those patterns to a comparable nearby group of practitioners, the authors found significant increases in many diagnostic and therapeutic services for the Copenhagen physicians after 1987. [51]

■ ". . . we find evidence of induced demand since doctors that are paid fee-for-service tend to lengthen duration of the treatment." [52]

In interpreting the results of the studies in these examples, it is therefore often difficult to separate the financial incentives from these other factors. Also, one should interpret the conclusions cautiously; correlation does not prove causation. Perhaps physicians who respond to certain incentives may be most likely to practice in areas having compensation systems with which they feel most comfortable, or they may seek locations having a growing demand for their services. Another important factor to consider is quality-of-care effects. Although certain payment methods appear to increase PID, it is unclear whether services were underutilized before the change or overutilized after incentives were added.

Payers, such as insurance companies and governments, who are aware of provider-induced demand have implemented different strategies to limit the costs that result from such behavior, such as:

- Decreasing fees

- Increasing or decreasing the number of providers

- Changing the payment method

- Reviewing utilization more carefully

- Implementing practice guidelines or other measures to reduce variations in care

The first and most common approach is reducing fees. This tactic is likely to fail unless both reduction in the number of patient visits and restriction of access to high-tech care are simultaneously implemented. (Recall that total costs are a function of price, volume, and intensity of service.)

Second, in attempts to introduce market competition and lower costs, payers sometimes encourage entry of more providers into each service area. The theory is that more participants will increase competition and lower prices. In the public sector, that means training more professionals, such as physicians, or allowing construction of more facilities in otherwise regulated markets. In the private sector, this tactic involves contracting with more providers. On the other hand, states have also attempted to control costs by regulating new construction through laws that require review of projects costing more than a specified amount—so-called certificate of need (CON) legislation. For reasons mentioned above, providers react to these conditions causing these tactics to become ineffective; increasing the number of physicians does not lower health care costs, and it frequently raises total expenditures.[53] Likewise, measures such as CON laws have not had a significant effect on controlling health care costs, as evidenced by repeal of many of these measures in the 1970s.[54] In fact, there is theoretical evidence that more hospitals in a concentrated geographic area will *increase* costs by duplicating technology to enhance their competitiveness, a paradox sometimes called a "medical arms race." (This topic is, in fact, a bit more complex.[55])

The third tactic to control PID is changing the payment method. Instead of paying providers on a per-item basis, methods such as capitation (paying a fixed amount per person, usually per month, for a specified set of services or products) or global payments per type of case *have* been successful in moderating overall cost increases—or at least making them more predictable.

Fourth, commercial insurance companies have often used utilization review to try to limit PID. These measures require providers to call the payer for permission to (1) perform a service (such as elective surgery or a high-cost diagnostic test), (2) prescribe a high-cost or non-formulary drug, or (3) order a medical device. Although payers claim they have scientifically determined criteria that will enable them to evaluate the appropriateness of the request, on further examination of this procedure one must question whether and how it is successful. Since most of the methods these companies use are proprietary, they have not been open to valid study. One fact is commonly known, however: well over 90 percent of requests are approved without further review. This piece of information should make us suspect that the "hassle factor" may be just as (or more) valuable a utilization-reduction technique than the actual criteria that companies use. In fact, in 1999 UnitedHealth Group, one of the largest health care companies in the United States, announced it had determined that it was spending $100 million per year on preauthorization activities and approving 99 percent of physician requests. Based on this finding, the company announced it was eliminating this process for most types of services. Other companies have also scaled back these activities for the same reason.

Finally, practice guideline and treatment protocol programs have had variable success in controlling cost.

LOCAL (SMALL AREA) VARIATIONS

In view of all these consumer and provider factors, it should come as no surprise that patterns of care differ among nations and even among different regions of a given country. The variations are, in fact, much more extreme than one might imagine. For example, utilization of services can vary dramatically from town to town. The research that spurred interest in this topic dates to a landmark 1973 article in *Science* by Wennberg and Gittelsohn[56] (see Table 4.3). The authors found marked differences in a wide variety of surgical procedures among different towns in a state that at that time had a population of 444,000. This study, as well as numerous others that followed over the years, concluded that these differences were *not* due to variations in illness patterns. It is also important to realize that areas with higher utilization or cost do not necessarily have better outcomes. As Fisher and Wennberg pointed out: "Increased spending is associated neither with increased use of services known to be effective in reducing morbidity [sickness] or mortality [death], nor with increased use of surgical procedures where patients' preferences are important."[57]

The following are some international examples of local area variations:

- In Ontario, after "controlling for population characteristics and access to care (including the number of hospital beds, and the density of orthopaedic and referring physicians), orthopaedic surgeons' opinions or enthusiasm for the procedure was the dominant modifiable determinant of area variation."[58]

- In Ontario, there was an "almost 10-fold difference between the areas" with the highest and lowest rated of tympanostomy tube placement. "[I]t was the opinion of primary physicians that predicted rates."[59]

- "Following cardiac rehabilitation, there is a considerable regional variation in the prescription of cardiovascular medication in Germany. Beta-Blockers and lipid-lowering agents are prescribed more frequently in the West and ACE inhibitors in the East. Even after adjustment for differences in patient characteristics, region of residence remains an independent predictor for the prescription of lipid-lowering agents and ACE inhibitors."[60]

- In the U.K., "[p]rescription rates for antiplatelet agents varied significantly between the RHAs [Regional Health Authorities] for both TIA [transient

TABLE 4.3. Local Area Variation

Variation in number of surgical procedures performed per 10,000 persons for the thirteen Vermont hospital service areas and comparison populations, Vermont, 1969. (Rates adjusted to Vermont age composition.)

Surgical Procedure	Lowest Two Areas		Entire State	Highest Two Areas	
Tonsillectomy	13	32	43	85	151
Appendectomy	10	15	18	27	32
Hemorrhoidectomy	2	4	6	9	10
Males					
Hernioplasty	29	38	41	47	48
Prostatectomy	11	13	20	28	38
Females					
Cholecystectomy	17	19	27	46	57
Hysterectomy	20	22	30	34	60
Mastectomy	12	14	18	28	33
Dilation and curettage	30	42	55	108	141
Varicose veins	6	7	12	24	28

Source: Wennberg, J., and Gittelsohn, A. "Small Area Variations in Health Care Delivery." *Science*, 1973, *182*, 1102–1108. Reprinted with permission from AAAS.

ischemic attack] and stroke patients. Antiplatelets were prescribed for 15%–25% of stroke patients and for 30% and 45% of TIA patients over the 5 years, depending on region."[61]

In summarizing the reasons for these discrepancies, Detsky states that there "are three main reasons why there might be variation in the use of diagnostic and therapeutic procedures: differences in health care systems, physicians' practice styles, and patient characteristics."[62] We have already discussed factors related to the last two reasons. To physician practice styles we can add three other reasons: physicians' own beliefs about effectiveness of care, their medical training, and their beliefs in their own abilities. An example of what is meant by health care system characteristic differences is the study by Fisher and others that found the regional "differences in Medicare spending are largely explained by the more inpatient-based and specialist-oriented pattern of practice observed in high-spending regions. Neither quality of care nor accesses to care appear to be better for Medicare enrollees in higher-spending regions."[63] For more extensive data on local area variations, an excellent resource is *The Dartmouth Atlas* (http://www.dartmouthatlas.org/).

SUMMARY

In this chapter we have examined how key factors—age, sex, race, income or socio-economic status, education, availability of care, and culture and patient beliefs—affect people's decisions to seek health care. Their demand is reduced by such factors as the increasing cost of health care, preventive measures they undertake, their efforts to avoid risky behavior, and their response to healthy lifestyle promotion. On the other hand, their demand for health care may be increased by provider-induced activities undertaken to increase provider income or to cope with the uncertainty of interpreting a medical condition. The great geographical variation in health care utilization by category suggests that provider-induced activities or norms play some role.

DISCUSSION QUESTIONS

1. You are the marketing manager for a national laboratory that has just come out with a blood test to screen for a rare genetic disease in fetuses of pregnant women. Because the test involves genetic screening, it is very expensive. Who are all the relevant stakeholders who will promote and block introduction of this test to this select population?

2. A newly popular type of insurance is a "consumer-directed health plan," where individuals have large deductibles to encourage prudent purchasing. Who is likely to sign up for these plans? From what you know about the RAND Health Insurance Experiment, is this approach likely to control health care costs? What are the drawbacks of such plans?

3. You are a territory manager for the cardiology division of a major medical device company. You notice that among the five largest cardiology groups in your area there is a threefold difference between lowest and highest use of your products. This finding is despite the fact that your competitor has not significantly penetrated this market. Using what you know about local area variations and physician behavior, what might explain this difference?

PART

2

ANALYZING THE MARKET

CHAPTER

5

STRATEGY AND MARKET PLANNING

LEARNING OBJECTIVES

In this chapter, we will address the following questions:

1. What are the main steps in building a strategic plan for a health care organization?

2. What goes into conducting an environmental analysis?

3. How can SWOT analysis and Five Forces Analysis enrich the strategic planning process?

4. What contents must be included in a marketing plan?

OPENING EXAMPLE

Humana Grows From a Small Startup to a Major Health Insurance Company

Humana Inc., headquartered in Louisville, Kentucky, is one of the nation's largest publicly traded health benefits companies, with approximately 6.4 million medical members located primarily in eighteen states and Puerto Rico.

In 1961, two young Kentucky lawyers, David A. Jones and Wendell Cherry—along with four friends—each invested $1,000 to achieve their vision of operating a nursing home business, which was called Heritage House. Together, Jones and Cherry had an uncanny ability to forecast changes and respond swiftly. By 1968, their company, called Extendicare, included seven nursing homes. An initial public offering that year generated money for further expansion.

That same year, the partners took another bold step and acquired their first hospital, Medical Center Hospital in Huntsville, Alabama, which was still under construction. By the time the Huntsville facility opened in 1970, Extendicare owned nine other hospitals. In 1972, it had divested itself of all nursing homes to concentrate on its growing hospital business.

Reflecting its new direction, Extendicare became Humana Inc. in January 1974. According to the company's annual report that year, the new name was selected "to project more truly the philosophy of the company, to stand out distinctively and to provide an identity with non-limiting connotations."

Through rapid growth and strategic acquisitions, Humana became the world's largest hospital company by the early 1980s, owning more than 80 hospitals in the United States and abroad. In 1982, Humana established its Centers of Excellence program, designating hospitals that offered unsurpassed specialty care within each center's geographic region.

More change was in store for the company. The hospital industry as a whole was evolving in response to cost and other pressures. As outpatient care increased and inpatient admissions declined, Humana created a family of flexible health insurance products in 1984. Called Humana Health Care Plans, the new offerings marked Humana's entry into the budding HMO industry.

Throughout the late 1980s, Humana's vertical integration approach helped the company keep hospital admissions up and insurance costs down. As both the hospital and insurance industries continued to evolve, Humana saw the need to separate its hospital and insurance divisions. So in 1993 Humana spun off its hospital operations into a new company called Galen Health Care Inc. Soon afterward, Galen merged with Columbia/HCA.

Following the split, Humana increased the number of those whom the company insured through both acquisitions and same-plan growth. Major acquisitions in the late

1990s included EMPHESYS Financial Group, Physician Corporation of America (PCA), and ChoiceCare.

In 2007 Humana purposely decreased the number of members it insures by strategically divesting nonessential business and operations to focus its energy and resources on its core business of health insurance and related services.

Source: Adapted from http://humana.com/corporatecomm/companyinfo/history.asp.

OVERVIEW: DEFINING THE ORGANIZATION'S PURPOSE AND MISSION

Every organization has to define the core purpose for its existence. That purpose is usually contained in its mission statement. Although health care organizations will commonly define their purpose as "providing health care services or products," they need to make a statement that is more specific and customer-outcome-oriented. A community hospital might say, "We make lives better for those who have been afflicted with illness." A health club might say, "We provide exercise, health information, and health products that will increase our members' chances of avoiding illnesses or disability."

To define its mission, the enterprise needs to address Peter Drucker's classic questions:[1] What is our business? Who is the customer? What is of value to the customer? What will our business be? What *should* our business be? As we address each of these elements, this chapter provides guidelines on developing a marketing strategy to achieve desired customer outcomes.

STRATEGIC PLANNING

Strategic planning starts with developing a definition of your business.

Business Definition

The business definition requires understanding of at least five elements:

- *History of aims, policies, and achievements.* In medical groups, physicians should understand why the group was formed, what processes have contributed to (or detracted from) its success, and what it has accomplished. Hospital employees should appreciate the origins of the organization, particularly if it is a nonprofit enterprise. Even successful medical product companies communicate this element to their employees and customers. For example, Johnson & Johnson presents its history and credo to explain "Our Company" on its Web site (http://www.jnj.com/our_company/index.htm). If members of the organization understand the organization's history, leaders can more predictably gauge how they will react to the process as well as the content of changes necessary for strategy implementation. Also, this understanding is critical to appreciating corporate culture—the shared values and beliefs of the firm's members.

- *Current preferences of owners and management.* One of the biggest obstacles to mission statement formulation is the inability of decision makers to agree on common, current preferences. This problem is especially pervasive in multispecialty medical groups in academic centers. For example, in this setting, managers are increasingly focused on physician financial productivity derived from providing patient care. Physicians who have substantial clinical responsibilities, however, often believe that their time is not appropriately rewarded, particularly when promotion depends on their research productivity. Medical product or pharmaceutical companies face a similar problem when they must choose where to devote research or sales support among divisions. The organization must therefore determine not only what services it seeks to provide, but also the relative importance of the mix of those services. These preferences must be clear and explicit before the firm writes a mission statement or embarks on a strategy formulation.

- *Market environment.* An environmental assessment is critical to mission statement formulation. Because of its importance, we discuss this element in detail in a following section.

- *Resources.* The organization's resources set constraints on the mission statement. These resources are both tangible, such as cash, plant, and equipment, and intangible, such as reputation and image.

- *Distinctive competencies.* The business should ask itself not only what it does well but also what it does better than other similar organizations. Such competencies are not only clinical, such as better surgical outcomes, but also operational, such as better coordination of care for patients who have complex illnesses, more efficient billing systems, or a more patient-friendly staff.

Organizations often define their business in terms of their output. For example, a hospital may say that it does knee and hip surgeries. But Theodore Levitt argued that market definitions of a business are superior to product definitions.[2] Levitt encouraged organizations to define their business in terms of needs, not products; outcomes, not outputs. Thus the hospital that does knee and hip surgery is producing or improving patient mobility; the cancer physician is there to produce hope.

Further, a business can be defined in terms of three additional dimensions: customer groups, customer needs, and technology.[3] Consider a small organization that defines its business as designing lighting systems for hospital operating rooms. Its customer group is hospitals, the customer need is bright lighting, and the technology is halogen bulbs.

Most businesses finish this part of the mission self-assessment with their *current* business definition. To fully realize the potential of a mission statement, however, the organization should also ask itself, what *should* our business definition be? The corollary to this question is, given our current resources, what can we do better? Answering these questions will help the firm not only to more clearly define its resources and distinctive competencies, but also to begin the process of strategy formulation and organizational improvement.

To *fully* explore an understanding of the business definition, however, leaders must pose a third essential question: what *could* our business be? A corollary to this question is, given realistic additional resources, what would our business look like and what could we accomplish? Answering these questions can help the organization begin the process of realistic goal setting and capital budgeting.

Customer Identification

Customer identification requires the firm to answer the following questions: Who are our customers? Where are they? What are their characteristics? Although we discuss customer definition elsewhere in this book, we augment that notion here to help formulate mission and strategy.

The quality expert J. M. Juran used "the word 'customers' to include *all persons who are impacted by our processes and our products*. Those persons include internal as well as external customers. . . . The term 'external customers' is used here to mean persons who are not a part of our company but who are impacted by our products. The term 'internal customers' means persons or organizations who are part of our company."[4]

Juran makes three additional important points about understanding the concept of a customer. First, when he refers to "products," he is including both goods *and* services. Thus he extends the idea of customer from the industrial production arena to the service sector, including the delivery of health care.

Second, although a business may have many customers, only a subset of them actually *uses* the product. Juran defines "the word '*user*' to designate *anyone who carries out positive actions* with respect to our product—actions such as further processing, sale, ultimate use, and so on." Thus, although suppliers are external customers, patients are both customers and users of health care services.

Finally, the business must prioritize the importance of its various customers. We can order the importance of our customers by using three categories: those who are most affected by what we do, those whom we *wish* to affect the most, and those who can help us further our business. The first category of customers is the natural recipients of our products; for example, patients who sustain sports injuries are the natural customers of orthopedic groups.

In the second category (those we wish to affect the most), firms either can diversify (along different service lines or in different geographic areas) or can seek unfulfilled mission objectives. For example, public health clinics may find that they are serving populations lacking proper immunizations. In the final category, hospitals can craft a symbiotic relationship with their important customers, such as health plans and physicians.

After a business has identified its customers and prioritized their importance, it must define its service area. Whereas medical products (such as pharmaceuticals and devices) have widespread distribution, one of the major characteristics of health *services* is that all health care is local. It is up to the service organization, however, to determine what the word *local* means to its business. Few medical groups draw on a national or international patient base, so geographic market definition will depend on such features as urban versus rural environment, number and distribution of local competitors, and availability of public transportation. For instance, because many residents of New York City depend exclusively on public transportation, proximity to a bus or train stop could be extremely important to a group's patients. On the other hand, many Californians are accustomed to traveling longer distances in their cars; therefore a facility's proximity to a highway exit may be very important to residents in that state.

Once the firm has determined the scope of its geographic coverage, it must define the segments of the market it seeks to serve. Market segmentation involves identifying a group of current or potential customers with similar characteristics. The characteristics can be determined by demographics, such as age or sex; service line, such as primary care, infertility services, or mental health; payer type, such as cash-only (as for aesthetic surgery), Medicare, or managed care; or other general preferences. We discuss segmentation in more detail in Chapter Eight.

When an organization identifies its customers, it often finds that their needs conflict. For example, both payers and patients are important customers for medical groups. Just as health plans may impose unreasonable constraints on the delivery of patient care, patients can express unrealistic demands for the provision of medical services. Balancing conflicting customer needs is a constant and difficult challenge for all health care firms. To meet this challenge, once an organization completes its customer identification, it may need to modify its business definition to help clarify priorities.

Value Proposition

For most businesses, value is defined as the best product or service one can obtain for a given price or, for a desired product or service, for the lowest price at which it can be obtained. Thus value is most often defined as a trade-off between cost and quality. Although these concepts of cost and quality are important in health care, as we mentioned in Chapter Two, a third dimension, *access*, must also be considered. Therefore, an appropriate *mix* of cost, quality, and access is essential for a firm to deliver customer value. That mix decision must then be reflected in the mission statement.

Of additional importance is managing a *value chain*. Porter proposed the concept as a tool for identifying ways to create customer value[5] (see Figure 5.1). Every organization performs a coordinated set of activities to design, produce, market, deliver, and support its products and services. The value chain identifies nine strategically relevant activities that create value and cost. These nine value-creating activities consist of five primary activities and four support activities.

The primary activities comprise bringing materials into the business (inbound logistics), converting them into final products and services (operations), shipping out final products and services (outbound logistics), marketing them to the target

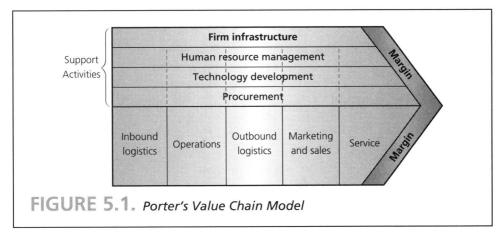

FIGURE 5.1. *Porter's Value Chain Model*

Source: Porter, M. E. *Competitive Advantage: Creating and Sustaining Superior Performance.* New York: Simon & Schuster, 1985.

market (marketing and sales), and servicing them (service). The support activities—procurement, technology development, human resource management, and firm infrastructure—are handled in specialized departments, which may be decentralized across the company. For example, several departments may do procurement and hiring.

The firm's task is to examine its costs and performance in each value-creating activity and to look for improvement opportunities. The company should also estimate its competitors' costs and performance standards as benchmarks against which to compare its own costs and performance. It should go further and study the "best of class" practices of the world's best organizations.[6]

Success depends not only on how well each department performs its work, but also on how well the various departmental activities are coordinated to conduct *core business processes*,[7] which include the following:

- *Market sensing.* Gathering market intelligence, disseminating it within the organization, and acting on the information

- *New offering realization.* Researching, developing, and launching new, high-quality offerings quickly and within budget

- *Channel bonding.* Developing strong partners on the supply and distribution side of the business

- *Customer acquisition.* Defining target markets and prospecting for new customers

- *Customer relationship management.* Building deeper understanding, relationships, and offerings to individual customers

- *Fulfillment management.* Receiving and approving orders, shipping goods or delivering services on time, and collecting payment

Strong organizations develop superior capabilities in managing and linking their core business processes. For example, consider Cardinal Health's value-added inventory management process, which supports its core business as a drug wholesaler:

FOR EXAMPLE

Getting medical supplies where they needed to go at Mountain View, California-based El Camino Hospital used to be a costly and labor-intensive process.

According to Ashley Hall, director of materials management at the hospital, the 395-licensed bed facility would receive bulk deliveries and store the supplies until they were needed. Those bulk orders would then be broken down and sent to central storage units, which would store them until they were divided into even smaller packages, and sent to the floors as necessary. Using this system, clerks would touch different supplies eight to 12 times.

El Camino decided it needed to automate the process in 2003 and began deploying supply chain management systems from Dublin, Ohio-based Cardinal Health Inc. The goal was to reduce the number of times the supplies were touched, limit the amount kept on hand and ease clinicians' concerns about having enough materials.

In the first 18 months the system was in use, El Camino saw more than $3 million in savings, and it has saved $2.5 million annually since then. "The cost savings is derived from a combination of inventory reduction, inventory holding costs, labor reduction, increased labor efficiencies for clinicians, and a reduction in distribution and handling fees from the distributor," Hall says.

When nurses need something, they go to the supply cabinet and log in using the computer attached to the storage system. Nurses request various supplies through the computer using the "take" button, which automatically tracks everything removed. They can also enter patient information to allow billing for specific items. Every 24 hours, the system takes a snapshot to see what supplies are needed and where. When the item reaches a set amount, the system automatically sends a message to re-order it. This automated process eliminates the need for a nurse having to remember what they used and having to restock or order new supplies. The hospital has seen some savings by reducing the number of full-time equivalent staff for stocking supplies, Hall says. The process used to take seven to eight employees and now it takes four.

Source: Adopted from "Supply Chain Mantra: 'Never Run Out'; Procurement System Enables Hospital to Cut Costs While Keeping Supplies Moving." Health Data Management, Oct. 2006, Supply Chain Technology, p. 70.

Given the three elements of business definition, customer identification, and value proposition, consider the following examples of mission statements from different types of health care organizations. These statements are not meant to illustrate best examples; you should analyze them in light of the needs of the particular organization using the criteria just described.

EXAMPLES OF MISSION STATEMENTS OF HEALTH CARE ORGANIZATIONS

Pfizer   We will become the world's most valued company to patients, customers, colleagues, investors, business partners, and the communities where we work and live.

Merck   The mission of Merck is to provide society with superior products and services by developing innovations and solutions that improve the quality of life and satisfy customer needs, and to provide employees with meaningful work and advancement opportunities, and investors with a superior rate of return.

Amgen   Amgen strives to serve patients by transforming the promise of science and biotechnology into therapies that have the power to restore health or even save lives. In everything we do, we aim to fulfill that mission. And every step of the way, we are guided by the values that define us.

Northwestern Memorial Hospital   Northwestern Memorial Hospital is an academic medical center where the patient comes first. We are an organization of caregivers who aspire to consistently high standards of quality, cost-effectiveness and patient satisfaction. We seek to improve the health of the communities we serve by delivering a broad range of services with sensitivity to the individual needs of our patients and their families.

American Medical Association   To promote the art and science of medicine and the betterment of public health.

American Hospital Association   To advance the health of individuals and communities. The AHA leads, represents and serves hospitals, health systems and other related organizations that are accountable to the community and committed to health improvement.

Boston Scientific   Boston Scientific's mission is to improve the quality of patient care and the productivity of health care delivery through the development and advocacy of less-invasive medical devices and procedures. This is accomplished through the continuing refinement of existing products and procedures and the investigation and development of new technologies that can reduce risk, trauma, cost, procedure time and the need for aftercare.

Medtronic   To contribute to human welfare by application of biomedical engineering in the research, design, manufacture, and sale of instruments or appliances that alleviate pain, restore health, and extend life.

Goal Setting

Once an organization has determined its mission, it should then formulate its goals. If the mission statement is a map indicating the direction in which the firm seeks to go, its goals are the milestones indicating how well the business is progressing on its journey. For goals to be meaningful, they must have at least the following five characteristics:

1. *Goals must be clearly tied to the mission statement.* For example, if a mission states that a medical group will improve quality of care as perceived by its patients, a goal should be to continuously improve patient satisfaction scores by using a valid assessment tool.

2. *Goals must be clearly defined.* Organizations should avoid such vague statements as "we want to be the best hospital in our area." More clearly defined goals might be to maximize profitability or provide a certain level of community service.

3. *Goals must be measurable.* Firms must be able to assign a numerical value to achievement of milestones in order to assess whether they are being reached. For example, profitability can be evaluated by such measures as return on equity or return on assets. Patient satisfaction can be measured by such indicators as minutes of waiting time or overall scores from patients who felt their physician listened fully to their problems.

4. *Goals must be prioritized.* There are three reasons for such prioritization. First, some goals are obviously more important than others. Given its mission, values, and resource constraints, an organization may be able to accomplish only so much in a certain time period. Second, some goals may conflict with one another. An example is managed care companies' desire in the 1990s to increase market share and profitability simultaneously. Finally, certain customers are more important than others. (Prioritizing customers does not mean one may discriminate against patients based on such factors as age, gender, race, and so on.)

5. *Goal setting must include a target time by which they must be achieved.* Goals must move from abstract concepts into something more tangible. Deadlines for goal achievement can specify either a target number, such as 92 percent patient satisfaction by year end, or a rate, such as 5 percent market share growth each year. If a particular rate of improvement is specified, setting deadlines is similar to the concept of improving "cycle time" in quality improvement initiatives. The aim of improving cycle time is to accomplish the same number of tasks or more in a shorter period. If overall patient satisfaction was improved by five percentage points in a year, an improvement goal might be to reach that milestone the following year in six to nine months.

Strategy

Although determining an organizational mission and goals are important, one must also have a plan for achieving them. This plan is the business strategy.

Besanko, Dranove, and Shanley begin their general text on strategy with a series of definitions:[8]

> The determination of the basic long-term goals and objectives of an enterprise, and the adoption of courses of action and the allocation of resources necessary for carrying out these goals.[9]
>
> The pattern of objectives, purposes or goals, and the major policies and plans for achieving these goals, stated in such a way as to define what business the company is in or should be in and the kind of company it is or should be.[10]
>
> What determines the framework of a firm's business activity and provides guidelines for coordinating activities so that the firm can cope with and influence the changing environment. Strategy articulates the firm's preferred environment and the type of organization it is striving to become.[11]

These definitions highlight certain key characteristics of organizational strategy. First, as we mentioned previously, although businesses are often involved in many *small* day-to-day decisions, strategy considers approaches to handling *major* issues with which the enterprise must deal now or in the future. Second, strategy involves setting the organizational direction for the medium to long term. These time frames, of course, are relative and vary by firm and industry. For example, pharmaceutical companies have very long-range plans with regard to new product development, often measured in decades. Smaller medical groups, on the other hand, have much shorter time frames, frequently measured in months or a year. Finally, useful strategies take into account that short-term decisions *do* need to be made. Strategy, therefore, provides a framework for making those decisions in the context of the organization's long-range goals.

Drafting a useful and appropriate strategy involves at least four steps: (1) environmental assessment (internal and external) and planning, (2) implementation of the strategy, (3) evaluation of the strategy's success, and (4) reassessment, given the feasibility a firm discovers in exploring its options. The complete planning, implementation, and control cycle is shown in Figure 5.2; it is the same process used to achieve many types of performance improvements.

Strategic planning occurs at four levels: corporate, division, strategic business unit (SBU), and product. The simple definition for a SBU is that division of the company closest to and most responsible for managing the product or service. As an example, consider an integrated health care delivery system comprising hospitals, ambulatory care centers, and long-term care facilities. At the corporate level, senior management designs a strategic plan to guide the whole enterprise. The hospital SBU

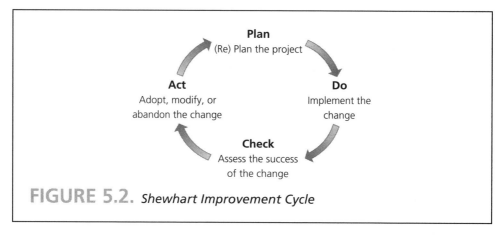

FIGURE 5.2. *Shewhart Improvement Cycle*

Source: Shewhart, W. A. *Statistical Method from the Viewpoint of Quality Control.* New York: Dover, 1930.

will have more specific strategies, such as providing oncology services. The specific product (service) within the unit, such as radiation therapy, may have its own plan.

Marketing plays a critical role in this process for products as well as services and organizations. For example, according to General Electric:

The marketing manager is the most significant functional contributor to the strategic-planning process, with leadership roles in defining the business mission; analysis of the environmental, competitive, and business situations; developing objectives, goals, and strategies; and defining product, market, distribution, and quality plans to implement the business's strategies. This involvement extends to the development of programs and operating plans that are fully linked with the strategic plan.[12]

The *marketing plan* is the central instrument for directing and coordinating the organization's resources to achieve the unit's objectives. This plan includes strategic and tactical elements. The *strategic marketing plan* defines the target market(s) and the value proposition that will be offered. The *tactical marketing plan* specifies the features and benefits of each product offering and the pricing, promotion, and place decisions.

Although planning occurs at each of the levels just described, they are "rolled up" from bottom to top, with senior management review and approval before ultimate implementation.

SWOT Analysis

One of the oldest and most popular methods used to assess the environment is determination of the organization's strengths, weaknesses, opportunities, and threats (SWOT analysis). Analyses of strengths and weaknesses provide an assessment of a

	Resources	Capabilities
Tangible	Cash, equipment, property	Clinical services
Intangible	Employee morale, favorable reputation	Patient satisfaction

FIGURE 5.3. *Examples of Resources and Capabilities*

firm's internal environment; consideration of opportunities and threats gives the firm an assessment of its external environment. We now consider each of these elements.

Strengths. Strengths have traditionally been divided into two categories: resources (what you have) and capabilities (what you do well). Both resources and capabilities can be tangible or intangible. Figure 5.3 provides some examples.

While these dimensions help a health care enterprise understand its current strengths, they should also be used to assess *potential* capabilities given current resources. This analysis is akin to answering the question "What *should* our business be?" during mission statement formulation. A final dimension of a strengths analysis entails evaluating the length of time they will last. In some respects, this projection involves linking consideration of strengths to an understanding of the opportunities and threats in the external environment (discussed in the following sections).

Weaknesses. Analysis of a firm's weaknesses can be conducted in a manner similar to analyzing its strengths; that is, the elements listed in Figure 5.3 for strengths may also be identified as weaknesses. For example, a medical group may lack cash and have a dysfunctional culture, a poor location, and higher-than-expected complication rates for procedures its physicians perform.

A firm should also assess its internal environment in three additional dimensions:

1. *Finances.* The organization must pick some key financial ratios that will indicate how well it is performing. Further, these ratios should be trended and benchmarked against industry standards.

2. *Performance capabilities.* The business must objectively assess how well it is performing those services that generate its operating revenue.

3. *Human resource capabilities.* This dimension includes not only obvious measures like staffing ratios and vacancies (such as in hospitals), but also intangible qualities like employee morale and corporate culture.

Exhibit 5.1 presents a tool for profiling the health care organization's major strengths and weaknesses.

EXHIBIT 5.1. **Checklist for Strengths and Weaknesses Analysis**

	Performance					Importance		
	Major Strength	Minor Strength	Neutral	Minor Weakness	Major Weakness	High	Medium	Low
Marketing								
1. Organization reputation	—	—	—	—	—	—	—	—
2. Market share	—	—	—	—	—	—	—	—
3. Customer satisfaction	—	—	—	—	—	—	—	—
4. Customer retention	—	—	—	—	—	—	—	—
5. Product quality	—	—	—	—	—	—	—	—
6. Service quality	—	—	—	—	—	—	—	—
7. Pricing effectiveness	—	—	—	—	—	—	—	—
8. Distribution effectiveness	—	—	—	—	—	—	—	—
9. Promotion effectiveness	—	—	—	—	—	—	—	—
10. Sales force effectiveness	—	—	—	—	—	—	—	—
11. Innovation effectiveness	—	—	—	—	—	—	—	—

(Exhibit 5.1 continued)

	Performance					Importance		
	Major Strength	Minor Strength	Neutral	Minor Weakness	Major Weakness	High	Medium	Low
12. Geographical coverage	——	——	——	——	——	——	——	——
Finance								
13. Cost or availability of capital	——	——	——	——	——	——	——	——
14. Cash flow	——	——	——	——	——	——	——	——
15. Financial stability	——	——	——	——	——	——	——	——
Operations								
16. Facilities	——	——	——	——	——	——	——	——
17. Economies of scale	——	——	——	——	——	——	——	——
18. Capacity	——	——	——	——	——	——	——	——
19. Able, dedicated staff	——	——	——	——	——	——	——	——
20. Ability to produce on time	——	——	——	——	——	——	——	——
21. Technical operations, skill organization	——	——	——	——	——	——	——	——
22. Visionary, capable leadership	——	——	——	——	——	——	——	——

(Exhibit 5.1 continued)

	Performance					Importance		
	Major Strength	Minor Strength	Neutral	Minor Weakness	Major Weakness	High	Medium	Low
23. Dedicated employees	—	—	—	—	—	—	—	—
24. Entrepreneurial orientation	—	—	—	—	—	—	—	—
25. Flexible, responsive	—	—	—	—	—	—	—	—

Source: Adapted from Kotler and Keller, *Marketing Management,* 12th ed. Upper Saddle River, N.J.: Prentice Hall, 2006, p. 55.

Opportunities. Three options are available to health care companies seeking to exploit environmental opportunities to augment its operations. The first is to achieve further growth within current business practices (intensive growth opportunities). The second is to build or acquire ventures that are related to current businesses (integrative growth opportunities). The third is to identify opportunities to add attractive businesses that are unrelated to current businesses (diversification growth opportunities). The firm may also want to take advantage of environmental opportunities to exit activities that no longer fit with its mission or strategy.

Intensive growth. Corporate management's first step should be to review opportunities to improve its existing businesses. Ansoff has proposed a useful framework for detecting new intensive growth opportunities—a "product–market expansion grid"[13] (see Figure 5.4).

The organization first considers whether it could gain more market share with its current offerings in its current markets (market-penetration strategy). Next it considers whether it can find or develop new markets for its current products (market development strategy). Then it considers whether it can develop new products of potential interest to its current markets (product-development strategy). As shown in Figure 5.4, there is a possible fourth strategy for a later date: diversification, whereby the organization reviews opportunities to develop new products for new markets.

How might an organization use these three major intensive growth strategies to increase its sales? Consider a health club, which is in the business of encouraging physical exercise and makes money by selling memberships. This business could enhance its market penetration strategy with any or all of these efforts:

	Current Products	New Products
Current Markets	1. Market-penetration strategy	3. Product-development strategy
New Markets	2. Market-development strategy	(Diversification strategy)

FIGURE 5.4. *Product-Market Expansion Grid*

(1) encouraging its current members to come to the gym more often (enhancing customer loyalty), (2) attracting competitors' customers, (3) convincing nonexercisers to join the club and start exercising.

How can the health club use a product-development strategy? It might first try to identify potential user groups in the current sales areas. For example, if the club finds it has been selling memberships primarily to women, it might create couples memberships to attract spouses or partners. It might also open additional branches or add new-product possibilities, such as Pilates or Tai Chi classes.

Integrative growth. To continue this example, a health club can also consider opportunities arising from integrating backward, forward, or horizontally. Backward integration might involve private labeling or selling home exercise equipment. An example of forward integration would be opening up a health food restaurant within the club. Horizontal integration can be achieved by acquiring one or more competitors.

Diversification growth. Diversification growth involves entering ventures that are unrelated to the present business. Three types of diversification are possible. First, the health club could invest in new services that have technological or marketing synergy with existing product lines (concentric diversification strategy), such as repairing exercise equipment for other health clubs. Second, the club might search for new products that could appeal to current customers, even though the new products are technologically unrelated to its current product line (horizontal diversification strategy), such as selling a line of vitamins. Finally, the organization might invest in a business that has no relationship to its current technology, products, or markets (conglomerate diversification strategy), such as opening a computer store.

Downsizing older businesses. Organizations must not only develop new businesses, they must also carefully prune, harvest, or divest old businesses in order to release needed resources and reduce costs. Reasons for business discontinuation include poor performance and lack of continued "fit" with current operations (regardless of profitability). For example, in 2006 Pfizer sold its consumer products division to Johnson & Johnson to focus on its pharmaceutical business. The sale included such household names as Listerine, Visine, and Neosporin.

Threats. An analysis of threats will yield those that are current and those that are projected. In considering threats, one must also look to their potential sources, such as competitors, suppliers, customers, technological change, or government (through laws and regulations). For instance, Christensen, Bohmer, and Kenagy[14] discuss threats from "disruptive innovations—cheaper, simpler, more convenient products or services that start by meeting the needs of less-demanding customers." They present the following example and explanation:

> *Imagine a portable, low-intensity X-ray machine that can be wheeled between offices on a small cart. It creates images of such clarity that pediatricians, internists, and nurses can detect cracks in bones or lumps in tissue in their offices, not in a hospital. It works through a patented "nanocrystal" process, which uses night-vision technology borrowed from the military. At 10% of the cost of a conventional X-ray machine, it could save patients, their employers, and insurance companies hundreds of thousands of dollars every year. Great innovation, right? Guess again. When the entrepreneur who developed the machine tried to license the technology to established health care companies, he couldn't even get his foot in the door. Large-scale X-ray equipment suppliers wanted no part of it. Why? Because it threatened their business models.*
>
> *What happened to the X-ray entrepreneur is all too common in the health care industry. Powerful institutional forces fight simpler alternatives to expensive care because those alternatives threaten their livelihoods [p. 102].*

In evaluating a firm's environment using a SWOT analysis, a few cautionary notes should be considered. First, although strengths, weaknesses, opportunities, and threats all need to be assessed, they are not all of equal importance to an organization. These four elements, therefore, should be prioritized by their current and potential impact. Second, these features need to be evaluated in the context of a specific time frame. For example, it is obvious that some opportunities have a limited availability. Also, some capabilities may become obsolete with introduction of new technology. Third, these elements must be evaluated in light of one another and their interdependence fully appreciated. For example, internal capabilities need to be evaluated in the context of the external environment.

A final comment about the SWOT analysis concerns the pitfalls of using this approach to analyze the environment. Even after an organization has clearly delineated its internal and external environments, it may not be able to match appropriate elements to achieve organizational success. For example, what if strengths do not allow a company to take advantage of an opportunity? Further, a SWOT analysis is a hit-or-miss process, since it does not provide a systematic means of analysis; it is easy to overlook important environmental factors. Finally, a SWOT analysis does not offer an approach to strategic implementation. SWOT analysis should therefore be supplemented by a Five Forces Analysis.

Five Forces Analysis

The Five Forces Analysis, developed by Michael Porter in his book *Competitive Strategy*,[15] has largely replaced the SWOT assessment in business school strategy courses and corporate planning. This method has at least five advantages over the SWOT assessment. First, in providing an understanding of the competitive environment, it is a more systematic and comprehensive approach to strategy than the SWOT analysis. Second, it can be used in a variety of settings, whether they are manufacturing or service companies, for-profit or nonprofit organizations. Third, by providing an analysis of each force's effect on industry profits, it furnishes an assessment of overall industry profitability. Fourth, this analysis identifies opportunities for success and threats to success. Finally, unlike the SWOT approach, it helps to generate strategic choices. The five forces can be summed up as follows:

1. Internal Rivalry
2. Threat of New Entrants
3. Threat of Substitute Products
4. Buyer Power
5. Supplier Power

We will discuss each of these five forces, using examples from the medical group sector.[16] Figure 5.5 displays this analytic framework.

Internal Rivalry. Internal rivalry is defined as competition among like firms in the same industry. Firms compete along a number of dimensions and it is useful to divide these dimensions into *non-price competition* and *price competition*. Non-price competition comprises three categories: products and services, promotion and branding, and access. We draw examples from medical groups, but one can infer how these principles apply to other health care sectors.

1. *Products and services.* The products and services a medical group offers are largely determined by its mission. For example, a group may be single specialty or multi-specialty. In the latter instance, the scope of services will obviously be determined by which specialties the group chooses to include. Product or service competition is determined not only by current offerings but also by the group's ability to adopt and offer new technology as it becomes available. Within this category, groups must determine which organizations are their competitors. For example, single specialty primary care groups do not compete with single specialty neurosurgery groups. Neurosurgery groups, however, may compete with orthopedic groups for specific services, such as back surgery. Primary care groups may compete directly with multi-specialty groups that incorporate primary care physicians.

2. *Promotion and branding.* Because of their usually small sizes, limited budgets, and small market niches, many medical groups have not, by and large, competed

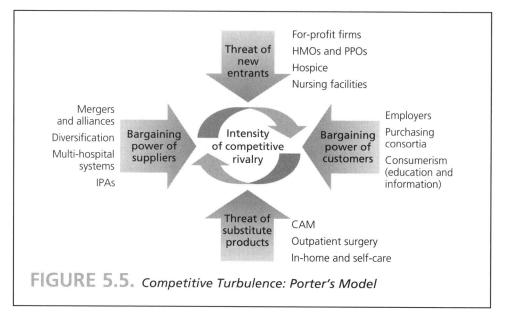

FIGURE 5.5. *Competitive Turbulence: Porter's Model*

Source: Health care adaptation of Michael Porter's Five Forces, *Competitive Strategy.* New York: Free Press, 1980. See also Besanko, Dranove, and Shanley, *The Economics of Strategy.* New York: Wiley, 2006.

on the basis of promotion and branding. However, perhaps the best example of successful branding with respect to medical groups is the Mayo Clinic. It is well known that before its Florida and Arizona satellites opened their doors, there were waiting lists for appointments. Because hospitals, health systems, and insurance companies often do such a good job of promoting themselves, many physicians and medical groups rely on these other firms' advertising and branding to bring their services to the public's attention. For example, many patients will choose physicians only because they are on staff at a particular hospital or have a contract with an insurance plan.

3. *Access.* With respect to medical services, access has four dimensions:

   a. *Location.* Not only must a medical group be physically located in a place proximal to its current and potential patients, but those patients must also be able to get to that location. Such features as travel time, highway access, proximity to public transportation, and parking are all important factors.

   b. *Delivery of services.* While location centers on how patients can get to the medical group, distribution analyzes how the group can reach out to its patients. Such outreach can be either actual or virtual. In the former case, one might look at such services as house calls or nursing home visits. These visits can be made by a physician or nurse practitioner/physician assistant.

In the virtual outreach category, one can look to such traditional methods as telephone calls or to web-based interventions, ranging from Web sites to telemedicine.

c. *Convenience.* Beyond the availability of place and delivery attributes, convenience focuses on delivery of the service when the patient needs or requests it. This feature, of course, involves a cost-benefit analysis. For example, availability outside a nine-to-five time frame is essential for pediatric practices, but other specialties may find that patients do not need or value office hours on evenings or weekends.

d. *Insurance contracting status.* To ensure sufficient patient volume, all health care service businesses must contract with enough insurance companies so that patients will seek them out. Many medical groups have used their contracting status to competitively promote themselves, as most patients cannot afford to pay for all of their medical services out of pocket. Further, many patients want to know that they can see the same practitioners regardless of the insurance their employer chooses on their behalf. Pharmaceutical companies face similar constraints when they seek to get their products on managed care formularies.

In summary, non-price competition involves the introduction of new or improved products, promotion or branding, and enhancement of access. Any of these strategies will increase fixed or marginal costs for providing services. In some industries, consumers are willing to pay more for non-price enhancements. In health care, however, because of the long-standing existence of insurance reimbursement, customers (which include payers and patients) may be more reluctant to pay extra.

We turn now to price competition. Because price wars often beget further price reductions, resulting in lower revenues, it can be an extremely destructive form of competition. Firms typically engage in this practice under three circumstances:

- First, they may lower their prices when the costs to their customers for switching providers are low. For example, medical groups may attract young, healthy patients (who have not established ongoing relationships with a physician) by contracting with managed care plans at discount rates. If, on the other hand, a patient has a chronic, complicated illness and has a long-standing, trusting relationship with a particular physician, the costs of changing sites of medical care would be high.

- Second, firms may also lower their prices when they seek to gain market share or avoid losing the market share they currently enjoy. With respect to medical groups, the situation has become particularly important in the environment of managed care. Groups have been forced to lower their charges, accept capitation, or both to maintain the ability to provide services to their current patients and stay attractive to potential new ones. Likewise, pharmaceutical companies will discount prices or offer larger volume-dependent rebates to managed care organizations in order to get or stay on their formularies.

■ Third, price lowering occurs in sectors in which the firms view themselves as independent actors rather than as part of a cohesive industry. Unlike airlines and breakfast cereal manufacturers (for whom the concept of price leaders and followers is well known), medical groups act quite independently from one another, and the individual physician practice sector is quite fragmented.

In addition to these three reasons why firms may lower prices, there are at least six environmental circumstances that encourage price reductions:

■ *Excess capacity.* When an industry has excess capacity, its member firms tend to lower their prices to cover marginal costs. In the health care field, this practice was especially evident when medical groups and hospitals priced their services to managed care organizations in order to cover marginal costs. Unfortunately for these organizations, the large shift to managed care left them with pricing that often did not adequately cover their *fixed* costs.

■ *The presence of many sellers.* When many sellers of services or products are present in an industry, the firms may act independently in their own interest and at the market's expense. In this environment, firms are unable to agree on correct pricing; this circumstance leads to divisions in the market. Further, these firms may feel it is easier to lower prices and gain market share because competitors will not follow suit. Clearly, this strategy is often a miscalculated one. The only major factor restraining firms in this environment is fear of a price war. Examples in this category include generic, over-the-counter medications.

■ *Absence of a history of cooperation and "facilitation" among firms.* In some sectors, certain firms are viewed as price leaders and price trend setters. Absent such price leaders, some industries foster implicit competition. In health care, rapid technological innovation has enabled firms to enter very profitable market segments in which such pricing history is lacking. In this setting, price competition frequently results. Ophthalmology groups providing vision correction surgery (LASIK) are facing this type of competition.

■ *Undifferentiated products or services.* When customers view products or services as undifferentiated—that is, interchangeable—and there are many providers and suppliers, firms tend to distinguish themselves by price competition. It is important to note that, in this category, much of the price competition in health care is due to lack of customer perception of substantial provider or supplier differentiation. Differentiating information, such as quality measures, is often either not available, difficult to understand, or not credible. Until this situation is corrected, payers will use price competition to sell their products, financed by extracting payment concessions from providers.

■ *Sellers can set prices secretly.* When negotiations between buyers and sellers are conducted in private—that is, prices are not publicly available—some firms may be likely to use pricing as a competitive strategy. For example, despite managed care claims that they give standard contracts to all medical groups in a given geographic area, many payment differentials do exist. Pharmaceutical companies face closer scrutiny, however, since they must offer lowest prices to their federal government clients (such as the Veterans Administration).

■ *Sales orders are large and infrequent.* In return for volume, many buyers naturally require discounted pricing. In the greater business community, this practice may occur when a firm negotiates for a large government contract. In the case of medical groups, such negotiations may occur when hospital-based physicians bid to supply their services to hospitals. Because of fraud and abuse laws, some of this bidding cannot be cash-based. It can, however, take the form of the provision of enhanced services or equipment. For example, a radiology group bidding to provide hospital services may purchase its own equipment, thus relieving the hospital of the need for large capital expenditures.

In summary, analysis of internal rivalry usually yields strategies that either enhance the product or service (usually resulting in price increases) or reduce prices. Unfortunately, the marketplace may force some firms, like medical groups, to adopt both strategies simultaneously, thereby often threatening their existence.

Threat of New Entrants. Markets with high profit margins obviously tend to attract entrants. New entrants, however, threaten the market in two ways. First, each firm in that sector will have a decreased market share and less business (unless the market is growing extremely rapidly and further entrants are limited). Second, with more sellers in the market there is an increased tendency to price competition. New entrants, however, must overcome certain barriers when they want to participate in a new sector. Some of these barriers are "naturally occurring," whereas others can be enhanced by existing firms as a competitive strategy to maintain their market position. These barriers are as follows:

■ *Economies of scale and scope.* Economies of scale not only give firms the opportunity to produce goods or services at a lower average cost, but also give them a chance to learn how to continuously improve their production. Such knowledge usually comes in the form of protected trade secrets and may be difficult for an entrant to rapidly copy. Similarly, a full scope of products and services is usually beyond the immediate capability of new entrants into a certain market. With respect to economies of scale and scope, therefore, unless a new entrant can gear up quickly, it will be at a significant disadvantage compared with established firms. It is noteworthy that this barrier has been less of a problem for manufacturers of generic medications than those seeking to produce copies of more complex biologicals, such as injectable hormones and antibodies.

■ *Capital requirements.* Some health care markets have very large capital requirements. For example, most medical groups have neither the space nor money to buy and maintain an MRI scanner. Many OB/GYN offices, however, have been able to buy and use ultrasound machines to enhance patient convenience and their own profitability. Low capital requirements in this respect have proved detrimental to traditional hospital-based radiology departments.

■ *Access to key resources or distribution channels.* With respect to medical service providers, a key, but often limited resource is skilled, specialized personnel; for example, radiology techs and pharmacists. Distribution channel problems also may exist, particularly for medical groups that seek to serve the homebound elderly and those who provide specialized services in rural areas.

■ *Legal restrictions.* Legal restrictions often present barriers to entry of new firms. In the general business world, such barriers are usually presented by patents and copyrights. Additional barriers in health care are created by requirements for licensure and certificates of need for hospitals anticipating large capital expenditures. Further, compliance with regulations is often very costly and time consuming and creates sector-specific barriers, as in the case of freestanding surgery centers and skilled nursing facilities.

■ *Branding.* Branding has generally not been a barrier to market entry for medical groups, and the reverse has occasionally been true. As mentioned earlier, Mayo Clinic's entry into the Florida and Arizona markets was facilitated by its brand image.

■ *Exclusive and/or long-term agreements with major customers.* An example of this barrier to entry is the provision of mental health services. Many managed care plans have exclusive arrangements with specialty companies to provide treatment of psychiatric and chemical dependency problems. New mental health groups and independent psychiatrists often find it difficult to enter markets that are highly penetrated by managed care organizations.

■ *Current firms with excess capacity.* As mentioned earlier, when existing firms have excess capacity, they tend to use price reductions as a competitive strategy. Therefore, when a market is profitable, if its current occupants have excess capacity even the perceived threat of a significant number of new entrants will drive prices down. Examples occur in markets that rely on expensive, high-tech equipment that is not being fully utilized, such as when actual or potential entrants announce the establishment of MRI services.

The characteristics of barriers to entry are never static and must constantly be reassessed. Laws, regulations, and new technologies can create, lower, or eliminate entry barriers. For example, when laws changed to enable procedures other than minor surgery to be performed outside the hospital, a whole new category of licensure was developed for freestanding surgicenters. Further, newer techniques in surgery, such as laparoscopic procedures, allowed for less invasive treatments. Advances in anesthesiology have also enhanced the safety of these procedures and reduced recovery time.

Substitutes and Complements. Substitutes are those products or services that "do the same thing" as those for which they replace. In health care, the most obvious examples come from the pharmaceutical industry. The degree to which substitutes are a threat depends on how close to the original the *customer* perceives them to be. Substitutes are particularly threatening when they represent new and desirable technology. Other examples of substitutes are nonsurgical treatments for surgical ones, for which symptom relief and outcomes are nearly equivalent. For example, as mentioned previously, medication has all but replaced surgery as treatment for peptic ulcer disease.

Complements are used *in conjunction with* the product or service. Rather than seeing complements as a competitive threat, they can often be viewed as opportunities. A classic example of complements is presented by diet and exercise along with medication to treat diabetes. The strategist therefore must ask, Which markets complement what I do and which markets do I complement? In answering these questions, hospitals have looked to ambulatory care and home care as complementary services. Attention to complements is particularly important because advances in one market tend to boost profits in its complementary markets. Returning to the freestanding surgery center example mentioned earlier, we note that anesthesia is a complementary service. Advances in shorter and safer anesthetics have enhanced the number of surgeries that can be safely performed on an outpatient basis.

Buyer Power. Two circumstances promote the power of buyers. First, *direct buyer power* is manifested when the buyer is so large that the seller cannot turn away business. The classic example is the defense industry, for which governments are the predominant purchasers. *Indirect buyer power* occurs when purchasers are motivated and able to shop around. Medical groups have confronted both direct and indirect buyer power in their dealings with managed care organizations. At first, these buyers formed only a minor portion of groups' business. As they grew, however, many groups faced situations in which a single health plan accounted for 20 percent or more of their revenue. Because the health plans know they have buyer power and can take business elsewhere, they often engage in "take it or leave it" negotiations with medical groups. Because buyer power assumes the existence of other similar firms that are available to buyers, this situation is similar to that of internal rivalry.

At this point, one must ask two fundamental questions. First, what would motivate customers to shop around? This question should be asked from the perspective of customers leaving you and going to your competitors as well as leaving your competitors and coming to you. Second, what would *enable* customers to shop around? For medical groups, such enabling strategies might include advertising, open houses and health fairs, and the offering of a variety of services via the Internet. For pharmaceutical companies, products may change payment status on formularies, requiring patients to spend more (or less) on each prescription.

An additional strategy to lessen buyer power is to diversify buyer strength; that is, to seek other buyers for existing services. This strategy is particularly important to hospitals and physicians who deal with few managed care plans and depend on one or two of them for a large portion of their businesses.

Supplier Power. To determine the extent to which suppliers can exert their power over a firm, one must answer three questions:

- How important is the product or service that the supplier provides?

- How many similar supplier competitors are there?

- How high is the cost of switching from one supplier to another?

With respect to hospitals and medical groups, consider the example of their information systems, which are critical to their operational and functional successes. Because of the large number of vendors in this sector, supplier power results not from the unique importance of the product or lack of competitors, but from the high cost of switching from one system to another. Other examples of supplier power include companies that sell unique, essential products, like vaccines. At the other end of the spectrum is a medical group's answering service. Such a service is critical; however, there are many similar suppliers and the switching cost is relatively low.

Limitations of Using the Five Forces

Although a Five Forces Analysis provides a good overview of an *industry*, it does have some limitations. First, it does not deal with the magnitude or growth of demand in an industry. A Five Forces Analysis assumes that demand is large enough for firms to be profitable under the most favorable competitive conditions. Second, the analysis focuses on the industry *as a whole* and not the individual firms in it. The model is therefore useful mainly for assessing the profitability of the *average* firm. Third, it does not explicitly account for nonmarket forces, such as the role of government (except as a supplier or buyer) or nongovernmental organizations (NGOs). Because government is a very important stakeholder, particularly in the health care field, some have considered it a sixth force in this analysis. Finally, a Five Forces Analysis is qualitative as opposed to quantitative. For example, the analysis may say that a threat to entry is high but it does not say exactly how high and, therefore, how likely it is that a potential competitor will enter the market. In this respect, it is most useful in assessing *trends*.

MARKETING STRATEGIES

Although the SWOT and five forces analyses can be useful in assessing a group's environment, they are less useful in deciding on implementation strategies that will enable the organization to survive and prosper. Using the environmental analysis gained from these two methods, however, firms can decide on appropriate marketing strategies. In this section we discuss three approaches.

Changing Forces

In certain cases, if the five forces are working against an organization, one can undertake to change one or more of them. One way to accomplish a change is through legislative initiatives. OB/GYNs in many states have successfully lobbied for laws that have increased their availability to women belonging to managed care plans. Another example involves turning buyer power into supplier power. Many medical groups have found that managed care plans have dictated financial conditions and threatened to pull large numbers of patients from the practice if an agreement on terms could not be reached. Some medical groups, however, have used their position as a provider to a substantial portion of a plan's patients to negotiate more favorable terms. A final example involves joint ventures that link buyers or suppliers so that mutual profitability is tied to one another. Medical groups have found that joint ventures with hospitals have often enhanced such a cooperative relationship, particularly if both parties are at risk for delivering services under managed care contracts.

Segmentation

Segmentation involves finding a part of the industry that is not as severely affected by the five forces. Hospitals are particularly adept at pursuing this implementation strategy. For example, after hospitals became subject to diagnosis related group (DRG)–based reimbursement, they sought to increasingly diversify into those health care segments that were less affected by reimbursement changes; for example, rehabilitation services, pediatrics, home health care, and skilled nursing facilities. Some medical groups have succeeded with a segmentation strategy by providing services not typically covered by traditional insurance, like cosmetic surgery or vision correction procedures. (We discuss segmentation, targeting, and positioning in more depth in Chapter Eight.)

Positioning

Positioning means developing a differential advantage from other firms that protects it (or at least insulates it) from the five forces. One way that firms have approached positioning is by focusing on a specific value proposition for targeted customers. Such an approach has been suggested by Porter[17] and Treacy and Wiersema.[18] (See the discussion about strategic implications for health care in Chapter Two to augment understanding of this section.) According to these latter two authors, this value-driven strategy depends on at least three propositions:

1. No company can succeed today by trying to be all things to all people.

2. Value comes from choosing customers and narrowing the operations focus to best serve those customers.

3. Customers are able to distinguish among the various kinds of value, and they generally won't demand them all from the same supplier.

Positioning involves choosing a particular value-driven strategy. The strategy a business chooses will depend on its mission and hence its target customers. Treacy and Wiersema distinguish among the following three positioning strategies:

- *Product leadership.* Companies that adopt this strategy are completely devoted to producing the best product or service. All organizational processes are subservient to this function. Startup biotech firms fit into this category.

- *Customer intimacy.* Firms that adopt this strategy truly realize that they cannot be all things to all people. They target specific customers and seek to add value by providing "total solution" products and services in a long-standing relationship. Many consulting companies adopt this approach.

- *Operational excellence.* Firms that adopt this positioning strategy aim to provide their products or services at a low price in a standardized, low-stress environment. Operationally excellent companies are neither product or service innovators nor leaders, nor do they necessarily develop long-lasting relationships with targeted key customers. Their profitability depends on high-volume sales and adoption of the philosophy "variety kills efficiency."[19]

The first two positioning strategies—product leadership and customer intimacy—provide a *benefit advantage* to customers, whereas the third strategy offers a *cost advantage*. The marketplace will favor benefit advantage organizations under at least three conditions. First, customers must be willing to pay a premium for the product or "total solution" relationship. Second, while quality really matters to customers, they need to learn about different competitors to be able to tell them apart. Finally, the product or service must be an *experience good*. This term means that customers are able to use a product or service that provides a benefit; they can evaluate its quality and the firm that provides it.

Assuming these three conditions exist, there are, at a minimum, three methods to achieve a benefit advantage in the eyes of the customer. First, the firm can actually demonstrate that the product or service is a market leader with respect to such features as quality, durability, ease of use, or access. Second, the firm can build a favorable customer perception of the product or service. Such a perception can come from branding, independent reviews (such as "quality report cards") or, most important in health care, word of mouth. (Is the care at Mayo Clinic in Rochester, Minnesota, truly so much better than at a more local university medical center?) Finally, the firm can convince customers that a commodity product or service (a *search good*, defined shortly) is really an *experience good*. The marketing of gasoline brands presents a prime example of this technique.

In contrast to product leaders and customer intimate firms, operationally excellent organizations offer *cost advantages* as opposed to benefit advantages. Customers will favor an operationally excellent company when they are price sensitive and the product or service is a *search good*—that is, a product or service whose customers either understand its quality or care so little about it that they don't require much more information than price to purchase it. Again, one can see the example of gasoline as a basic search good (though many companies would like to try to position it in the minds of customers as an experience good). With respect to maintaining a cost advantage, a firm can take the following actions:

- *Exploit economies of scale (number of similar type services or products), scope (number of different, but related, products or services), or know-how.* Know-how is the equivalent of proprietary business methods and the accumulated learning that tells a firm what will or will not work.

- *Obtain access to low-cost inputs.* Such inputs may be labor costs, rent, or even enhanced customer order entry via e-commerce solutions. For example, Wal-Mart sells its goods (including prescription and over-the-counter medications) in large, no-frills warehouse spaces. Mail-order branded pharmaceutical suppliers employ similar operational tactics.

- *Implement process improvements.* These improvements can either simplify the delivery of a service or enhance the efficiency of a manufacturing process. Although it may seem obvious, it must be stated that one of the ways to improve processes is to eliminate non-value-added steps that increase the probability for error and increase cost. Operations research and process engineering have been particularly useful in achieving efficiencies in this area. Although not always competing on price, hospitals have used these process improvement methods to achieve this benefit.

- *Exploit the efficient organization of the vertical supplier-customer chain.* A classic example of this technique is just-in-time delivery of goods that will enable a firm to reduce inventory costs. Hospitals have used this method with respect to very expensive items such as pacemakers and implantable defibrillators.

- *Standardize all processes as much as possible.*

Limits to the Value-Driven Strategy: The Example of Medical Groups. Many companies have thrived using the market leader model just described; however, many medical groups find themselves in markets that are highly penetrated with managed care and face extensive regulation, both of which prohibit successful implementation of measures that this model requires. In this section, we explain the reasons for this situation.

First, with respect to being product (or service) driven, in the medical field all customers expect to receive the best product at all times. These customers include patients, payers, and the legal system. Although all providers are expected to achieve near-perfection, only those such as academic medical centers (AMCs) can reap the benefit of differentiating themselves from their competitors based on perceived quality.

Second, operational excellence (which enables lower prices) is valued only by some of the medical groups' customers. Obviously, many payers are pressing groups to accept lower prices. Most patients, on the other hand, are shielded from substantial financial risk by third-party payers. This latter situation is changing, however, with patients now responsible for increasing out-of-pocket expenses for traditional health plans and the emerging consumer-directed plans with their high annual deductibles. Medical groups are therefore experiencing mounting patient pressures to lower their prices. The overall effect is that the marketplace is demanding not the best product at the lowest *possible* price, but the best product *at* a low price. In a world of managed care, groups are forced to become operationally excellent organizations, whereas the marketplace is demanding product excellence. But as the market leader model states, superior performance in both of these attributes cannot exist simultaneously in a truly great organization.

At a time when the marketplace is demanding the best product at a low price, medical groups are also expected to deliver comprehensive and coordinated services to their patients. This activity is really a "customer intimacy" or "total solution" imperative. However, several environmental forces are working against the groups.

First, health plans are purchasing disease management services from independent firms with which a patient's medical group may not have a relationship, thus increasing the likelihood of fragmentation of services.

Second, patients are demanding more freedom to choose their medical providers, and legislatures are supporting this initiative by passing laws mandating managed care plans to provide more open access to primary care physicians and specialists. For example, many states have passed "any willing provider" laws that require managed care plans to contract with any physician (or even pharmacy) who will accept an agreement that is offered to other existing providers. This situation means that the patient's primary providers are challenged to work with others with whom they have no ongoing relationship (and who may practice at different hospitals) while at the same time attempting to provide the highest level of coordinated care.

In the short run, these groups need to conduct a comprehensive environmental analysis to determine an optimum *mix* of these three strategies. Such a tactic will not produce *the* optimal strategy but will lead to formulation of the best a group can accomplish in its current environment.

REASSESSMENT OF MISSION STATEMENT

After an organization has evaluated its environment and assessed its strategic options, it should return to its original mission statement to see if it is still desirable and feasible. This reassessment can have three effects. First, it can validate the reasons for the statement and the organization's purpose. Second, it can also cause the organization to more realistically evaluate its purpose. For example, a hospital may find that the environment is more hostile or resources more constrained than first realized. The mission statement must then be revised accordingly. Finally, and in contrast, after conducting an environmental analysis and formulating a strategic plan, a firm may find that it can accommodate a broader mission than it first considered. In summary, the strategic planning process requires perpetual periodic evaluations of an organization's mission, goals, and strategies as well as the interplay among those elements.

Vision and Values

In their book *Built to Last: Successful Habits of Visionary Organizations*, Collins and Porras found three commonalities shared by eighteen successful companies.[20] First, each held a distinctive set of values from which they did not deviate. Thus IBM has adhered to the principles of respect for the individual, customer satisfaction, and continuous quality improvement throughout its history; Johnson & Johnson holds to the principle that its first responsibility is to its customers, its second to its employees, its third to its community, and its fourth to its stockholders.

Second, successful organizations express their purpose in enlightened terms. Xerox wants to improve office productivity and Monsanto wants to help end hunger in the world. According to Collins and Porras, an organization's core purpose should not be confused with specific business goals or strategies and should not be simply a description of an organization's product line.

Third, successful organizations have developed a vision of their future and act to implement it. A business often presents its vision and values along with its mission statement. In the following examples, note how vision and value statements are more action-based than mission statements (which describe "who we are"). Again, these statements are not necessarily best practices; you should analyze their usefulness for the individual organization.

FOR EXAMPLE

Northwestern Memorial Hospital Vision

To be the regional hospital of choice that is recognized as having the most satisfied patients, the best possible clinical quality and outcomes, and the best physicians and employees.

Amgen Values

Be Science-Based, Compete Intensely and Win

Work in Teams

Create Value for Patients, Staff and Stockholders

Trust and Respect Each Other

Ensure Quality

Collaborate, Communicate and Be Accountable

Be Ethical

Boston Scientific Values Statement

The growth and success of our organization is dependent upon the shared values of our people. They understand that business exists to serve the customer. We must learn, understand and live by a unified set of values that will guide us in a continually changing medical environment:

To provide our people with a strong understanding of our mission and shared values

To think like our customers and work hard on their behalf

To pay relentless attention to business fundamentals

To bring a commitment to quality and a sense of urgency to everything we do

To rely on one another, to treat each other well and to put the development and motivation of our people at the top of our priority lists

To encourage innovation, experimentation and risk-taking

To recognize bureaucracy as an archenemy and not allow it to inhibit our good sense of business and creative spirit

To provide shareholders with an attractive return through sustained high-quality growth

To recognize and reward excellence by sharing Boston Scientific's success with our employees

STRATEGIC ALLIANCES

Because health care organizations are discovering that now, more than ever, they need strategic partners if they hope to be successful, many form alliances with other firms that complement or leverage their capabilities and resources. Alliances, however, are fraught with problems, and many fail.

We here offer some examples of types of alliances. Although alliances achieve common benefit for both parties, they are not merely one company hiring another to perform a service, though both must financially profit from the transaction.

- *Product or service:* One organization licenses another to produce its product or service, or two organizations jointly market their complementary service. The most common example in health care is pharmaceutical companies that license their products to firms having a stronger presence in other countries.

- *Promotional:* One organization agrees to promote another organization's product or service. Many small pharmaceutical companies use larger firms' sales forces to sell their products. In return, the promoting company gets to augment or complement its own portfolio.

- *Logistics:* One organization offers logistical services for another organization's products or services. For example, Abbott Laboratories warehoused and delivered 3 M's medical and surgical products to hospitals across the United States. In this case, the logistics provider derives a benefit of economies of scale for handling its own products.

- *Pricing:* One or more organizations join in a special pricing collaboration. An HMO can work with a national health club to offer lower rates for their members who sign up with the club. Both can achieve greater market share from this arrangement.

As these examples indicate, health care organizations need to be creative about finding partners who complement their strengths and offset their weaknesses.

MARKETING PLANNING

After the environmental assessment and mission check are completed, marketing managers must develop a marketing plan: a written document that summarizes what the firm has learned about the environment and describes how the organization plans to reach its objectives within the frame of the broader strategic plan.[21] Marketing plans are becoming more customer- and competitor-oriented, better reasoned, and more realistic than they were in the past. The plans draw inputs from all the company's functions and are team-developed.

The Composition and Content of a Marketing Plan

Marketing planning is done differently in different organizations. The plan is variously called a *business plan*, a *marketing plan*, and sometimes a *battle plan*. Most marketing plans cover one or a few years; they vary in length from under five to over fifty pages. Some organizations adhere strictly to their plans, whereas others see them as only a rough guide to action. The most frequently cited shortcomings of current marketing plans are lack of realism, insufficient competitive analysis, and a short-run focus. What, then, characterizes a useful marketing plan?

Sample Marketing Plan Content

1. *Executive summary and table of contents:* The marketing plan should open with a brief summary of the main goals and recommendations, which enables senior management to grasp the plan's major thrust. The table of contents outlines the rest of the plan and all the supporting rationale and operational detail.

2. *Environmental analysis:* This section presents relevant background data on sales, costs, profits, the market, competitors, channels, and the key forces operating in the environment. How is the market defined, how big is it, and how fast is it growing? What are the relevant technological, political, economic, social, and legal influences? How can the chief competitors be characterized? Who buys the product or service, why, when, where, and how? A detailed description of customer and competitive behavior is critical. Pertinent historical information can be included to provide context.

3. *Opportunity and issue analysis:* In this part, management reviews the main opportunities found in the SWOT analysis and identifies the key issues likely to affect the organization's attainment of its objectives.

4. *Objectives:* In this portion, the marketer outlines the plan's major financial and marketing goals, expressed in sales volume, market share, profit, and other relevant terms.

5. *Marketing strategy:* In this section the marketer defines the target segments —the groups and their needs that the market offerings are intended to satisfy. The marketer then establishes the offering's competitive positioning, which will create the tactics to accomplish the plan's objectives. These activities are carried out with inputs from other organizational areas, such as purchasing, operations, sales, finance, and human resources, to ensure that the business can provide proper support for effective implementation. The marketing plan should be specific about the branding and customer strategies that will be employed.

6. *Action programs:* The marketing plan must specify the activities for achieving the business objectives. Each marketing strategy element must be elaborated to address what will be done, when, and by whom; how much it will cost; and how progress will be measured.

7. *Financial projections:* This portion details the financial impact of the *action program*. On the revenue side, it shows the forecasted sales volume in units

and average price, and on the expense side, the expected costs of operations, distribution, and marketing, broken down into finer categories. Once approved, the budget is the basis for developing plans and schedules for material procurement, operations, employee recruitment, and marketing activities.

8. *Implementation controls:* The last section outlines the controls for monitoring and adjusting the plan. Typically, the goals and budget are spelled out for each month or quarter, so management can review each period's results and take corrective action when needed. A number of different internal and external measures are needed to assess progress and suggest possible modifications. (Chapter Fifteen describes the key metrics for diagnosing and tracking progress.) Some organizations include contingency plans outlining the steps management should take in response to specific major developments.[22]

A good marketing plan can be an invaluable tool in achieving marketing goals. Here are some questions to ask in evaluating a plan:

- Is the plan simple, easy to understand, and actionable?

- Is the plan specific? Are its objectives concrete and measurable? Does it include specific actions and activities, each with specific dates of completion, specific persons responsible and specific budgets?

- Is the plan realistic? Are the sales goals, expense budgets, and milestone dates realistic? Has a frank and honest self-critique been conducted to raise and resolve possible concerns and objections?

- Is the plan complete? Does it include all the necessary elements?[23]

SUMMARY

The marketing process involves an exploration of creating, communicating, and delivering superior value. The value chain is a tool for identifying key activities that create customer-perceived value and costs in a specific business.

Strong organizations develop competencies and superior capabilities in managing core business processes such as customer acquisition and retention, new services, and new product development. Managing these core processes means creating a marketing network in which the organization works closely with all parties in the value chain. High-performance businesses achieve marketplace success by improving critical business processes and aligning resources, competencies, and capabilities.

Market-oriented strategic planning is the managerial process of developing and maintaining a viable fit between the organization's objectives, skills, and resources and its changing market opportunities. The aim of strategic planning is to shape the organization's businesses and offerings so that they yield target profits and growth. Corporate headquarters sets the strategic-planning process in motion. Corporate strategy establishes the framework within which the divisions and business units prepare their strategic plans. Setting a corporate strategy entails four activities: defining the corporate mission, establishing strategic business units (SBUs), assigning resources to each SBU based on its market attractiveness and business strength, and planning new businesses while downsizing older businesses.

Marketing planning for individual business units and service entities entails the following activities: defining the business mission, analyzing external opportunities and threats, analyzing internal strengths and weaknesses, formulating goals, developing strategy, crafting supporting programs, implementing the programs, gathering feedback, and exercising control.

To ensure its success, each service level within a business unit must contribute to developing the overall marketing plan for the organization. This plan is one of the most important outputs of the marketing process.

DISCUSSION QUESTIONS

1. Academic medical centers (AMCs) have in their mission statements purposes that include research, teaching, and patient care. Can you think how each component may complement and conflict with the others?

2. A competitor of your pharmaceutical company is about to launch a product that will challenge one of your very profitable medications. At a marketing strategy meeting, one colleague recommends a preemptive price reduction to maintain market share. Discuss the pros and cons of this suggestion.

3. Choose a medical device, such as a home diagnostic machine, coronary artery stent, or wheelchair, and describe the industry structure using Porter's model.

CHAPTER

6

HOW HEALTH CARE BUYERS MAKE CHOICES

LEARNING OBJECTIVES

In this chapter, we will address the following questions:

1. What are the main stages in the consumer buying decision process?

2. What are the main characteristics, roles, and stages influencing the organization's buying process?

OPENING EXAMPLE

Hospital Drug Buying Reacts to Market Changes   A doctor at Watauga Medical Center, in Boone, North Carolina, wanted to prescribe the sleep aid drug Lunesta to his hospital patients. Several patients had found this drug helpful and wanted the physician to prescribe it. The doctor felt strongly about giving his patients this option, so he decided to make a request to add Lunesta to the hospital formulary. The drug formulary is the set of those drugs that the hospital regularly stocks and that are purchased through the hospital's group purchasing organization. The Watauga Medical Center drug buying process is, as at most hospitals, based on three overarching criteria: safety, cost, and efficacy. Modifications in the formulary are accomplished through the hospital's Pharmacy and Therapeutics (P&T) Committee.

The pharmacy department at Watauga Medical Center continually monitors the Food and Drug Administration (FDA) for new drugs to add to the formulary. Significant differences in the safety, efficacy, or cost profile of a new product will be criteria for formulary action. Typically, new drugs are reviewed and considered for the formulary if they have received FDA approval for new symptoms, are designated as fast-track priority drug approvals, or have been shown to address diseases with high levels of incidence in the hospital's primary market. These drugs are brought to the attention of the appropriate medical specialty group at the Medical Center to determine their interest in reviewing the drug. If the drug is rated as having little or no therapeutic gain by the FDA, no action is initiated by the hospital P&T Committee. Alternatively, the P&T Committee will evaluate a new drug if a request is made by a staff physician, the pharmacy director, or another staff clinician. Such was the case with Lunesta.

The pharmacy department first conducted an extensive literature search using the Web to identify evidence-based studies evaluating Lunesta. The scientific literature was analyzed by pharmacy clinicians, and a recommendation was made to the P&T Committee based the analysis. The recommendation was that Lunesta *not* be added to Watauga Medical Center formulary because (1) there were no studies to document an advantage in efficacy or safety over the sleep aid Ambien that was already on the formulary, (2) there were multiple drug interactions to monitor versus few for Ambien, and (3) there was no economic advantage over Ambien.

As always, Lunesta could be obtained for specific patients by the physician writing "dispense as written" on drug orders, but prescribing drugs not on the formulary usually results in a delay in obtaining them. Not so long ago, a hospital pharmacist could call a local commercial pharmacy for a drug not on the hospital pharmacy shelf, and it would be delivered to the hospital, repackaged, and given to the patient in a few hours. With the growth of electronic medication administration systems, however, most drugs are now dispensed on the hospital floor through an ATM-like machine that requires an identity card, a bar code, and an extensive electronic verification to ensure accuracy and reduce dispensing errors. This systematic strategy certainly has important benefits for patient safety, but it also may curtail flexibility in meeting the needs of physicians and patients who prefer drugs not on the hospital formulary.

With more patients learning about different drug brands from commercial and internet media and asking their doctor to prescribe them, hospital formularies are under increasing pressure to buy carefully and balance cost, effectiveness, safety, and the doctors' preferences.

Health care marketers need to gain an in-depth understanding of consumer and business buying behavior. Studying potential buyers provides clues for improving or introducing products or services, setting prices, devising channels, crafting messages, and developing other marketing activities. Marketers are also always looking for emerging trends that might suggest new marketing opportunities. This chapter first explores the psychology of individual health care buying dynamics, complementing the information in Chapter Four. We then examine the purchasing dynamics of organizational buyers.

OVERVIEW: KEY PSYCHOLOGICAL PROCESSES

Four key psychological processes—motivation, perception, learning, and memory—fundamentally influence consumer responses to marketing stimuli.

Motivation: Freud, Maslow, Herzberg, Prochaska

A person has many needs at any given time. Some needs are *biogenic;* they arise from physiological states of tension such as hunger, thirst, or discomfort. Other needs are *psychogenic;* they arise from psychological states of tension such as the need for recognition, esteem, or belonging. A *motive* is a need that is sufficiently pressing to drive the person to act. Three of the best-known theories of human motivation—those of Sigmund Freud, Abraham Maslow, and Frederick Herzberg—carry quite different implications for consumer analysis and marketing strategy.

Sigmund Freud assumed that the psychological forces shaping people's behavior are largely unconscious and that a person cannot fully understand his or her own motivations. Applying this to consumer responses, when a person examines specific brands, he or she will react not only to their stated capabilities, but also to other, less conscious cues. Shape, size, weight, material, color, and brand name can all trigger certain associations and emotions. A technique called *laddering* can be used to trace a person's motivations from the stated instrumental ones to the more terminal ones. Then the marketer can decide at what level to develop the message and appeal.

Abraham Maslow sought to explain why people are driven by particular needs at particular times.[1] Why does one person spend considerable time and energy on personal safety and another on pursuing the high opinion of others? His theory is that human needs are arranged in a hierarchy, from the most pressing to the least pressing. In order of importance these needs are physiological, safety, social, esteem, and self-actualization. A consumer will try to satisfy his or her most important needs first; when that need is satisfied, the person will try to satisfy the next most pressing need. Maslow's theory helps marketers understand how various products fit into the plans, goals, and lives of consumers. The very poor, for example, will not undertake self-actualization health activities, like exercise or weight loss, until their basic needs for food and shelter are met. The Meals On Wheels program for seniors focus on physiological needs, and services like sports medicine and psychological counseling appeal to higher social, esteem, and self-actualization needs.

Frederick Herzberg developed a two-factor theory that distinguishes *dissatisfiers* (factors that cause dissatisfaction) and *satisfiers* (factors that cause satisfaction).[2] The absence of dissatisfiers is not enough; satisfiers must be present to motivate a purchase. For example, a physician with a poor bedside manner would be a dissatisfier. Yet the presence of a pleasant bedside manner would not act as a satisfier or motivator of a purchase because it is not a source of intrinsic satisfaction. Solving the patient's health problem would be a satisfier. In line with this theory, marketers should avoid dissatisfiers that might unsell their products. They should also identify and supply the major satisfiers or motivators of purchase because these satisfiers will make the major difference as to which brand consumers will buy.

Psychologists James Prochaska and Carlo DiClemente at the University of Rhode Island developed the Stages of Change theory in 1982 when they were studying how smokers were able to give up their habits or addiction.[3] The idea behind the Stages of Change model is that behavior change does not happen in one step; rather, people tend to progress through different stages on their way to successful change. The rationale behind "staging" people was to tailor therapy to a consumer's needs at a particular point in the change process. As a result, the four original components of the Stages of Change theory (precontemplation, contemplation, action, and maintenance) were identified and presented as a linear process of change. Since then, a fifth stage (preparation for action) has been incorporated into the theory, as well as ten processes that help predict and motivate individual movement across stages. The stages are no longer considered to be linear but seem to be cyclical and vary for each individual.

The Stages of Change model has been applied to a broad range of behaviors including weight loss, injury prevention, and overcoming alcohol and drug addiction. Expecting behavior change by simply telling someone who, for example, is still in the precontemplation stage that he or she must go to a certain number of AA meetings in a certain time period may be counterproductive because the person is not ready to change. Each person must decide when a stage is completed and when it is time to move on to the next stage (see Table 6.1).

TABLE 6.1. **Prochaska and DiClemente's Stages of Change Model**

Stage of Change	Characteristics	Techniques
1. Pre-contemplation	Not currently considering change: "Ignorance is bliss"	Validate lack of readiness
		Clarify: decision is theirs
		Encourage reevaluation of current behavior
		Encourage self-exploration, not action
		Explain and personalize the risk
2. Contemplation	Ambivalent about change: "Sitting on the fence"	Validate lack of readiness
	Not considering change within the next month	Clarify: decision is theirs
		Encourage evaluation of pros and cons of behavior change
		Identify and promote new, positive outcome expectations
3. Preparation	Some experience with change and is trying to change: "Testing the waters"	Identify and assist in problem solving re: obstacles
	Planning to act within 1 month	Help patient identify social support

(Table 6.1 continued)

Stage of Change	Characteristics	Techniques
		Verify that patient has underlying skills for behavior change
		Encourage small initial steps
4. Action	Practicing new behavior for 3–6 months	Focus on restructuring cues and social support
		Bolster self-efficacy for dealing with obstacles
		Combat feelings of loss and reiterate long-term benefits
5. Maintenance	Continued commitment to sustaining new behavior	Plan for follow-up support
	Post–6 months to 5 years	Reinforce internal rewards
		Discuss coping with relapse
6. Relapse	Resumption of old behaviors: "Fall from grace"	Evaluate trigger for relapse
		Reassess motivation and barriers
		Plan stronger coping strategies

Source: Prochaska, DiClemente, and Norcross, *American Psychologist*, 1992.

Perception

A motivated person is ready to act, yet *how* that person actually acts is influenced by his or her view or perception of the situation. *Perception* is the process by which an individual selects, organizes, and interprets information inputs to create a meaningful picture of the world.[4] Perception depends not only on the physical stimuli, but also on the stimuli's relation to the surrounding field and on conditions within the individual. The key point is that perceptions can vary widely among individuals exposed to the same reality because of three perceptual processes: selective attention, selective distortion, and selective retention.

The average person may be exposed to over five thousand ads or brand communications a day, and almost all of these stimuli will be screened out—a process called selective attention. Thus marketers have to work hard to attract consumers' attention. Through research, marketers have learned that people are more likely to notice stimuli that relate to a current need; this is why people who want to quit smoking are more apt to notice ads for smoking cessation products like Nicorette gum. Furthermore, smokers are more likely to notice stimuli that they anticipate, such as Nicorette gum on sale in a drugstore. Smokers are also more likely to notice stimuli whose deviations are large in relation to the normal size of the stimuli, such as an ad offering "buy one, get one free" for a pack of Nicorette gum instead of one offering $.50 off.

Even noticed stimuli do not always come across in the way the senders intended. *Selective distortion* is the tendency to twist information into personal meanings and interpret information in a way that fits our perceptions. Consumers will often distort information to be consistent with their prior brand and product beliefs.[5] Selective distortion can work to the advantage of marketers with strong brands when consumers distort neutral or ambiguous brand information to make it more positive. In other words, a pain reliever may seem to work faster, or a wait in a hospital emergency department may seem shorter, depending on the particular brands involved.

People forget much information to which they are exposed but will tend to retain information that supports their attitudes and beliefs. Because of *selective retention*, we are likely to remember good points mentioned about a product we like and forget good points about competing products. Selective retention again works to the advantage of strong brands, and it also explains why marketers repeat messages to ensure that the information is not overlooked.

Health Belief Model

Related to perception, the *health belief model* (HBM) was developed in the 1950s by social psychologists and subsequently expanded.[6] The HBM states that recognizing a personal health behavior threat is affected by three factors: general health values (including interest and concern about health), specific health beliefs about vulnerability to a particular health threat, and beliefs about the consequences of the health problem. According to the HBM, an individual who perceives a health threat and then takes action to prevent a health problem has most likely:

- *Perceived susceptibility.* The individual perceived the likelihood of having an experience or a condition that would negatively affect health.

- *Perceived seriousness.* The person believed that a disease or condition would noticeably affect him or her physically, emotionally, financially, or psychologically.

- *Perceived benefits of taking action.* The person believes that positive outcomes will result from addressing the health problem.

- *Perceived barriers to taking action.* Counterbalancing the first three beliefs is the contemplation that the treatment or preventive measure may be inconvenient, expensive, unpleasant, painful, or upsetting.

- *Perceived cues to action.* These types of internal and external actions and reminders may be needed for the desired behavior to occur.

- *Perceived efficacy.* This is the individual's assessment of ability to adopt the desired behavior.

Marketers using the Health Belief Model conduct market research to identify each of these five elements (susceptibility, seriousness, benefits, barriers, and perceptions of effective cues to action) before developing marketing strategies.

Consider the following example that applies this model. The National High Blood Pressure Education Program conducted market research and learned that more than sixty-five million American adults, or one in three, have high blood pressure, and fewer than 30 percent are controlling their condition.[7] The Program was interested in influencing desired behaviors by increasing blood pressure monitoring and compliance with recommended lifestyle and medication plans. Research respondents pointed to perceived susceptibility, seriousness, and barriers such as these:

- "It is hard for me to change my diet and to find the time to exercise."

- "My blood pressure is difficult to control."

- "My blood pressure varies so much, it's probably not accurate."

- "Medications can have undesirable side effects."

- "It's too expensive to go to the doctor just to get my blood pressure checked."

- "It may be the result of living a full and active life. Not everybody dies from it."

Using this research along with the Health Belief Model, the National Heart, Lung and Blood Institute developed marketing strategies that projected the following concepts:[8]

- You don't have to make all of the changes immediately. The key is to focus on one or two at a time. Once they become part of your normal routine, you can go on to the next change. Sometimes, one change leads naturally to another. For example, increasing physical activity will help you lose weight.

- You can keep track of your blood pressure outside of your doctor's office by taking it at home.

- You don't have to run marathons to benefit from physical activity. Any activity, if done at least thirty minutes a day over the course of most days, can help.

The marketing program began in 1972, when less than one-quarter of the American population knew of the relationship between hypertension, stroke, and heart disease. In 2001, more than three-quarters of the population was aware of this connection. One important result has been that virtually all Americans have had their blood pressure measured at least once, and a substantial percent of the population has it measured yearly.

Learning

When people act, they learn, and most human behavior is learned. Learning involves changes in an individual's behavior arising from experience. Theorists believe that learning is produced through the interplay of drives, stimuli, cues, responses, and reinforcement. A *drive* is a strong internal stimulus that impels action. *Cues* are minor stimuli that determine when, where, and how a person responds.

Suppose you go to a Minute Clinic to get a flu shot. If your experience is rewarding, your response to a flu vaccine and the Minute Clinic will be positively reinforced. Later, when you have a cough, you may assume that because Minute Clinic provided fast, effective service in the past, you will receive the same care for your present illness. In other words, you *generalize* your response to similar stimuli. A countertendency to generalization is *discrimination*, in which a person learns to recognize differences in sets of similar stimuli and adjust responses accordingly. For example, you would not go to a Minute Clinic if you thought you were having a heart attack, because you discriminate in your decision making on the basis of perceived severity of illness. Applying learning theory, marketers can build demand for a product by associating it with strong drives, using motivating cues, and providing positive reinforcement.

Memory

Cognitive psychologists distinguish between *short-term memory* (STM)—a temporary repository of information—and *long-term memory* (LTM)—a more permanent repository. All the information and experiences that individuals encounter as they go through life can end up in their long-term memory.

Most widely accepted views of LTM structure involve some kind of associative model formulation.[9] For example, the *associative network memory model* views LTM as consisting of a set of nodes and links. *Nodes* are stored information connected by *links* that vary in strength. Any type of information—verbal, visual, abstract, or contextual—can be stored in the memory network. A spreading activation process from node to node determines the extent of retrieval and what information can actually be recalled in any given situation. When a node becomes activated because external information is being encoded (such as when a person reads or hears a word or phrase) or internal information is retrieved from LTM (as when a person thinks about some concept), other nodes are also activated if they are sufficiently strongly associated with that node.

Following this model, consumer brand knowledge in memory can be conceptualized as consisting of a brand node in memory with a variety of linked associations. The strength and organization of these associations will be important determinants of the information that can recalled about the brand. *Brand associations* consist of all brand-related thoughts, feelings, perceptions, images, experiences, beliefs, attitudes, and so on that become linked to the brand node. Marketing can be seen as making sure that consumers have the right types of product and service experiences such that the right brand knowledge structures are created and maintained in memory. Some organizations create mental maps of consumers that depict their knowledge of a particular brand in terms of those key associations that are likely to be triggered in a marketing setting and their relative strength, favorability, and uniqueness to consumers.

Encoding. *Memory encoding* refers to how and where information gets into memory. The amount or quantity of processing that information receives at encoding refers to how much a person thinks about the information; the nature or quality of processing refers to the manner in which a person thinks about the information. Both quantity and quality of processing are important determinants of the strength of an association.[10] In general, the more attention is placed on the meaning of information during encoding, the stronger the resulting associations in memory will be.[11] Also, the ease with which new information can be integrated into established knowledge structures depends on such characteristics as simplicity, vividness, and concreteness. Repeated exposures to information provide greater opportunity for processing and the potential for stronger associations; however, the exposure must first be persuasive and involving.

Retrieval. *Memory retrieval* refers to how information is pulled out of memory. According to the associative network memory model, the strength of a brand association increases the likelihood that that information will be easily accessible and can be recalled by "spreading activation." Successful recall of brand information by consumers depends on more than the initial associative strength of that information in memory. Three factors are particularly important. First, *other* product information in memory can produce interference effects. It may cause the brand information to be either overlooked or confused. In a market in which all hospital television ads seem the same, with doctors offering health advice, consumers can easily confuse hospital brands. Second, the time elapsed since exposure to information at encoding affects the strength of a new association; the longer the time delay, the weaker the association.

Finally, information may be "available" in memory (that is, potentially recallable) but may not be "accessible" (that is, unable to be recalled) without the proper retrieval cues or reminders. The particular associations for a brand that come to mind depend on the context in which the brand is considered. The more cues linked to a piece of information, the greater the likelihood that the information can be recalled. Thus marketing messages displayed *inside* a hospital convey information at that moment, but they also remind consumers of information conveyed outside the hospital.

THE BUYING DECISION PROCESS: THE FIVE-STAGE MODEL

Basic psychological processes play an important role in our understanding of how consumers actually make their buying decisions. Market-led organizations try to fully understand the consumers' buying decision process—all their experiences in learning, choosing, using, and even disposing of a product.[12] Marketing scholars have developed a five-stage buying decision model shown in Figure 6.1. Starting with problem recognition, the consumer then passes through information search, evaluation of alternatives, purchase decision, and post-purchase behavior. Clearly, the buying process starts long before the actual purchase and has consequences long afterward.[13] Although the model implies that consumers pass sequentially through all five stages in buying, consumers sometimes skip or reverse some stages. The model provides a good frame of reference, however, because it captures the full range of considerations that arise when a consumer faces a highly involving new purchase.[14]

Problem Recognition

The buying process starts when the buyer recognizes a problem or need. The need can be triggered by internal or external stimuli. With an internal stimulus, a consumer's physiological need—hunger, thirst, sex—rises to a threshold level and becomes a drive. Alternatively, a need can be aroused by an external stimulus. The external cue can be personally delivered; for example by a friend, a spouse, or a salesperson; or it can be nonpersonal, such as a magazine article, an ad, e-mail, or another external source.

External cues can be either marketer-controlled or non-marketer-controlled. A very important marketing task is to survey consumers to learn the major types of triggering cues that will stimulate their interest in the particular product class. Marketing strategies can then be developed to trigger consumer interest. For example, many hospitals spend heavily on television advertising to promote their heart and cancer services. This spending can increase consumer awareness and even preference

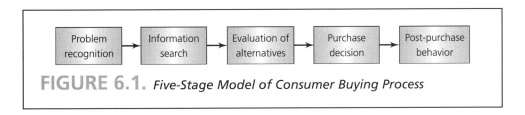

FIGURE 6.1. *Five-Stage Model of Consumer Buying Process*

for these services, but market research indicates that the leading reason heart and cancer inpatients select a hospital is a physician's recommendation.[15]

Information Search

An aroused consumer facing a buying decision will be inclined to search for information, but the effort placed on searching will depend on the product class and the perceived level of information need. Product marketers need to understand the *information neediness* of their target market: how much information the consumer is likely to gather before making a buying decision for this particular product. They also need to know the *information sources* consumers will use to obtain information and what will be their relative influence.

Information Neediness. Buyers vary greatly in their information-gathering behavior. Some individuals collect much information about their purchases across many product classes, and certain product class categories generate more information-gathering behavior across all types of individuals. For example, some buyers would not think of purchasing a car or appliance without first consulting *Consumer Reports* magazine, and most people interested in buying a new car will also collect comparison product and pricing data on several models and dealers.

Information gathering can be divided into two categories. The "softer" one is called *heightened attention;* at this level a person simply becomes more receptive to information about a product. A consumer thinking about getting rid of his eyeglasses may start noticing newspaper ads for LASIK eye surgery. If this interest grows, he may undertake an *active information search* wherein he talks with friends who have had the procedure, searches online, makes notes on differences among service providers, and gets a recommendation for an ophthalmologist from his primary care physician or friends. How much effort he expends depends on the strength of the need, the amount of information the consumer has, the ease of obtaining additional information, and the satisfaction derived from the search. (With regard to this latter dimension, marketers should be aware of a category of searchers who derive pleasure exclusively from searching; they are low-probability buyers. Although they themselves may not buy, they can act as an important information resource for those who are ready to make a purchase.) More information gathering is conducted with more complex, high-risk, and important buying decisions. Consumers will gather little information for getting a flu shot, but they will ask many questions about where to have elective surgery, who will perform it, and how much it will cost.

Perceived Information Availability. Perceptions of what information is available also affect purchase behavior. Three models of purchase behavior have been established, based on information neediness and perceived information availability (see Table 6.2).[16]

In the *low-involvement model*, consumers who face low risk and simple purchase decisions do not gather much information. They believe that there is minimal information of value available that will help to differentiate alternative choices. For

TABLE 6.2. **Models of Purchase Behavior**

	Low-Involvement Model	Learning Model	Dissonance Attribution Model
Information Neediness	Low	High	High
Perceived Information Availability	Low	High	Low

example, a new employee who is required to have a pre-employment physical before starting work neither needs nor seeks information on alternative providers of the exam, does not believe that there is much information of value on a routine physical, and believes that all providers will perform similarly. Many preventive services and some early disease diagnostic services are in this model.

In the *learning model*, consumers collect information, analyze it, form attitudes about alternatives, and then decide what to buy. Economists refer to this process as the *rational man hypothesis* because anyone exhibiting this behavior appears to act rationally. For example, a family helping a senior couple move to an assisted living facility would develop a list of facilities in the area; obtain referrals from residents, hospital social workers, and physicians; and visit the facilities and take tours. This systematic process would provide the information needed to allow the family to rank the different alternatives and select the best facility. The learning model assumes that the purchase decision is important, high-risk, and complex, so the buyer wants plenty of information. The model also assumes that the buyer perceives information is readily available and believes the information will allow the buyer to distinguish among purchase alternatives.

The *dissonance attribution model* is similar to the learning model in that the purchaser views the buying decision as high-risk or important but does not perceive information to be available that can be used to distinguish among alternatives. The purchaser is faced with an important decision and arbitrarily decides on a purchase. After the purchase, the buyer may decide the purchase was a wise or unwise decision and may even seek information on the purchase choice. This buying behavior may sometimes appear to be irrational. An example of the dissonance attribution model is the way in which many consumers select a personal physician. The physician-patient relationship is obviously very personal and can potentially impact life-or-death decisions. Typically, a physician should be selected based on evaluation of his or her competence, trustworthiness, and likeability. Most consumers are unable to objectively differentiate physicians based on these criteria before choosing; they may therefore obtain opinions from family and friends, consult the Yellow Pages of the phone book, or select a doctor based on office location or contracting status with their insurance plan. An example of a recent innovation to help prospective patients choose a physician is RateMDs.com, a consumer Web site that records and reports on consumer experiences (see Field Note 6.1).

FIELD NOTE 6.1.

Web Site Offers Consumers a Free Forum to Rate and Help Select a Doctor RateMDs.com (http://www.ratemds.com) allows users to rate their doctors in three categories: punctuality, helpfulness, and knowledge. Users can also write a short comment about their experiences with their doctors. RateMDs.com was founded by software engineers Joanne Wong and John Swapceinski and went online February 1, 2004. "Having visited several doctors in the past few years, I became frustrated with the treatment I received, and the lack of comparative information available for choosing a physician," said Wong. "We decided the time was right to allow patients to 'give their doctors a checkup.'" RateMDs.com cofounder John Swapceinski said, "The tremendous popularity of our site has demonstrated the unmet demand for professional services information, and what service is more important than medical service? It can literally be a matter of life and death." Visitors to the site can praise or pan their doctors by leaving feedback, and research other doctors by reading the comments left by previous visitors. The site is free of charge to all users.

Information Sources. The health care marketer must be very knowledgeable about common information sources that consumers use and their relative influence on the purchase decision. These information sources fall into four groups:

- *Personal.* Family, friends, neighbors, acquaintances
- *Commercial.* Advertising, Web sites, salespeople, dealers, packaging, displays
- *Public.* Mass media, consumer-rating organizations
- *Experiential.* Handling, examining, using the product or testing the service

Although the consumer usually receives the *most* information about a product from commercial, marketer-dominated media, the most *influential* information comes from personal recommendations or publicly available independent authorities. The two categories of sources provide complementary functions; commercial media inform, whereas personal or expert sources legitimize or enhance the evaluation process. For example, physicians often learn of new drugs from commercial sources but turn to other doctors for legitimizing opinions (see Figure 6.2).

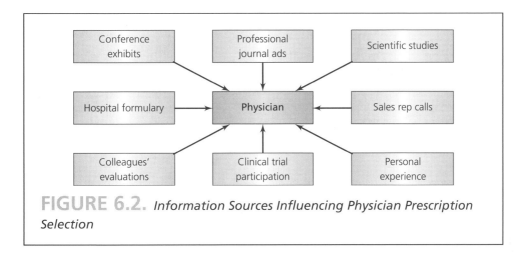

FIGURE 6.2. *Information Sources Influencing Physician Prescription Selection*

Field Note 6.2 demonstrates how the Internet is becoming an increasingly powerful and useful consumer tool.

FIELD NOTE 6.2.

On-line Medical Web Sites Compete   Currently the best-known and most used Web site for medical information is WebMD.com, which draws more than forty million unique users a month to its network of consumer sites. The site lists health news of the day, the top twelve health topics for men and women, the most common treatments, how to find a doctor, symptom checking, and so on.

Other Web sites include NIH.gov (from the National Institutes of Health), Yahoo Health, Mayoclinic.com, and About.com Health (owned by the New York Times Company). Google and other search engines enable users to type in a word or phrase, such as ''sore throat,'' and instantly find relevant information about potential causes and risks, treatments and tests, and alternative medicines.

In 2007 Stephen Case, founder of AOL, along with several notable investors including Colin Powell and Carly Fiorina, launched a new site called RevolutionHealth.com. He hopes that in the ensuing five years the site will become as dominant in health care information as Starbucks is in coffee or Nike in fitness. The site sorts 1,500 medical conditions by the ailment or treatment. It contains related comments from experts and from other users of the site, as well as a directory of doctors by specialty and location, along with short reviews by patients. Information is featured from the Mayo Clinic, Cleveland Clinic, and Harvard Medical School, which also have their own Web sites. Users can create their own pages within RevolutionHealth.com for collecting personal and general information, which they can keep private or share as they choose. As the site is free, the main revenue comes from advertising that, it is hoped, will not influence any objective content. Revolution Health.com's likelihood of passing up WebMD depends upon how innovative and distinctive its features are.

Source: Milt Freudenheim, "AOL Found Hopes to Build New Giant Among a Bevy of Health Care Web Sites," *New York Times*, Apr. 16, 2007.

Once a consumer faces a set of choices—say, choosing a health care plan—she goes through a successive set of screening decisions The individual consumer will come to know only a subset of the *total set* of brands available (*awareness set*), some of which will meet initial buying criteria (*consideration set*). As the consumer gathers more information, only a few will remain as strong contenders (*choice set*) from which she makes a final choice.[17] An organization must strategize to get its brand into the prospect's awareness set, consideration set, and choice set. The organization must also identify the other brands in the consumer's choice set so that it can plan the appropriate competitive appeals.

A marketer's task is therefore to interview consumers and ask what sources of information they sought or received in the course of the buying process. This research is valuable if a substantial percentage of consumers engage in active search and show some stable patterns of using the information sources. Additional questions for consumers include the type of information that came from each source and the influence of each information source on the final decision. This consumer information can be used to create effective marketing communications content, select the most appropriate media vehicles, and manage word of mouth.

Evaluation of Alternatives

Although much has been written about subliminal decision making, the most current models view the process as cognitively oriented, meaning that consumers form judgments largely on a conscious and rational basis.

In attempting to satisfy a need, the consumer is also looking for certain benefits from the product solution; each product is viewed as a bundle of attributes with varying abilities to deliver these benefits. Naturally, the attributes that are of interest to buyers vary by product. For example, the attributes sought in a travel medicine clinic might be up-to-date knowledge of disease incidence in foreign countries, web access to information, 24x7 access to an affiliated physician in the country being visited, and an affordable service subscription price. Thus the job of marketers is to segment these customers according to the attributes that are most important to each group.

Evaluations often reflect beliefs and attitudes that consumers acquire through experience and learning. These beliefs and attitudes in turn influence buying behavior. A *belief* is a descriptive thought that a person holds about something. Just as important as beliefs are attitudes. An *attitude* is a person's enduring favorable or unfavorable evaluation, emotional feeling, and action tendencies toward some object or idea.[18] People have attitudes toward almost everything: religion, politics, clothes, music, food, and health care products and services.

Because attitudes economize on energy and thought, they can be very difficult to change, and a company is well-advised to fit its product into existing attitudes rather than to try to change attitudes.

The consumer arrives at attitudes, judgments, and preferences toward various brands through an attribute evaluation procedure, developing a set of beliefs about where each brand stands on each attribute.[19] According to the *expectancy-value model* of attitude formation, consumers evaluate products and services by combining their brand beliefs—the positives and negatives—according to importance. This model assumes high *consumer involvement*—that is, the level of engagement and active processing a consumer undertakes in response to a marketing stimulus.

For example, suppose Margaret has narrowed her choice set to four pediatric practices for her children on the basis of five attributes: location convenience, office hours, network affiliation with specialists at an academic medical center, physician empathy, and costs. If one pediatric practice dominated the others on all the criteria, we could predict that Margaret would choose it. However, not all practices have the same benefits in terms of these attributes. The task of the marketing manager is to segment potential customers into groups with the same or similar preferences and enhance the attractiveness of the practice by one or several of the following steps:

- Expand office hours to include nights and weekends (real positioning).

- Alter consumer beliefs about the brand (psychological repositioning).

- Alter consumer beliefs about competitors' brands (competitive depositioning).

- Alter the importance of weights (to persuade buyers to attach more importance to the attributes in which the brand excels).

- Call attention to neglected attributes (such as commitment to the community).

- Shift the buyer's ideals (to persuade buyers to change their ideal levels for one or more attributes).[20]

Purchase Decisions

In the fourth stage, the consumer forms preferences among the brands in the choice set and may also form an intention to buy the most preferred brand. At least three factors can intervene between a purchase intention and a purchase decision. The first is the *attitudes of others*. Suppose Margaret prefers pediatric practice A, but her closest friends strongly recommend practice B; Margaret's purchase probability for practice A will be somewhat reduced. The extent to which another person's attitude reduces the preference for an alternative depends on two factors: (1) the intensity of the other person's negative attitude toward the consumer's preferred alternative and (2) the consumer's motivation to comply with the other person's wishes.[21] The more intense the other person's negativism and the closer the other person is to the consumer, the more the consumer will adjust his or her purchase intention. Conversely, a buyer's preference for a brand will increase if someone he or she respects favors the same brand strongly.

Related to the attitudes of others is the role played by information intermediaries who publish their evaluations or recommendations. Examples include The Leapfrog Group (http://www.leapfroggroup.org), a voluntary organization of large employers who aim to mobilize "employer purchasing power to alert the health industry that big leaps in health care safety, quality, and customer value will be recognized and rewarded. Among other initiatives, Leapfrog works with its employer members to encourage transparency and easy access to health care information as well as rewards for hospitals that have a proven record of high quality care."

The second factor is *unanticipated situational factors* that may arise to change the purchase intention. Margaret might lose her job, her husband might lose his, some other purchase might become more urgent, or a practice staff member might be rude to Margaret. Marketers know that such unanticipated factors in the *critical contact situation* can have a significant influence on the final decision. These factors explain why preferences and even purchase intentions are not completely reliable predictors of purchase behavior.

A consumer's decision to modify, postpone, or avoid a purchase decision is also heavily influenced by *perceived risk*, such as the amount of money at stake, the amount of attribute uncertainty, and the amount of consumer self-confidence.[22] A heart valve replacement would be considered a high perceived risk purchase, given the expense, the pain, and the possibility of life-threatening complications. In contrast, going to a dermatologist to treat a plantar wart has a relatively low perceived risk, because it is a low-cost purchase with little discomfort and a fairly certain outcome.

Consumers develop routines for reducing risk, such as decision avoidance, information gathering from friends and professionals, and preference for recognized names. Regarding this last factor, because many health care purchases have high perceived risk, consumers often show preference for a particular brand. This simple, sometimes automatic approach of buying the "recognized brand" can present a challenge to local health care providers. For example, a patient in Chicago may choose the Mayo Clinic for a routine operation that could be easily done in a local community hospital or academic medical center—with lower travel cost, a shorter waiting time, and the same outcome. Marketers must deeply understand the factors that provoke a feeling of risk in consumers, then provide information and support that will reduce the perceived risk.

Post-Purchase Behavior

After the purchase, the consumer may experience dissatisfaction that stems from the product experience not matching expectation, finding the same product at a lower price, or hearing favorable things about other brands in the same category.[23] The

marketer therefore must realize that the customer does not stop seeking information after the sale is complete; marketing communications must supply beliefs and evaluations that reinforce the consumer's choice and help him or her feel good about the brand. To successfully accomplish this task, marketers must monitor post-purchase satisfaction, post-purchase actions, and post-purchase product uses.

Cognitive dissonance theory holds that almost every purchase is likely to lead to some post-purchase discomfort; the magnitude of the discomfort and what the consumer will do about it are the key issues marketers must address. For example, dissatisfied consumers may try to reduce their dissonance by abandoning the service or returning the product, or they may try to reduce the dissonance by seeking information that will confirm its high value (or avoid information that may disconfirm its high value). The consumer's coping style and tendency toward cognitive dissonance also play roles. Some consumers tend to magnify the gap between expectation and performance when the product is not perfect, and they will be highly dissatisfied. Other consumers tend to minimize the gap and will feel less dissatisfied.

The importance of post-purchase satisfaction suggests that product claims must truthfully represent the product's likely performance. Some sellers might even understate performance levels so that consumers experience higher-than-expected satisfaction with the product.

Health care organizations can take positive steps to help buyers feel good about their choices. A pediatric practice can send warm, introductory letters to new patients; solicit customer suggestions for improvements; offer child health information that will address common questions and concerns; provide information through the channel the consumer prefers—for example, through e-mail or the practice Web site; place ads showing satisfied practice consumers; and provide channels for speedy redress of customer grievances.

One potential opportunity to increase frequency of product use arises when consumers' perceptions of their usage differ from the reality. For example, many people underestimate the time since their last preventive care visit to their physician or dentist. In this case, consumers must be persuaded of the merits of more regular usage, and any potential hurdles to increased usage must be overcome. In terms of the latter, product or service designs and packaging can make the product more convenient and easier to use. The pediatric practice can communicate regularly with consumers explaining the need for routine vaccinations, physicals, and seasonal reasons for visiting the practice (illnesses in the winter and injuries in the summer). It can also offer more convenient hours to minimize the perceived barrier of waiting for the physician.

ORGANIZATIONAL BUYING AND DECISION MAKING

From the individual, we now turn to how organizations make their purchase decisions. Webster and Wind define *organizational buying* as the decision-making process by which formal organizations establish the need for purchased products and services and identify, evaluate, and choose among alternative brands and suppliers.[24] Organizational buying differs from the consumer market in a number of significant ways.

Three Types of Markets

There are three types of organizational markets: the business market, the institutional market, and the government market.

The Business Market. The *business market* consists of all the organizations that acquire goods and services used in the production of other products or services that are sold, rented, or supplied to others (see Chapter Three for a description of the major health care market segments that this market comprises).

More dollars and items are involved in sales to business buyers than to consumers. Consider the process of producing and selling a simple wheelchair. Metal and fabric companies must sell materials to distributors, who sell materials to wheelchair manufacturers, who sell wheelchairs to wholesalers, who, in turn, sell them to retailers, who finally sell the chairs to consumers. Business markets have several other important characteristics that contrast sharply with those of consumer markets:

- *Fewer, larger buyers.* The business marketer normally deals with far fewer and much larger buyers than the consumer marketer does. For example, the fate of McKesson, a large drug wholesaler, depends on getting contracts from major pharmaceutical manufacturers.

- *Close supplier-customer relationship.* With the smaller customer base and the power of the larger customers, suppliers are frequently expected to customize their offerings to individual business customer needs. For example, pharmaceutical benefit management (PBM) companies will supply their health plan customers with highly customized drug benefit schemes that match the plan's price positioning strategy.

- *Professional purchasing.* Trained purchasing agents follow formal policies, constraints, and requirements when buying. Many of the buying instruments—such as proposals, and purchase contracts—are not typically found in consumer buying. A part of this category comprises hospitals that buy through group purchasing organizations (GPOs).

- *Multiple buying influences.* More people typically influence business buying decisions. Because purchasing committees for major goods often consist of technical experts and even senior management, business marketers have to send well-trained sales representatives and teams to deal with these sophisticated buyers. HSS, a medical coding software company, pairs salespeople with systems engineers to explain technical details to hospital information systems specialists.

- *Multiple sales calls.* With more people involved in the selling process, it takes multiple sales calls to win most business orders, and some sales cycles can take years. A study by McGraw-Hill found that it takes four to four-and-a-half calls to close an average industrial sale. In the case of capital equipment sales for large projects, it may take multiple attempts to fund a project, and the sales cycle—between quoting a job and delivering the product—is often measured in years.[25]

■ *Derived demand.* Because demand for business goods is ultimately derived from the demand for consumer goods or services, business marketers must monitor the buying patterns of ultimate consumers. For instance, in responding to the demand from their employer customers for lower-priced insurance premiums, insurers have responded with "consumer-directed" health plans that have lower premiums but higher deductibles.

■ *Inelastic demand.* Total demand for many business goods and services is inelastic. The demand for drugs purchased by hospitals is only somewhat affected by changes in reimbursement and capital market performance, because physicians require an adequate supply to effectively treat hospital patients.

■ *Fluctuating demand.* Demand for business goods and services tends to be more volatile than the demand for consumer goods and services. Because of the need to project trends, a given percentage increase in consumer demand can lead to a much larger percentage increase in the demand for plant and equipment necessary to produce additional output. On the other hand, negative customer news can drop demand to zero, as occurred for Merck's Vioxx when reports started to link the drug with unexpected deaths.

■ *Geographically concentrated buyers.* More than half of U.S. business buyers are concentrated in seven states: New York, California, Pennsylvania, Illinois, Ohio, New Jersey, and Michigan. This geographical concentration of producers helps to reduce selling costs. Warsaw, Indiana, is the backbone of the global market for replacement hips, knees, and shoulders. Warsaw probably controls about 40 percent of the worldwide orthopedics business, and suppliers head there on sales calls.

■ *Direct purchasing.* Business buyers often buy directly from manufacturers rather than through intermediaries, especially items that are technically complex or expensive such as imaging equipment and information systems.

The Institutional Market. The health care *institutional market* consists of hospitals, nursing homes, prisons, and other institutions that must provide health care goods and services to people in their care. Many of these organizations are characterized by fixed budgets and captive clienteles. For example, being the food supplier of choice for the nation's hospitals means big business.

When hospitals decide on food purchases for patients, the objective is not profit, because the food is provided as part of the total service package; however, poor food will cause patients to complain and hurt the hospital's reputation. The hospital purchasing agent has to search for institutional food suppliers whose quality meets or exceeds a certain minimum standard *and* whose prices are low. Many food companies set up a separate division to sell to institutional buyers because of these buyers' special needs and characteristics. For instance, Heinz produces, packages, and prices its ketchup differently to meet the requirements of these customers.

The Government Market. The U.S. government buys goods and services valued at $200 billion, making it the largest customer in the world. Over twenty million individual contract actions are processed every year, according to the General Sources Administration Procurement Data Center. Although most items purchased are between $2,500 and $25,000, the government also makes purchases, such as for technology, in the billions. Because their spending decisions are subject to public review, government organizations require considerable documentation from suppliers. Suppliers are therefore subject to excessive paperwork, bureaucracy, regulations, decision-making delays, and shifts in procurement personnel, all of which increase the cost of doing business. In addition to these costs, governments require the lowest prices. The reasons many companies conduct business with governments are to help cover fixed costs and receive the endorsement that enables them to access private contracts more easily.

Buying Situations

Business buyers face many decisions in making a purchase, among which are the complexity of the problem being solved, the newness of the buying requirement, the number of people involved, and the time required. Patrick Robinson and others distinguish three types of buying situations: straight rebuy, modified rebuy, and new task.[26]

- *Straight rebuy.* The purchasing department reorders on a routine basis (such as office supplies, sutures) and chooses from suppliers on an approved list. The suppliers make an effort to maintain product and service quality and often propose automatic reordering systems to save time. "Out-suppliers" attempt to offer something new or to exploit dissatisfaction with a current supplier, often trying to get a small order and then enlarge their purchase share over time.

- *Modified rebuy.* The buyer wants to modify product specifications, prices, delivery requirements, or other terms. The modified rebuy usually involves additional participants on both sides. The "in-suppliers" become nervous and have to protect the account, whereas the out-suppliers see an opportunity to propose a better offer to gain some business.

- *New task.* A purchaser buys a product or service for the first time (for example, a medical office building, a new security system). The greater the cost or risk, the larger the number of participants and the greater their information gathering—and therefore the longer the time a decision takes.[27] New-task buying passes through several stages: awareness, interest, evaluation, trial, and adoption.[28] Communication tools' effectiveness varies at each stage. Mass media are most important during the initial awareness stage, salespeople have their greatest impact at the interest stage, and technical sources are most important during the evaluation stage.

The business buyer makes the fewest decisions in the straight rebuy situation and the most in the new-task situation. In the new-task situation, the buyer has to determine product specifications, price limits, delivery terms and times, service terms, payment terms, order quantities, acceptable suppliers, and the selected supplier. Different participants influence each decision and the order in which these decisions are made varies. This new-task situation is the marketer's greatest opportunity and challenge. Because of the complicated selling involved in new-task situations, many companies use a *missionary sales force* consisting of their most effective salespeople.

Systems Buying and Selling

Many business buyers prefer to buy a total solution to their problem from one seller. This practice, called *systems buying*, originated with government purchases of major weapons and communications systems. The government would solicit bids from *prime contractors* who would assemble the package or system. The winning contractor then bid out and assembled the system's subcomponents from other contractors.

Sellers have increasingly recognized that buyers like to purchase in this way, and many have adopted systems selling as a marketing tool. One variant of systems selling is *systems contracting*, wherein a single supplier provides the buyer with his or her entire requirement of MRO (maintenance, repair, operating) supplies. This offering lowers the buyer's costs because the seller manages the customer's inventory and less time is spent on supplier selection. The seller benefits from reduced procurement and management costs, price protection over the term of the contract, and lower operating costs because of a steady demand and reduced paperwork. Systems selling is a key industrial marketing strategy in bidding to build large-scale industrial projects, such as hospitals, medical office buildings, pharmaceutical manufacturing plants, and laboratories.

Decision Makers in the Business Buying Process

As might be expected, the key decision maker for a business purchase varies by the type of transaction. Purchasing agents are influential in straight-rebuy and modified-rebuy situations. The new-buy situations can be more complex. For example, in addition to finance personnel, physicians, nurses, and technical experts in laboratory or information systems are often involved in the purchase decision of complex and expensive medical equipment and supplies.[29]

Buying Center

Webster and Wind call the decision-making unit (DMU) of a buying organization the *buying center*. It is composed of "all those individuals and groups who participate in the purchasing decision-making process, who share some common goals and the risks arising from the decisions."[30] The buying center includes organizational members who play any of these seven roles in the purchase decision process:

1. *Initiators.* People who request that something be purchased, including users or others in the organization.

2. *Users.* Those who will use the product or service; often users initiate the buying proposal and help define product requirements.

3. *Influencers.* People who influence the buying decision, including clinical and technical personnel, who often help define specifications and also provide information for evaluating alternatives.

4. *Deciders.* Those who decide on product requirements or on suppliers.

5. *Approvers.* People who authorize the proposed actions of deciders or buyers.

6. *Buyers.* People who have formal authority to select the supplier and arrange the purchase terms. Buyers may help shape product specifications, but their major role is selecting vendors and negotiating terms. In more complex purchases, the buyers might include high-level managers.

7. *Gatekeepers.* People who have the power to prevent sellers or information from reaching members of the buying center; examples are purchasing agents, receptionists, and telephone operators.[31]

Several individuals can occupy a given role (for example, there may be many users or influencers), and one individual may occupy multiple roles.[32] A purchasing manager, for example, often occupies simultaneously the roles of buyer, influencer, and gatekeeper: he or she can determine which sales reps can call on other people in the organization; what budget and other constraints to place on the purchase; and which firm will actually get the business, even though others (deciders) might select two or more potential vendors who can meet the organization's requirements. The typical buying center has a minimum of five or six members, and often has dozens, including people outside the organization, such as government officials, consultants, technical advisors, and members of the marketing channel.

Buying Center Influences. Buying centers usually include several participants with differing interests, authority, status, empathy, and persuasiveness. Each participant is likely to give priority to very different decision criteria. For example, engineering personnel may be concerned primarily with maximizing the actual performance of the product; production personnel may be concerned mainly with ease of use and reliability of supply; financial personnel may focus on the economics of the purchase; purchasing may be concerned with operating and replacement costs; union officials may emphasize safety issues; and so on.

Business buyers also respond to subconscious influences when they make their decisions. Each carries personal motivations, perceptions, and preferences, which are influenced by the buyer's age, income, education, job position, personality, attitudes toward risk and culture. Based on these and other factors, buyers exhibit different buying styles. For example, some prefer to conduct rigorous analyses of competitive proposals before choosing a supplier whereas others may pit the competing sellers against one another. Occasionally, buyers know exactly which company will win the bid, but they go through a selection process for the sake of appearances.

Webster cautions that ultimately, individuals, not organizations, make purchasing decisions.[33] Individuals are motivated by their own needs and perceptions in attempting to maximize the rewards (pay, advancement, recognition, and feelings of achievement) offered by the organization. Personal needs motivate the behavior of individuals, but organizational needs legitimate the buying decision process and its outcomes. People are buying solutions to two problems: the organization's economic and strategic problem and their own personal problem of obtaining individual achievement and reward. In this sense, industrial buying decisions are both rational and emotional, as they serve both the organization's and the individual's needs.[34]

Buying Center Targeting. To target their efforts properly, business marketers must answer the questions: Who are the major decision participants? What decisions do they influence? What is their level of influence? What evaluation criteria do they use? Consider the following example:

FOR EXAMPLE

A company sells nonwoven disposable surgical gowns to hospitals. The hospital personnel who participate in this buying decision include the vice president of purchasing, the operating-room administrator, and the surgeons. The vice president of purchasing analyzes whether the hospital should buy disposable gowns or reusable gowns. If the findings favor disposable gowns, then the operating-room administrator compares various competitors' products and prices and makes a choice. This administrator considers absorbency, antiseptic quality, design, and cost, and normally buys the brand that meets the functional requirements at the lowest cost. Surgeons influence the decision retroactively by reporting their satisfaction with the particular brand.

The business marketer is not likely to know exactly what kind of group dynamics take place during the decision-making process, although whatever information he or she can discover about personalities and interpersonal factors is useful. Small sellers concentrate on reaching the *key buying influencers*. Larger sellers go for *multilevel in-depth selling* to reach as many participants as possible. Their salespeople virtually "live" with high-volume customers. Companies will have to rely more heavily on their communications program to reach hidden buying influences and keep current customers informed.[35] Business marketers must periodically review their assumptions about buying center participants. For years, Kodak, which sold X-ray film to hospital lab technicians, did not notice that the decision was increasingly being made by professional administrators. As sales declined, Kodak hurriedly revised its market target strategy.

In defining target segments, four types of business customers can often be identified, with corresponding marketing implications:

- *Price-oriented customers* (transactional selling). Price is everything.

- *Solution-oriented customers* (consultative selling). They want low prices but will respond to arguments about lower total cost or more dependable supply or service.

- *Gold-standard customers* (quality selling). They want the best performance in terms of product quality, assistance, reliable delivery, and so on.

- *Strategic-value customers* (enterprise selling). They want a fairly permanent sole-supplier relationship with the supplier.

Risk-and-gain sharing can be used to offset requested price reductions from customers. For example, suppose Medline, a hospital supplier, signs a hospital agreement promising $350,000 in savings over the first eighteen months in exchange for a tenfold increase in the hospital's share of supplies. If Medline achieves less than this promised savings, it will make up the difference; if it achieves substantially more than this promise, it participates in the extra savings. To make such arrangements work, the supplier must be willing to help the customer to build a historical database, reach an agreement for measuring benefits and costs, and devise a dispute resolution mechanism.

Stages in the Buying Process

Business buying passes through eight stages, called *buy phases*, as identified by Robinson and Associates in the *buy grid* model.[36] In modified-rebuy or straight-rebuy situations, some stages are compressed or bypassed. For example, in a straight-rebuy situation, the buyer normally has a favorite supplier or a ranked list of suppliers and the supplier search and proposal solicitation stages would be skipped. The sections that follow examine the stages of a typical new-task buying situation.

Problem Recognition. The buying process begins when someone in the organization recognizes a problem or need that can be met by acquiring a good or service. The recognition can be triggered by internal or external stimuli. Internally, problem recognition commonly occurs when an organization decides to develop a new product and needs new equipment and materials, or a machine breaks down and requires new parts, or purchased material turns out to be unsatisfactory, or a purchasing manager senses an opportunity to obtain lower prices or better quality. Externally, the buyer may get new ideas at a trade show, see an ad, become subject to a new regulation, face changes in reimbursement for a health care product or service, or receive a call from a sales representative offering a better product or a lower price. Business marketers can stimulate problem recognition by direct mail, Web site search optimization, e-mail, telemarketing, and calling on prospects.

General Need Description and Product Specification. Next, the buyer must determine the needed item's general characteristics and required quantity. For standard items this is simple, but for complex items the buyer will work with others—engineers, users—to define characteristics like reliability, durability, or price. Hospitals interested in purchasing a new information system typically form multidisciplinary buying committees. These committees include system users and influencers. The committee usually has management, clinical, financial, technical, information systems, physician, engineering, facilities, outside consultant, and executive management representation, and decision making is based on group consensus.

The buying organization now develops the item's technical specifications. Often, the company will use *product-value analysis*, a cost-reduction approach in which components are studied to determine if they can be redesigned or standardized or made by cheaper production methods. The PVA team will examine the high-cost components in a given product and identify overdesigned components that last longer than the product itself. Tightly written specifications will allow the buyer to refuse components that are too expensive or that fail to meet specified standards. Suppliers can use product value analysis as a tool for positioning themselves to win an account.

Supplier Search. The buyer next tries to identify the most appropriate suppliers through trade directories, contacts with other companies, trade advertisements, and trade shows. Business marketers also put products, prices, and other information on the Internet.[37] E-procurement involves more than acquiring software; it requires changing purchasing strategy. Many types of purchases can be made directly and safely on the Internet. If the information is rich enough to satisfy the buyer, there is no further stage to purchasing. When this is not the case, the buyer proceeds to request proposals from some of the business buyers he has identified on the Web. The supplier's task is to get listed in major online catalogs or services, develop a strong advertising and promotion program, and build a good reputation in the marketplace.

After evaluating each company, the buyer will end up with a short list of qualified suppliers. More professional buyers have forced suppliers to change their marketing to increase their likelihood of making the cut. Consider the following example:

FOR EXAMPLE

Misys is a UK-based health information systems company that sells software and hardware to hospitals, physicians, and home health care companies. Misys encounters prospects by having salespeople "cold call" hospital chief information officers, chief financial officers, chief medical officers, and home care executive directors. The salespeople attempt to start calling as high on the organization chart as possible to get the attention of decision makers. At the Healthcare Information and Management Systems Society (HIMSS) and other trade shows, Misys also meets prospects who are on a reconnaissance mission to find companies that can help solve their information system problems. Hospitals learn of Misys through reports from KLAS, a health information system consulting company that rates different software applications. Prospects can then visit Misys and other potential suppliers on the Web to learn more about product capabilities. Finally, referrals from other Misys customers are a source of prospects, and these referred prospects have the highest statistical likelihood of becoming Misys customers.

Proposal Solicitation. In this stage, the buyer invites qualified suppliers to submit proposals. When the item is complex or expensive, the buyer will require a detailed written proposal from each qualified supplier. After evaluating the proposals, the buyer will invite a few suppliers to make formal presentations. Business marketers must be skilled in researching, writing, and presenting proposals. Their written proposals should be not just technical documents, but marketing documents that describe value and benefits in customer terms. Oral presentations should inspire confidence, positioning the company's capabilities and resources so that they stand out from the competition.

If Misys is selected to present a proposal, they will usually join three to seven other companies that are invited to prepare proposals. The objective of the hospital in this stage is to whittle down the list of competitors. A common tool to accomplish this objective is the *request for proposal* (RFP), which describes in detail all of the specifications needed for a project or product. Companies that respond to the RFP often face strict rules in regard to completing the document, including reply deadlines and rules for limiting contact with key personnel in the buyer's organization. Sometimes companies will enlist the help of a preferred supplier or consultant in authoring the RFP. Although company policy may require an RFP process, many are conducted with the winner a foregone conclusion—for example, this is estimated to be the case for as many as 60 to 70 percent of hospital RFPs.

Supplier Selection. Before selecting a supplier, the buying center will specify desired supplier attributes and indicate their relative importance. It will then rate each supplier on the attributes to identify the most attractive one. Business marketers need to do a better job of understanding how business buyers arrive at their valuations. Anderson, Jain, and Chintagunta conducted a study of the principal means business marketers use to assess customer value and found eight different *customer value assessment* (CVA) methods.[38] Although companies tended to use the simpler methods, the more sophisticated ones promise to produce a more accurate picture of customer-perceived value.

The choice and importance of different attributes vary with the type of buying situation.[39] Delivery reliability, price, and supplier reputation are important for routine-order products. For procedural-problem products, such as a copying machine, the three most important attributes are technical service, supplier flexibility, and product reliability. For political-problem products that stir rivalries in the organization (such as the choice of a computer system), the most important attributes are price, supplier reputation, product reliability, service reliability, and supplier flexibility.

Despite moves toward strategic sourcing, partnering, and participation in cross-functional teams, buyers still spend a large portion of their time haggling with suppliers on price. Marketers can counter the request for a lower price in several ways. They may be able to show evidence that the life-cycle cost of using their product is lower than that of competitors' products. They can also cite the value of the services the buyer now receives, especially if those services are superior to those offered by competitors. As part of the buyer selection process, buying centers must also decide how many suppliers to use. Companies are increasingly reducing the number of suppliers.

Order-Routine Specification. After selecting suppliers, the buyer negotiates the final order, listing the technical specifications, the quantity needed, the expected time of delivery, return policies, warranties, and so on. In the case of maintenance, repair, and operating (MRO) items, buyers are moving toward blanket contracts rather than periodic purchase orders. A *blanket contract* establishes a long-term relationship in which the supplier promises to resupply the buyer as needed, at agreed-upon prices, over a specified period of time. Because the seller holds the stock, the blanket contract is sometimes called a *stockless purchase plan*. The buyer's computer automatically sends an order to the seller when stock is needed. Blanket contracting leads to more single-source buying and ordering of more items from that single source; out-suppliers have difficulty breaking in unless the buyer becomes dissatisfied with the in-supplier's prices, quality, or service.

Companies that fear a shortage of key materials are willing to buy and hold large inventories. For example, hospital pharmacies experience temporary drug shortages regularly, and these shortages create a cascading effect in the search for other drugs as substitutes. These shortages have become more commonplace because drug wholesalers no longer have a financial incentive to carry large inventories. As a result, hospital pharmacies need to anticipate market demand for drugs, load their inventories accordingly, and continue to balance the cost of holding the drugs with controlling costs.

Performance Review. In the final stage of the buying process, the buyer periodically reviews the performance of the chosen supplier(s) using one of three methods:

- Contact the end users and ask for their evaluations.

- Rate the supplier on several criteria using a weighted score method.

- Aggregate the cost of poor supplier performance to come up with adjusted costs of purchase, including price.

The performance review may lead the buyer to continue, modify, or end the relationship with the supplier. To keep customers, the supplier should assess the same variables that are monitored by the product's buyers and end users. For example, because Misys states that using its software will reduce a hospital's accounts receivable cycle by a certain number of days, the customer will monitor this measure for the first ninety days to ensure that this claim is substantiated. If there is a discrepancy, the hospital's contract may call for a pricing modification or other change.

Business Relationships: Risks and Opportunities

Building strong business relationships depends on how the buyer perceives the supplier's credibility. Corporate credibility refers to the extent to which customers believe that a firm can design and deliver offerings that satisfy their needs and wants. Corporate credibility relates to the reputation that a firm has achieved in the marketplace, and it is the foundation for a strong business relationship. It is difficult for a firm to develop strong ties with another firm unless it is seen as highly credible based on these three factors:

- *Corporate expertise.* The extent to which a company is seen as able to make and sell products or conduct services

- *Corporate trustworthiness.* The extent to which a company is seen as motivated to be honest, dependable, and sensitive to customer needs

- *Corporate likeability.* The extent to which a company is seen as likable, attractive, prestigious and dynamic

Buvik and John note that in establishing a customer-supplier relationship, there is tension between safeguarding and adaptation.[40] Vertical coordination can facilitate stronger customer-seller ties but at the same time may increase the risk posed to the customer's and supplier's specific investments. *Specific investments* are those expenditures tailored to a particular company and value chain partner (such as investments in company-specific training, equipment, and operating procedures or systems).[41] Specific investments help firms grow profits and achieve their positioning.[42] Yet they also entail considerable risk to both customer and supplier. Transaction theory from economics maintains that because these investments are partially sunk (and to that extent cannot be recovered), they lock in the investing firms to a particular relationship. A buyer may be vulnerable to holdup because of switching costs; a supplier may be more vulnerable to holdup in future contracts because of dedicated assets or expropriation of technology or knowledge.

Another concern arises when buyers cannot easily monitor supplier performance. *Opportunism* can be thought of in terms of "some form of cheating or undersupply relative to an implicit or explicit contract."[43] It may involve blatant self-interest and deliberate misrepresentation that violates contractual agreements. An information systems company that demonstrates software functionality during the sales process, but knows that its technology cannot possibly deliver this functionality, hurts itself as well as tarnishes the entire industry through this form of opportunism. Opportunism is a concern because firms must devote resources to oversight that otherwise could be allocated to more productive purposes. Contracts may become inadequate to govern supplier transactions when supplier opportunism becomes difficult to detect, firms make specific investments in assets that cannot be used elsewhere, and contingencies are harder to anticipate. A joint venture (versus a simple contract) is more likely when the supplier's degree of asset specificity is high, monitoring the supplier's behavior is difficult, and the supplier has a poor reputation.[44] A supplier with a strong reputation will try to avoid opportunism to protect its valuable intangible asset.

SUMMARY

The starting point for marketing planning is to understand how members of the target market make their buying decisions. We examined separately the decision influences and processes of both individual consumers and business organizations.

Individual consumers' choices are influenced by their cultural, social, and personal factors, as well as their psychological processes of motivation, perception, learning, and memory. At least five roles—initiator, influencer, decider, buyer, and end user—may be played out in the buying process. A single individual buyer may go through five stages in buying a product or service: problem recognition, information search, evaluation of alternatives, purchase decision, and post-purchase behavior.

Organizations such as for-profit firms, institutions, and government agencies also must make buying decisions to obtain the inputs for their operations. Those who sell to business buyers will deal with far fewer customers and face more professional buyers, and other factors will be different from those that affect consumer buyers. The business buying process varies depending on whether the situation is one of a straight buy, rebuy, or new task. In simpler situations the buying center will consist of a purchasing agent who will do the buying; in more complicated situations a number of people will participate in the buying process. The buying process consists of problem recognition, general need description and product specification, supplier search, proposal solicitation, supplier selection, order routine specification, and performance review. Business marketers work hard to establish relations, often by making specific investments tailored to the buyer, which improves the relationship, but carries some risk.

DISCUSSION QUESTIONS

1. The Kate B. Reynolds Foundation made a three-year grant to establish a clinic in a medically underserved, low-income neighborhood. What can be done to draw in low-income people to use this clinic, given their likely needs and concerns?

2. Most needs for health care services and products seem tied to the physiological and safety needs shown in Maslow's hierarchy of needs pyramid. Describe the types of health care needs that could be related to the upper levels of Maslow's pyramid—the social, esteem and status, and self-actualization levels.

3. Media stories have recently focused on the obesity epidemic in the United States. If most health behavior is learned, how would you recommend that consumers learn to (a) avoid becoming obese in the first place or (b) change their health behaviors if they are currently obese?

4. Pharmaceutical companies hire contract research organizations (CROs) to outsource portions of their clinical research functions. Many of the large "big pharma" companies prefer making provider agreements with the five largest CROs. Smaller competing CROs, however, frequently have the same or better clinical research capabilities and charge lower fees. As the chief marketingofficer of one these smaller CROs, how would you convince a big pharma company to use your services?

CHAPTER

7

USING MARKET INFORMATION SYSTEMS AND MARKETING RESEARCH

LEARNING OBJECTIVES

In this chapter, we will address the following questions:

1. What are the main components of a health care marketing information system?

2. What systems help health care organizations maintain and use their internal records?

3. What methods can health care organizations use to gather and respond to marketing intelligence on opportunities and threats?

4. What are the main methods for conducting reliable marketing research?

5. How can a health care organization improve its research tools and sources?

OPENING EXAMPLE

Blue Cross Blue Shield Investigates the Effectiveness of Its Advertising in Selling Its Health Plan   In late 2000, a large Blue Cross/Blue Shield (BCBS) health care plan in the Midwest decided to examine the effectiveness of its advertising campaign. This branding campaign, consisting of TV, radio, and print ads, was intended to position the health plan favorably among a specifically targeted segment of prospective plan members.

Health plans rely on actuaries to forecast the health risk and medical costs of plan members. If a health plan attracts a larger number of low risk members with high loyalty, its profit is larger. Conversely, if a health plan attracts a larger number of high risk members, and fails to maintain loyalty among the lower risk members, profits will be lower. Attracting and retaining higher risk members is referred to as "adverse selection" and is something health plans work to minimize.

This BCBS plan was targeting consumers to reduce the health plan's risk of adverse selection. One of the key goals of the research was to gather evidence to show that the advertising supported this outcome. By using a random telephone survey of 1,200 consumers in a four state region, the Plan looked at levels of unaided recall, aided recall, and preference. *Unaided* recall refers to asking consumers an open-ended question about remembering an advertisement but does not mention possible choices. An example of an unaided recall question is "Do you recall any ads for health plans?" An *aided* recall question usually follows an unaided question and does offer choices: "Do you recall any advertisements for: Blue Cross-Blue Shield, Aetna, or Cigna?". A *preference* question asks which plan is preferred. If a consumer has a relatively high level of advertising recall, and a positive attitude or preference for a particular product, then the consumer is more likely to purchase that product if it meets a need.

This BCBS research study incorporated the Profiles of Activities and Attitudes Toward Healthcare (PATH) Model. The PATH Model is unique in that it provides a multidimensional picture of health care consumer priorities, behaviors and attitudes. The PATH Model identifies nine distinct segments based on thinking and behavior among adults that are independent of any demographic, geographic, or socioeconomic factors. These patterns of thinking and behavior describe consumer health care preferences and actions that predict response to marketing communications as well as medical risk levels. By analyzing the ad recall and preference levels across adults based on their PATH type, the health plan was able to evaluate its positioning with consumers who had lower medical risk, lower costs, and higher plan loyalty.

This marketing research study showed that the branding campaign had *not* been successful in attracting consumers with the lower risk PATH types. In particular, the findings revealed that ad recall and brand preference levels among the most desirable consumer types were below average. To compound the problem, the research also revealed that both ad recall and plan preference levels were higher among consumers with PATH types linked to above average medical costs and higher levels of plan loyalty. This represented a double adverse selection outcome. The advertising was helping to both attract and retain higher risk members.

Based on the findings of this research study and the insights revealed by the PATH model, BCBS started afresh and created an advertising campaign more favorably tailored to those adults with lower risk and higher loyalty. Follow-on research confirmed the health plan's success at targeting and appealing to the consumers it wanted to meet its marketing objectives. A few percentage point increases in the representation of PATH types with lower risk and higher loyalty translated into millions of dollars of reduced risk, longer retention of high margin members, and less resources spent on new member recruitment.

OVERVIEW: THE NEED FOR MARKET INFORMATION

The PATH market research helped the Blue Cross/Blue Shield health plan create more effective advertising that led to a more valuable membership mix and increased profitability. Many health care organizations are not as market-driven. Managers in these organizations are often not aware of the capabilities or the range of market research tools available. Interestingly, although physicians always begin patient care with a highly structured and documented patient history and physical exam, most doctors do not apply this same evaluative rigor to making marketing decisions. Often, intuition is the basis for such choices as selecting a location for a satellite office, offering a new medical service, or determining how to increase patient visits. A doctor would not prescribe a drug for an illness by forgoing a thorough patient evaluation and instead relying on guesswork and hoping for the best. Likewise, making management decisions without appropriate market research is perilous to the financial success of the organization.

The health care marketing environment is changing at an accelerating rate, so the need for real-time market information is greater than at any time in the past.

Technology is creating radical shifts in treatment outcomes, locations, costs, and prices. Regulations are decreasing in certain markets and increasing in others. Reimbursement changes frequently. Managers need more information more quickly. Additionally, consumers are becoming increasingly savvy in selecting health care providers and treatments; this push is being fueled largely by the information explosion of the Internet.

To reduce business risk and predict the needs and preferences of both purchasers and users of health care, sellers of health care services and products must turn to marketing research. As sellers attempt to increase their use of branding, product differentiation, advertising, and promotion, they require information on the cost-effectiveness of these marketing tools. The seven characteristics of good market research practice are as follows:[1]

1. *Scientific method:* Effective marketing research uses the principles of the scientific method: careful observation, formulation of hypotheses, prediction, and testing.

2. *Research creativity:* At its best, marketing research develops innovative ways to solve a problem: for example, a hospital catering to heart patients collected consumer demographic and disease interest data through its Web site, then used the data to contact the consumers, inviting them to join an affinity "club" with member meetings and discounts related to heart health.

3. *Multiple methods:* Marketing researchers shy away from overreliance on any one method. They also recognize the value of using two or three methods to increase confidence in the results.

4. *Interdependence of models and data:* Marketing researchers recognize that data are interpreted from underlying models that guide the type of information sought.

5. *Value and cost of information:* Marketing researchers show concern for estimating the value of information against its cost. Costs are typically easy to determine, but the value of research is harder to quantify. It depends on the reliability and validity of the findings and management's willingness to accept and act on those findings.

6. *Healthy skepticism:* Marketing researchers show a healthy skepticism toward glib assumptions made by managers about how a market works. They are alert to the problems caused by "marketing myths."[2]

7. *Ethical marketing:* Marketing research, ethically conducted, benefits both the sponsoring company and its customers. The misuse of marketing research can harm or annoy consumers, increasing their resentment at what they regard as an invasion of their privacy or a disguised sales pitch.

THE COMPONENTS OF A MODERN MARKETING INFORMATION SYSTEM

In today's information-focused society, organizations with superior information enjoy a competitive advantage. The organization can choose its markets better, develop superior offerings, and execute more effective marketing planning.

Health care companies' information systems have quite a wide range of capabilities. Some companies, such as health plans and pharmaceutical firms, have developed marketing information systems that rapidly provide management with valuable detail about customer wants, preferences, and behavior. These systems derive data from diverse sources that range from disease patterns and prevalence to pricing of existing products against competitors' brands. At the other end of the spectrum may be a physician's office that lacks any data compiling capability, keeps paper-based charts, and outsources all of its billing. Still other organizations in the middle of this range may have departments that limit their work to routine patient or customer satisfaction tracking or the occasional community survey.

The marketing manager's role here is to act as the primary two-way conduit between the decision makers in the health care organization and the environment. This manager not only gathers and synthesizes the information that others request, but also suggests what information should be acquired to make more informed decisions at both the operational and strategic levels. To meet these needs, organizations design marketing information systems (MIS), which we define as *people, equipment, and procedures to gather, sort, analyze, evaluate, and distribute needed, timely, and accurate information to decision makers*.

The data for the MIS can come from many sources; for example, internal company records, marketing intelligence activities, marketing research, and marketing decision support analysis. The organization's MIS should balance managers' wants and needs with what is economically feasible. To accomplish this goal, an internal MIS committee should interview a cross-section of managers to discover the firm's information needs. The following are some important questions that must be answered:[3]

1. What decisions do you regularly make?
2. What information do you need to make these decisions?
3. What information do you regularly get?
4. What special studies do you periodically request?
5. What information would you want that you are not getting now?
6. What information would you want daily? Weekly? Monthly? Yearly?
7. What magazines and trade reports would you like to see on a regular basis?
8. What topics would you like to be kept informed of?
9. What data analysis programs would you want?
10. What are the four most helpful improvements that could be made in the present marketing information system?

INTERNAL RECORDS SYSTEM

Examples of internal data that can be useful for health care companies include

- Inpatient admissions patient visits and procedure volume
- Revenue, costs, and margins
- Product sales, procedure volumes
- Prices

- Inventory levels
- Receivables and payables

HEALTH CARE SERVICES: THE CLINICAL AND FINANCIAL SYSTEMS

One important problem many health care organizations face is fragmentation and lack of interoperability among its functional information systems. For example, the heart of the internal records system for any health care service organization resides in the clinical and financial functions, which are often not integrated. Further, even given a single function, like billing or charting patient clinical data, there may be a mix of automated and manual systems, unnecessary duplication of data entry, or wasteful decentralization of inputs. For example, if one follows a patient through a hospital, how many times is the unique registration number manually entered into the system? How often is the patient asked about medications or allergies? Many larger and financially sound hospitals are seeking to remedy these problems by implementing enterprise-wide information systems that will integrate this disparate information and reduce redundancy.

For most health services marketing managers, however, finding, reconciling, and ensuring the accuracy of the clinical and financial data is often a challenge. Table 7.1 describes potential uses of internal records for health care providers. It should be noted that internally generated information will rarely be used alone in making marketing decisions.

HEALTH CARE PRODUCTS: THE ORDER-TO-PAYMENT CYCLE

An increasing number of companies are using the Internet and their proprietary intranets to improve the speed, accuracy, and efficiency of the order-to-payment cycle. In health care product companies, sales representatives, dealers, and customers dispatch orders to the company by fax, e-mail, or on-line communications. The sales department prepares invoices and transmits copies to appropriate departments. Computerized warehouses fill these orders quickly. Out-of-stock items are back ordered. Shipped items are accompanied by shipping and billing documents that are sent to the ordering departments.

For example, Allegiance Healthcare supplies hospital purchasing departments with computers so that the hospitals can electronically transmit their orders. The timely arrival of orders enables Allegiance to cut inventories, improve customer service, and obtain better terms from suppliers for higher volumes.

THE MARKETING INTELLIGENCE SYSTEM (MIS)

Whereas the internal records system supplies results data, the marketing intelligence system supplies external environmental data. These data can come from such

TABLE 7.1. Examples of Internal Records Supporting Health Care Marketing Applications

Marketing Application	Data and Information	Location of Data
Heart Center Marketing Plan	Primary care referral data over the past three years, current baseline use, and capacity of the facility	Physician call center, billing department, personnel staffing records
Service-Line Profitability Analysis	Admissions data sorted by ICD-9CM diagnosis Charge master pricing data	Admissions department, health information management department, patient accounting department
Physician Billing Service Market Share Analysis	Number of physician clients Number of practice clients Number of medical specialties served	Client service department Finance department Coding department
Health Plan Member Profitability Forecast	New member volume trends Premium revenue trends Medical cost trends	Sales department Finance department Actuarial department
Hospital Information System Sales Performance Analysis	Number of referrals Number of sales calls Sales closed to sales call ratios	Marketing call center Field sales management Finance department

secondary sources as books, newspapers and trade publications or can be gathered from primary sources by researching competitors; talking to customers, suppliers, and distributors; and conducting primary marketing research.

The concept of collecting and analyzing market intelligence may be alien to some sectors of the health care market but is routine for others. For example, physicians may not want to admit that they have competitors; pharmaceutical companies, however, take competitors extremely seriously. Collecting and analyzing marketing intelligence is not unethical. An important component of market intelligence is understanding the strengths and weaknesses of competitors. Leonard Fuld, president of Fuld & Company, published a side-by-side comparison of what constitutes good market and competitive intelligence and how it contrasts with some negative perceptions of intelligence gathering (see Table 7.2).[4]

A health care organization can take several steps to improve the quality of its marketing intelligence. First, it can train those in the organization who are closest to the customer to identify customer needs and potential market trends. Although salespeople often are best positioned to fulfill that function, anyone in the organization can contribute to a better understanding of customers, including phone operators, maintenance staff, and other employees with direct customer contact. In addition to training employees to identify opportunities, the organization must also give them the means and appropriate channels to communicate the information. For example, if a

TABLE 7.2. What Is Competitive Intelligence?

Market Competitive Is . . .	Market Competitive Is Not . . .
1. **Information that has been analyzed to the point where you can make a decision.**	**Spying.** Spying implies illegal or unethical activities.
2. **A tool to alert management to early warning of both threats and opportunities.**	**A crystal ball.** There is no such thing as a true forecasting tool. Intelligence does give organizations good approximations of reality, near- and long-term.
3. **A means to deliver reasonable assessments.** Competitive intelligence offers approximations and best views of the market and the competition. It is not a peek at the rival's financial books.	**Database search.** Databases offer just that—data. They certainly do not replace human beings who need to make decisions by examining the data and applying their common sense, experience, analytical tools, and intuition.

(Table 7.2 continued)

4. Comes in many flavors. A research scientist sees it as a heads-up on a competitor's new R&D initiatives. A salesperson considers it insight on how his or her company should bid against another firm in order to win a contract. A senior manager believes intelligence to be a long-term view on a marketplace and its rivals.	**The Internet or rumor chasing.** The Internet is primarily a communications vehicle, not a deliverer of intelligence. You can find hints at competitive strategy, but you will also uncover rumors disguised as fact, or speculation dressed up as reality.
5. A way for companies to improve their bottom line.	**Paper.** Think face-to-face discussion or a quick phone call if you can, rather than paper delivery. Unfortunately, many managers think that by spending countless hours on computer-generated slides, charts and graphs, and footnoted reports, they have delivered intelligence.
6. A way of life, a process. If a company uses competitive intelligence correctly, it becomes a way of life for *everyone* in the organization—not just the strategic planning or marketing staff. It is a process by which critical information is available for anyone who needs it.	**A job for one smart person.** At best, the director of marketing keeps management informed and ensures that others in the organization become trained in ways to apply this tool.
7. Part of all best-in-class companies. Best-in-class organizations apply competitive intelligence consistently. The Malcolm Baldrige Quality Award, the most prestigious total quality award for American corporations, includes the gathering and use of external competitive information as one of its winning qualifications.	**An invention of the 20th century.** Competitive intelligence has been around as long as business itself. The 19th century British financier Nathan Rothschild cornered the market on British government securities by using carrier pigeons to receive early warning of Napoleon's defeat at Waterloo.

(Table 7.2 continued)

8. Directed from the executive suite. The best-in-class intelligence efforts receive their direction and impetus from the CEO. While the CEO may not run the program, he dedicates budget and personnel; most important, he promotes its use.	**Software.** Software does not in and of itself yield intelligence. It collects, contrasts, and compares. True analysis is a process of people reviewing and making sense of the information.
9. Seeing outside yourself. Organizations that successfully apply competitive intelligence gain an ability to see outside themselves. Competitive intelligence pushes the not-invented-here syndrome out the window.	**A news story.** While media reports may yield interesting sources for the competitive intelligence analyst to interview, they are not always the most timely or specific enough for critical business decisions.
10. Both short- and long-term. A company can use intelligence for many immediate decisions, such as how to price a product or place an advertisement. At the same time, you can use the same set of data to decide on long-term product development or market positioning.	**A spreadsheet.** Intelligence comes in many forms, only one of which is a spreadsheet or some quantifiable result. Management thinking, marketing strategy, and ability to innovate are only three among a host of issues that rely on a wide range of subjective, non-numeric intelligence.

Source: Fuld, ''What Competitive Intelligence Is and Is Not!'' [http://fuld.com/Company/CI.html], March 2007.

pharmaceutical sales representative finds out from physicians that two local hospitals are merging and will be consolidating drug purchases, what method does she use and to whom does she communicate this information to make sure it gets to the right people in a timely fashion? To encourage such communication, the drug firm could set up a reward program for those who exchange valuable intelligence. An organization could also identify those who are in a position to gather intelligence about competitors and industry trends, such as salespeople who call on the organization and also on their competitors, experts who speak at professional association meetings, and exhibitors at trade shows who also work with their competitors.

Secondary data sources are also useful. For example, marketers can access free e-mail subscriptions to daily news pertaining to health care market changes. Two sources of these e-mail services are HealthLeaders magazine (www.healthleadersmedia .com), which delivers daily links to news articles in publications across the nation, and America's Health Insurance Plans (www.ahip.org).

Companies can also collect competitive intelligence from other publicly available information about competitors. For example, valuable information can be obtained by purchasing competitors' products; attending their open houses; exhibiting at trade shows; reading their published reports (including financial filings, if they are publicly traded firms); attending stockholders' meetings; talking to their employees, dealers, distributors, suppliers, and freight agents; and collecting their ads.

The organization can set up an advisory panel made up of its representative, largest, most outspoken, or most sophisticated customers. For example, Hitachi Data Systems, which sells data storage technology to health care organizations, holds a three-day meeting with its customer panel of twenty members every nine months. They discuss service issues, new technologies, and customers' strategic requirements. The discussion is free-flowing, and both parties gain: Hitachi gains valuable information about customer needs, and the customers feel more bonded to a company that listens closely to their comments.[5]

Another advisory panel could include industry experts. For example, medical device manufacturers have scientific advisory panels made up of physicians or engineers to recommend product innovations or marketing techniques to enhance customer satisfaction. The organization can purchase information from outside suppliers such as the A.C. Nielsen Company, Press Ganey, IMS, or Information Resources, Inc. These research firms can often gather more and better data at a much lower cost than the company could manage on its own, and they can provide industry-wide comparisons for benchmarking.

Regardless of the sources, organizations should balance internal access to this intelligence with the need to keep it safe and secure. Such tools as read-only files and password-protected intranets can help achieve this balance. A number of different types of software programs are available to meet the needs for organizing and distributing market intelligence. Such software can perform the following sample tasks:[6]

- *Organize, analyze, and distribute competitor information.* This software is useful for short, up-to-date reports that compare products or services, profile companies and key people, and the like, so that others in your company who "just want to use the information" can easily get the reports via a browser, without ever having to learn how to use a new piece of software. Example: STRATEGY! software (www.strategy-software.com).

- *Organize information about your competitive environment for easier analysis.* A relational database will help meet this need. Examples: STRATEGY! software (www.strategy-software.com); Wincite Systems (www.wincite.com).

- *Monitor competitors' Web sites automatically.* If a competitor's Web site changes, the tool will let you know and show you *only* what has changed since the last time you saw it. Examples: Copernic Tracker (www.copernic.com/en/products/tracker).

- *Search for and compile very specific information automatically from the Internet.* Useful, for example, to find any discussion about Pfizer happening anywhere on the Internet, including expressions of dissatisfaction that may occur in chat groups, and so on. Example: WebQL Software (www.caesius.com).

- *Provide and facilitate a competitor intelligence (CI) workflow system, or portal solution.* This software is useful if you need a system specifically designed for organizations where top executives post key intelligence questions to their analysts. The analysts can then compile documents for analysis and commentary. Examples: Cipher Systems (www.cipher-sys.com).

- *Furnish a decision-support software.* This software helps ask questions of a group trying to arrive at a specific decision in a disciplined way. Example: Wisdombuilder (www.wisdombuilder.com).

- *Establish a database that is designed and built to meet exact structural expectations that you have already identified.* This software is useful if you have an idea of exactly what you need in terms of how your market information should be structured in a relational database framework. Example: Wincite, (www.wincite.com); alternatively, a contractor can provide custom software and database programming.

- *Use the work product solely for your own benefit.* This software compiles information about people, products, and companies that are most important to you; it is not intended to generate reports or share with others. Example: Microsoft Excel (www.microsoft.com/excel).

- *Track and understand what people are saying about your company, products, or services.* Consulting and technology services can be used to monitor what is being said about your brand and competitors' brands on the Internet. Example: Brandpulse by Intelliseek (www.intelliseek.com).

MARKETING RESEARCH SYSTEM

We define *marketing research* as the systematic design, collection, analysis, and reporting of data and findings relevant to a specific marketing situation facing the company.

Marketing research acts as a risk reduction tool. Managers can verify assumptions, gain new insights into consumers and competitors, and recognize emerging market opportunities. It is the primary job of the marketing researcher to identify and analyze market data and information and to offer the perspective of the customer.

Preview of the Marketing Research Process

Alan Andreasen recommends that we begin our research journey with the end in mind. He calls this "backward research" and states, "The secret here is to start with the decisions to be made and to make certain that the research helps management reach those decisions."[7]

As an overview, here are eight areas of questions that must be answered when planning a research project:

1. *Purpose:* What decisions will this research will help inform? What are the questions that you need this research to help answer?

2. *Informational objectives:* What specific information do you need to make this decision or answer these questions?

3. *Audience:* From whom do you need the information? Whose opinion matters?

4. *Technique:* What is the most efficient and effective way to gather this information?

5. *Sample size, source, and selection:* How many respondents should you survey, given your desired statistical confidence levels? Where will you get names of potential respondents? How do you select (draw) your sample from this population to ensure your data are representative of your target audience for the research?

6. *Pretest and fielding:* Who will pretest the survey instrument (such as a questionnaire, focus group discussion guide) and conduct the research, and when?

7. *Analysis:* How will data be analyzed and by whom, to meet the planners' needs?

8. *Report:* What information should be included in the report, and what format should be used for reporting?

Exploratory Marketing Research

After considering these questions and reviewing internal records systems and market intelligence systems, exploratory research will help the marketer more fully understand the organization's marketing decisions in the context of the environment. Exploratory research includes secondary data gathering, as well as surveying primary sources, such as interviewing individuals and groups.

Secondary Data Research. Secondary sources are publicly available data that have been previously collected. The appendix at the end of this chapter shows a sample of the rich variety of available secondary data sources.[8] Data obtained in this fashion provide a starting point for analysis and offer the advantages of low cost and ready availability.

Although secondary data are likely to provide many useful ideas and findings, the researcher must be careful in making inferences. These data were often collected for purposes and under conditions that might be different from those the researcher desires and, thus, might limit their usefulness. Because researchers may find that the secondary data still leave many questions unanswered, they may need to collect primary data, through either observation or interviewing.

Primary Marketing Research

Primary marketing research is defined as data that is collected for the first time and is customized to fit a specific need.

Primary data are most often collected in five ways: informal observation, focus groups, qualitative surveys, quantitative surveys, and behavioral research. The most appropriate choice of a methodology hinges on cost-benefit trade-offs and the questions the study is intended to answer. In determining which method is best, the organization should ask itself: How soon does it need the information? How critical is the information to making the *next* decision? What resources (money, time, and personnel) can it afford to devote? Is there a better way to get the information at a lower cost?

Observational Research. New data can be gathered by observing the relevant actors and settings. Northwestern Memorial Hospital in Chicago regularly contracts with professional "mystery shoppers" who pose as hospital patients. These researchers visit Northwestern's competitors—as well as Northwestern itself—and note how they are treated by registration clerks, nursing staff, physicians, and others. They also listen and observe how employees respond to each other and listen to surrounding patients tell stories and make comments. This exploratory research can yield some useful hypotheses about how patients feel about different hospitals and their services.

Focus Group Research. Focus group research is very popular among health care service organizations because it is relatively low cost. A focus group is a gathering of eight to ten people who are invited to spend a few hours with a skilled moderator to discuss a product, service, organization, or other marketing entity. The participants should be representative of the market segments related to the research focus (for example, women likely to use maternity services, primary care physicians with above-average cardiology referral volume, or key opinion leaders in oncology research). The moderator needs to be objective, knowledgeable on the issue, and skilled in group dynamics. The moderator encourages free and easy discussion, hoping that the group dynamics will reveal deep feelings and thoughts, while at the same time focusing the discussion on the subject in a neutral fashion. Critics have argued that although focus groups have an advantage in bringing many people together at the same time, they could potentially suffer from "group think" and distort individual opinions. A skilled focus group moderator significantly reduces this risk.

Focus group research is a form of qualitative research whose conclusions cannot be projected to the entire market.[9] To be able to project results to the *entire* market, researchers much conduct *quantitative* research studies based on statistically valid and reliable methods, using randomized samples of sufficient size (see the following section on survey research). Focus groups provide directional data if participant response patterns emerge over the course of at least four or five groups. Ideally, the results from the focus group research are followed by a form of quantitative research to statistically test the hypotheses and conclusions. Focus groups follow a structured discussion guide and often include:

- Free associations (to learn top-of-mind thoughts and feelings about a specific topic)

- Conceptual mapping (to graphically map concepts and their associative meanings maps)

- Perceptual mapping (to identify a brand's strengths and weaknesses on selected key attributes relative to the competition)

- Mind mapping (a technique to capture free associations on paper in a nonlinear way)

- Concept statement testing (often used to measure resonance with an advertisement or new product concept)

- Story telling

The discussion—which is recorded through note taking, captured on audiotape or videotape, or observed by researchers behind a one-way mirror—is subsequently studied to understand consumer beliefs, attitudes, and behavior. Findings are analyzed, conclusions are synthesized, and the results of the groups along with next steps are reported and presented.

The Pros and Cons of On-Line Focus Groups

On-line focus groups and web-based surveys are two recent innovations in qualitative research. Using a secure DSL line and a chat-mediated, web-based virtual room, respondents with access to personal computers and web browsers are recruited, based on research specifications. Because the respondents cannot see one another, they tend to speak very freely. In addition, respondents who would be quiet in a traditional focus group tend to come out more in this situation. Clients are able to witness the entire session from their own PCs. In the privacy of the researcher's virtual backroom, clients can communicate with one another from different locations, as well as with the moderator. The respondents do not see these backroom communications. The entire session is automatically recorded and a verbatim transcript is available immediately.[10]

The disadvantages of on-line focus groups are many. The security of the internet focus group is not nearly as tight as it is with live sessions. As a result, in the internet environment you never know who is really talking, as opposed to a live situation in which participants must have photo identification to be considered for the group.

The inability to view body language is also a drawback because the nonverbal response of a participant in a focus group is as important as what the participant says in terms of determining the participant's feelings toward a particular topic under discussion. Although the internet focus group technique is not nearly as encumbered by the problems of one person influencing the other, there is not the same sense of community and sharing of information in this milieu as in a live group discussion. Further, the moderator becomes more of a "traffic cop" in the internet environment, whereas in a live focus group this individual is integral to the flow and dynamics of the group setting.

Another important benefit of traditional focus groups that does not exist with the internet version is the ability to show external stimuli to the people in the groups to obtain their reactions. An example is storyboards for a new advertising campaign or a new packaging design for a household product. Although it is possible to send images over the Internet to people to get their reactions, in the current state of the technology there can be major problems in terms of both the quality of the ultimate image that is downloaded and the speed with which it is received. Further, the image is only two-dimensional in the internet world, whereas with in-person focus groups, the stimuli can be three-dimensional and involve other senses such as touch, sound, or taste.[11] For example, taste-testing a liquid medication additive for texture and palatability obviously cannot be accomplished on-line.

Individual In-Depth Interview Research. Another type of research is the individual in-depth interview. Here a skilled interviewer spends one or two hours with one interviewee posing probing questions. The assumption is that the interviewee may not be fully conscious of the reasons for his or her behavior or may have erected many defenses against honest or complete answers. The interviewer may use projective techniques such as word associations or filling in the blanks to gain a deeper understanding of the person's perceptions, preferences, and decision processes. The interviewer may interview several such persons on this one-to-one basis until some common insights are discovered and further interviews are unnecessary. Although less efficient than focus groups, in-depth interviews are more private and can elicit different insights.

Survey Research. Surveys are best suited for descriptive research. Organizations undertake surveys to learn about people's knowledge, beliefs, preferences, and satisfaction, and to measure their magnitudes in the general population. Here are several examples of survey techniques:

- Customized questionnaires that are organization-specific; for example, to determine public views of a particular hospital, pharmaceutical company, product or service

- Industry questionnaires with added organization-specific questions; for example, to determine the position of the organization, product, or service in the marketplace

- Questions to an ongoing consumer panel run by itself or an independent marketing research firm

- A mall intercept study that asks people in a shopping mall to volunteer to answer research questions

Surveys can be either qualitative or quantitative. Small sample surveys of twenty-five to two hundred respondents—that may or may not use random samples—can yield helpful information by using the telephone, mail, or on-line interviewing. Qualitative survey data can be directional, but cannot be used to draw conclusions about the entire market. The key is to identify consistencies in the patterns of responses that may be used to identify marketing hypotheses.

Sampling plan. The first question to be answered in primary marketing research is, who does it make the most sense to interview? Designing a sampling plan calls for three decisions:

- Sampling unit: Who is to be surveyed?

- Sample size: How many people should be surveyed?

- Sampling procedure: How should the respondents be chosen?

Sampling unit: Who is to be surveyed? The marketing researcher must define the target population that will be sampled. Should we base our survey more on the opinions of "heavy users" of our services, or should we give more weight to those who have less experience whom we would like to recruit? If the survey will use a random sampling, then a sampling frame must be developed so that everyone in the target population has an equal or known chance of being sampled.

Sample size: How many people should be surveyed? The "real" answer to a survey question can be found if everyone in the market answers a question. Sampling is done because asking every member of a market a series of questions is not feasible. Although it is often assumed that the larger the sample the better, the most important element of a sample is not its size, but its variability. For example, the answer given to the question "What color is a clear sky?" is highly likely to be "blue" and have a low level of variability. In contrast, the answer to the question "What are the main problems of the U.S. health care system?" has a much higher variability. For technical reasons, the closer the result is to 50 percent, the larger the confidence range is around that result. Because there is no one confidence range for a sample of a particular size, most researchers talk in terms of the maximum sampling error (the error when the observed percentage result is 50 percent) when selecting a sample size for study.

Table 7.3 can be read in the following manner: in a random sample of 400 interviews, if an observed percentage result is 50 percent, the chances are approximately 95 in 100 that a range of ±5 percent (45 percent to 55 percent) includes the true percentage results in the entire population. As a rule of thumb, the minimum recommended sample size for a random sample is 200.

TABLE 7.3. **Range of Sampling Errors (Plus and Minus) Due to Sample Size (95 Percent Confidence Level)**

Sample Size	Percentage Result Obtained			
	50 Percent	40 Percent or 60 Percent	30 Percent or 70 Percent	20 Percent or 80 Percent
25	+20.0	+19.6	+18.3	+16.0
75	11.5	11.3	10.5	9.2
100	10.0	9.8	9.2	8.0
150	8.2	8.0	7.5	6.6
200	7.1	7.0	6.5	5.7
400	5.0	4.9	4.6	4.0
600	4.1	4.0	3.8	3.3
1,000	3.2	3.1	2.9	2.6
3,000	1.8	1.7	1.7	1.5

Sampling procedure: How should the respondents be chosen? A computerized random number generator is one method for selecting participants for a survey using a random sample. When the cost or time involved in probability sampling is too high, marketing researchers will take non-probability samples. The following list describes three types of probability sampling and three types of non-probability sampling. Some marketing researchers believe that non-probability samples are very useful in many circumstances, even though they do not allow sampling error to be measured. For example, pharmaceutical companies conduct sample opinion research from "thought leaders" in the relevant clinical discipline.

Probability Sample

■ *Simple random sample:* Every member of the population has an equal chance of selection.

- *Stratified random sample:* The population is divided into mutually exclusive groups (such as age groups), and random samples are drawn from each group.
- *Cluster (area) sample:* The population is divided into mutually exclusive groups (such as city blocks), and the researcher draws a sample of the groups to interview.

Non-Probability Sample

- *Convenience sample:* The researcher selects the most accessible population members.
- *Judgment sample:* The researcher selects population members who are good prospects for accurate information.
- *Quota sample:* The researcher finds and interviews a prescribed number of people in each of several categories.

Questionnaires. *Questionnaire content*. A questionnaire consists of a set of questions presented to respondents. Because of its flexibility, the questionnaire is by far the most common instrument used to collect primary data. Questionnaires need to be carefully developed, tested, validated, and debugged before they are administered on a large scale. For example, numerous studies have shown that opinions about institutions are very different from those about individuals: "How do you feel about physicians?" and "How do you feel about *your* physician?" elicit very different responses.

Questionnaire development. The research questions should reflect the study's research issues, which in turn are based on the marketing decisions being considered. The questionnaire developer should exercise care in the wording and sequencing of questions. The survey must use simple, direct, unbiased wording and be pretested with a sample of respondents. A few general rules are: (1) the lead question should attempt to create interest, (2) difficult or personal questions should be asked toward the end, and (3) the questions should flow in a logical order.

Marketing researchers distinguish between closed-end and open-end questions. Closed-end questions specify all the possible answers and provide answers that are easier to interpret and tabulate. Open-end questions allow respondents to answer in their own words and often reveal more about how people think. They are especially useful in exploratory research, in which the researcher is looking for insight into how people think and feel about a product or issue rather than in measuring how many people think a certain way.

Methods of contact to administer questionnaires. In preparing a questionnaire, the researcher carefully chooses how the survey respondents will be reached: through mail, telephone, personal, or on-line interview.

The *mail questionnaire* is the best way to reach people who would not give personal interviews or whose responses might be biased or distorted by the interviewers. Mail questionnaires require simple and clearly worded questions. Unfortunately, the response rate is usually low or slow.

A majority of hospitals rely on mail questionnaires for patient satisfaction data. Questionnaires are mailed to all discharged patients, and because they do not have an incentive to return the survey, the rate of return is often less than 30 percent; a high level of nonresponse bias in the data occurs if the rate of return is less than 70 percent. The results, therefore, represent a convenience sample, not a random sample. Although most of the responses in this type of survey are very positive (and thus of little true statistical value), the extremely dissatisfied patients who are often motivated to respond may serve as a good disaster check and signal to improve service.

Telephone interviewing is the best method for gathering information quickly. The interviewer is able to clarify questions if respondents do not understand them, and the response rate is typically higher, around 85 percent, depending on the quality of the sample. The main drawback is that the interviewers have only a limited time before the respondent loses interest in the survey or simply hangs up the phone. Telephone interviewing is getting more difficult because of answering machines, caller ID, and people's general suspicions of telemarketing. Using this method in the business-to-business environment works well if the interviewee is paid.

Personal interviewing, or in-depth interviewing (IDI), is the most versatile method. The interviewer can ask more questions and record additional observations about the respondent, such as dress and body language. However, personal interviewing is the most expensive method and requires more administrative planning and supervision than the other three. It is also subject to interviewer bias or distortion.

Personal interviewing takes two forms. In *arranged interviews*, respondents are contacted for an appointment, and often a small payment or incentive is offered. *Intercept interviews* involve stopping people at a shopping mall or busy street corner and requesting an interview. Intercept interviews have the drawback of being non-probability samples, and they must not require too much time.

Market researchers are using *on-line interviewing* more frequently because it provides information faster than traditional research techniques. On-line techniques include the following:

- Including a questionnaire on the organization's Web site and offering an incentive for responses.
- Placing a banner on some frequently visited sites (such as Yahoo!), inviting people to answer some questions and enter a drawing to win a prize.
- Entering a target chat room and seeking volunteers for a survey.

In collecting data on-line, however, the company must recognize that because the participants are self-selected, the responses are not representative of a target population. The opinions of consumers who do not use the Internet or who do not want to answer a questionnaire are missing. Still, the information can be useful for exploratory research in suggesting hypotheses that might be investigated subsequently in a more scientific survey.

Behavioral Research. Behavioral research focuses on measures of actual behavior to describe health care consumers. Product scanning in grocery store check-outs collects data representing purchase behaviors. In a health care context, the number of visits to a doctor's office, the number of visits to an emergency department, and the number of prescription refills all represent measures of behavior. Behavioral research focuses on what happens, but it cannot explain *why* something happens.

THE PATH MODEL: UNDERSTANDING THE HEALTH CARE CONSUMER

Attitudinal research, also referred to as psychographics, focuses on measures of attitudes, opinions, and interests. It attempts to identify the "why" behind the observed behavior. In health care, the Profiles of Activities and Attitudes Toward Healthcare (PATH) Model is a hybrid between the two approaches. PATH takes measures of *described* behavior (for example, "I regularly participate in active or competitive sports") and beliefs (for example, "Doctors often prescribe drugs to patients without knowing all the side effects") and uses these measures to infer health priorities. Health priorities are more relevant than attitudes, because priorities are what actually shape our behavior. Behavior indicates priorities.

PATH has been linked to health care trends including prevalence of disease, claims rates, patient satisfaction, loyalty, response to interventions, communications, and adherence levels. For example, PATH is used in hospital marketing communications to attract patients with specific diseases. It is also used by health plans to avoid adverse selection and increase member loyalty. Additionally, PATH is used in demand management and disease management interventions to improve outcomes among employees or consumers with chronic conditions, such as diabetes, hypertension, or cancer.

The PATH Model essentially identifies and explains the dynamics of consumer health buying behavior. It is the most researched, tested, validated, and applied consumer behavior model in the field. Its efficacy stems from the fact that up to 45 percent of an individual's actual health service utilization can be explained by health-related perceptions and attitudes.[12]

Here is how the PATH model works:

1. Consumers answer a twenty-question questionnaire.

2. The questionnaire results are entered into the PATH Model algorithm.

3. The questionnaire responses are evaluated across eleven health care dimensions that have been found to be most predictive of health care attitudes and behavior.

4. Consumers are classified into the nine PATH groups.

The nine PATH types and the eleven health care dimensions are shown in Figure 7.1. The relationships between PATH classifications and health care management applications are shown in Figure 7.2.

Collecting Research Data

The data collection phase of marketing research is generally the most expensive and the most prone to error. In the case of surveys, four major problems arise: (1) some respondents will not be reachable and must be recontacted or replaced, (2) some respondents will refuse to cooperate, (3) some respondents will give biased or dishonest answers, and (4) some interviewers will be biased or dishonest. Yet data collection methods are rapidly improving, thanks to computers and more sophisticated telecommunications. For example, computers now automate the key activities of a telephone interviewing facility. Computer-assisted telephone interviewing systems, or CATI, support interviewers in conducting interviews. The software manages the questionnaire, skip patterns are executed exactly as intended, responses are within range, and there are no missing data. CATI systems also allow survey responses to be entered directly into electronic databases and manual data entry is eliminated.

Analyzing the Information

The next step in the marketing research process is to extract findings from the collected data. The researcher tabulates the data and computes frequency distributions, averages and measures of dispersion for the major variables. The researcher also applies some advanced statistical techniques and decision models in the hope of discovering additional findings. The following are several quantitative tools used in marketing decision support systems.

1. *Multiple regression:* A statistical technique for estimating a "best fitting" equation, showing how the value of a dependent variable varies with changing values in a number of independent variables. *Example:* A pharmaceutical company can estimate how unit sales are influenced by changes in the level of company advertising expenditures, sales force size, and price.

2. *Discriminant analysis:* Classifies an object or persons into two or more categories. *Example*: A large pharmacy retail chain can determine the variables that discriminate between successful and unsuccessful store locations.

3. *Factor analysis:* Determines the few underlying dimensions of a larger set of intercorrelated variables. *Example:* A medical device company is interested in isolating those personality traits of its salespeople that are most likely to lead to success in selling sophisticated, complex, customized equipment to orthopedic surgeons.

4. *Cluster analysis:* Separates objects into a specified number of mutually exclusive groups so that the groups are relatively homogeneous. *Example*: An

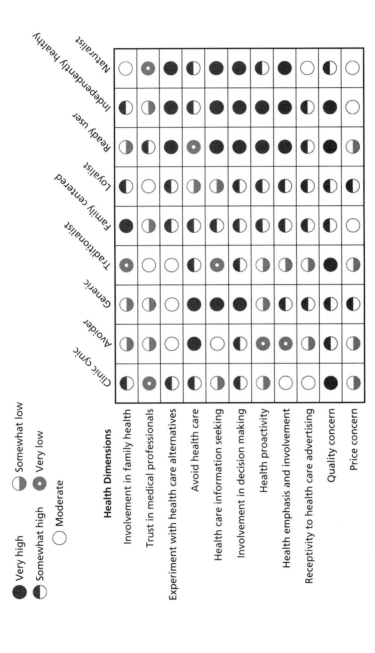

FIGURE 7.1. *Nine PATH Profiles and Eleven Dimensions*

Source: PATH Institute, Fontana, Calif.

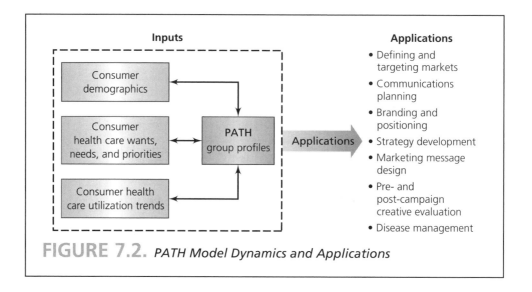

FIGURE 7.2. *PATH Model Dynamics and Applications*

academic medical center marketing researcher wants to classify a set of cities into four distinct groups to decide where to expand its world-renowned services.

5. *Conjoint analysis:* Respondents' ranked preferences are deconstructed to determine the inferred utility function for each attribute and their relative importance. *Example:* A health plan can determine the total utility delivered by different combinations of benefits for a given premium.

6. *Multidimensional scaling:* Produces perceptual maps of competitive products or brands. Objects are represented as points in a multidimensional space of attributes in which their distance from one another is a measure of dissimilarity. *Example:* A health information systems company wants to see where its brand is positioned in relation to competitive brands.

Presenting the Findings and Conclusions

As the second-to-last step, the researcher presents the findings that are relevant to the major marketing decisions facing management. Health care service organizations often find that they have a high volume of data but lack a focused analysis committed to actionable decisions.

Making the Decision

The managers who commissioned the research need to weigh the evidence, understanding that the findings could suffer from a variety of errors. If their confidence in the findings is low, they may decide against introducing the new service or product. They may even decide to study the issues further and do more research. The decision is theirs, but the hope is that if the new product or service is introduced to the market, the research will provide them with insight to make the launch successful, and measure ongoing results.

MARKETING DECISION SUPPORT SYSTEM

A growing number of organizations are using a *marketing decision support system* (MDSS) to help their marketing managers make better decisions. An MDSS is a coordinated collection of data, systems, tools, and techniques with supporting software and hardware with which an organization gathers and interprets relevant information from its own business and the environment and turns it into a basis for marketing action.[13] Sometimes referred to as a "marketing information dashboard," key indicators of marketing and business performance are automatically updated and made available on managers' computer desktops.

Suppliers of Marketing Research

Companies generally budget marketing research at 1 percent to 2 percent of total revenue. Most large health care product companies have their own marketing research departments, which often outsource data collection and reporting, using third parties to ensure study confidentiality and to minimize bias. If the research participants know that, for example, the medical device manufacturer Boston Scientific is sponsoring the study, the participants' personal feelings and biases about the company and its products will likely influence their responses.

Health care service companies are less likely to have their own research departments because market research is often a low priority. Hospitals, for example, may contract with an outside research company to conduct patient satisfaction research. They may also subscribe to a market research service that provides regular information based on secondary data about the hospital environment. The research data received from the latter source is not usually tied to specific marketing decisions, and its accuracy, value, and cost-effectiveness can be questionable. Also, to be useful, there must be a group of comparable organizations for benchmarking purposes.

If health care firms choose to outsource their marketing research, there are numerous choices. The *GreenBook® Worldwide Directory of Marketing Research Companies and Services*, published by the New York Chapter of the American Marketing Association, lists seventeen health care categories, out of a total of over four hundred categories that represent thousands of market research companies globally. These companies fall into three major categories:

1. *Syndicated service research firms.* These firms specialize in collecting continuous consumer and trade information, which they sell in the form of standardized product reports on a subscription fee basis to all clients. The Advisory Board, based in Washington, D.C., provides health care market study reports based on the collective interests of their health care clients. By sharing the financial burden of conducting this wide-ranging, often qualitative research, the Advisory

Board members can purchase this information at a lower price than if they commissioned it individually.

2. *Custom marketing research firms.* These types of firms develop research studies based on the needs of specific clients. The cost of conducting this type of research depends on the type of research conducted (qualitative, quantitative, psychographic, and so on), the number of interviews or research participants involved, and the level of analytical sophistication needed. The cost and scope of custom marketing research can be scaled to help make low to high risk and return marketing decisions.

3. *Specialty-line marketing research firms.* These firms provide specialized services to other marketing research firms and to organizations' marketing departments. The best example is a field service firm—such as the Telephone Centre in Greensboro, North Carolina—that sells telephone and on-line interviewing services to clients who are capable of preparing their own questionnaires, gathering their own data, conducting analysis, and reporting results.[14]

Overcoming Barriers to the Use of Marketing Research

In spite of the rapid growth of marketing research, many companies still fail to use it sufficiently or correctly, for several reasons:[15]

■ *A narrow conception of the research:* Many managers see marketing research as a fact-finding operation. They expect the researcher to design a questionnaire, choose a sample, conduct interviews, and report results, often without a careful definition of the problem or of the decisions facing management. When fact-finding fails to be useful, management's idea of the limited usefulness of marketing research is reinforced.

■ *Uneven caliber of researchers:* Some managers view marketing research as little more than a clerical activity and treat it as such. Less competent marketing researchers are hired, and their weak training and deficient creativity lead to unimpressive results. The disappointing results reinforce management's prejudice against marketing research. Management continues to pay low salaries to its market researchers, thus perpetuating the problem.

■ *Poor framing of the problem:* In the famous case when Coca-Cola introduced the New Coke brand after much research, its failure was largely due to not setting up the research problem correctly. The issues concerned how consumers felt about Coca-Cola as a brand and the longer-term taste of the product—not a quick taste-test in isolation.

■ *Late and occasionally erroneous findings:* Managers want results that are cheap, accurate, conclusive, and fast—but good marketing research takes time and money. Managers need to recognize that they will trade off accuracy if speed and price are their highest priorities.

■ *Personality and presentational differences:* Differences between the styles of line or operations managers and marketing researchers often get in the way of productive relationships. To a manager who wants concreteness, simplicity, and certainty, a marketing researcher's report may seem abstract, complicated, and tentative. Yet in more progressive organizations, marketing researchers are increasingly being included as members of the product management team, and their influence on overall strategy is growing.

DEVELOPING A MARKETING RESEARCH PLAN: APPLICATION AND EXAMPLE

Developing a plan is the first step in an effective marketing research study. The purpose of a marketing research plan is to ensure that the needs of all the organization's stakeholders are being met and that the marketing research results and process are clearly communicated and approved. The example illustrates how a physician practice used marketing research to increase its market share.

1. Background

The Background section of the plan briefly provides an overview of the situation. It can include changing environmental or market conditions, product innovations, corporate vision, or other events or circumstances that have prompted the need for marketing research. The following sample would be prepared as part of a contract with an outside consulting firm.

FOR EXAMPLE

Regional Radiology (RR) had an opportunity to expand its imaging services in a new geographic market segment by leasing office space to provide four-slice CT imaging services. RR had forecast that the proposed office would break even with eight hundred scans annually or approximately 3.2 scans per day. There were no other office locations currently being considered for evaluation.

2. Marketing Research Recommendation

The research recommendation includes three sections: (a) marketing decisions, (b) research objectives, and (c) research methodology.

a. Marketing Decisions. Thinking through the decisions to be made with the research results will lead to a higher likelihood of action being taken; however, the marketing problem should not be defined too narrowly in the context of the research study.

- Should Regional Radiology invest in the equipment, space, and staff to open a satellite office in this new location?
- If they do invest, which specific area referring physicians should RR target?
- Based on referring physician preferences, what would be the best approach for building awareness, trial, and preference for this new CT imaging service?
- What other related services could RR potentially provide to meet the needs of referring physicians (for example, ultrasound or MRI)?

b. Marketing Research Objectives. This section of the research plan focuses on the research data and information that must be collected to support the marketing decisions. In this particular situation, the marketing decision to establish, or not establish, a new satellite office relied on analyzing the data elements listed below.

- Profile specific physicians likely to refer patients to the new CRR office.
- Estimate the total number of CT imaging referrals by area physicians.
- Identify and rank the factors most important in referral decisions and in changing referral patterns.
- Measure levels of satisfaction with imaging center competitors.
- Estimate referral share percentage by competitor among survey respondents.
- Identify related market opportunities for CRR.
- Specify strategies to build CRR referrals.

c. Marketing Research Methodology. The selection of the best research methodology depends on the nature of the research needed and the available budget. The marketing manager needs to balance the cost of the research with its value. Secondary research should always be conducted first. If the secondary research is unable to provide the data needed to make the marketing decisions, primary research should be considered.

Selecting a primary research methodology calls for decisions on the data sources, research approaches, research instruments, sampling plan, and contact methods.

d. Work Plan. The work plan, based on the marketing decisions and research issues, details the process and workflow needed to complete the market research project.

e. Schedule and Costs. The final step estimates the time and money to complete the project.

FOR EXAMPLE

Phase I. We will review the area population growth projections and other secondary market data that RR has already collected. We will develop a sampling plan to complete telephone interviews based on the RR list of referring physicians and physician extenders. We expect to complete ten interviews in the four targeted zip codes, based on our preliminary review of the list, but we are interested in completing additional interviews if possible.

A questionnaire will be developed, incorporating the research issues that will help us collect the information needed to make the best marketing decisions. We will work closely with RR to refine the survey instrument to ensure that it captures the data needed. The questionnaire will be pretested to identify any opportunities to improve clarity and execution.

Phase II. We will look up the telephone numbers of the prospective physician respondents and contact them by phone to obtain their fax numbers. We will then send a fax advising them that we will be conducting a telephone survey and requesting their participation. To prepare the physicians for the interview, the letter will include the survey topics. As an incentive for participation, the physician will be offered a $50.00 honorarium for completing the five-to-seven-minute interview.

We will phone each physician to schedule an interview. Additionally, we will leave a toll-free phone number for the physicians to call us, if they wish, to arrange an interview appointment. The respondents will *not* know that CRR is sponsoring this study.

Phase III. We will tabulate and analyze the data and write a detailed report that includes study conclusions, findings, and indicated actions. A written report will be delivered along with a summary presentation.

FOR EXAMPLE

We anticipate that the Phase I sampling plan and questionnaire development process can be completed within one week from proposal approval. The field work of Phase II can be completed in two weeks. The Phase III analysis, reporting, and presentation stage will be completed within one week from the conclusion of the field work. The entire study will be completed within four weeks.

We estimate the cost of such a study is about $10,000 including all questionnaire development, sample, honoraria, analysis, reporting, and the on-site presentation. Of course, the exact amount will vary by location and scope of work.

FORECASTING AND DEMAND MEASUREMENT

One major reason for undertaking marketing research is to identify new market prospects by measuring and forecasting the size, growth, and profit potential of each opportunity. Sales forecasts, based on demand estimates, are used by finance departments, to plan for the needed cash for investment and operations; by manufacturing, to establish capacity and output levels; by purchasing, to acquire the right amount of supplies; and by human resources, to hire the needed number of workers. Although marketers are responsible for preparing the sales forecasts based on estimates of demand, managers need to define what they mean by market demand. The first step is to determine which market to measure.

Which Market to Measure?

In determining the size of a market, we offer some working definitions about the number of buyers who might exist for a particular offer. Let us start with the definition of *market:* the set of all actual and potential buyers of a firm's offer.

The *potential market* is the set of consumers who profess a sufficient level of interest in a market offer; but consumer interest is not enough to define a market. Potential consumers must have enough income and must have access to the product. The *available market* is the set of consumers who have interest, income, *and* access to a particular offer.

For some products, the company or government may restrict sales to certain groups. For example, many drug sales require a prescription from a physician. In this case, the eligibles constitute the *qualified available market:* the set of consumers who have interest, income, access, and qualifications for the particular market offer.

A company can go after the whole available market or concentrate on certain segments. The *target market* is the part of the qualified available population the organization decides to pursue. (We discuss this concept in depth in Chapter Eight.) An academic medical center, for example, might decide to concentrate its marketing and distribution effort on the East Coast, while an urban community hospital will typically focus on a radius of five to ten miles. Finally, the *penetrated market* is the set of consumers who are buying the company's product. The medical center may care for patients in its target market as well as those from other parts of the United States and the world.

Demand Measurement

Once the organization has defined its market, the next step is to estimate market demand. *Market demand* for a product or service is not a fixed number but a function of the total volume that would be bought by a defined customer group in a delineated geographical area during a given time period in a distinct marketing environment using a specific marketing program. The market demand measurement is not a fixed number, but is a function of the stated conditions.

The dependence of total market demand on underlying conditions is illustrated in Figure 7.3 (a). The horizontal axis shows different possible levels of industry marketing expenditure in a given time period. The vertical axis shows the resulting demand level. The curve represents the estimated market demand associated with varying levels of industry marketing expenditure.

Some base sales (called the *market minimum*, labeled $Q1$ in the figure) take place without any demand-stimulating expenditures. Higher levels of industry marketing expenditures yield higher levels of demand, first at an increasing rate, then at a decreasing rate. Marketing expenditures beyond a certain level do not stimulate much further demand, suggesting an upper limit to market demand called the *market potential* (labeled $Q2$).

The level of industry marketing significantly affects the total size of an *expansible market*. In Figure 7.3 (a), the distance between $Q1$ and $Q2$ is relatively large. In a relatively *nonexpansible market*—one not much affected by the level of marketing expenditures—the distance between $Q1$ and $Q2$ is relatively small. Organizations operating in a nonexpansible market must accept the market's size (the level of *primary demand* for the product class) and try to win a larger *market share* (the level of selective demand for the organization's service or product).

The market demand curve shows alternative current forecasts of market demand associated with different possible levels of industry marketing effort in the current period. Because only one level of industry marketing expenditure will actually occur, the market demand corresponding to this level is called the *market forecast*. The market forecast shows *expected* market demand, not maximum market demand.

Market potential is the limit approached by market demand as industry marketing expenditures approach infinity for a given marketing environment. The phrase "for a given market environment" is crucial. The market demand for many products is higher during prosperity than during recession, as illustrated in Figure 7.3 (b). Organizations cannot do anything about the position of the market demand

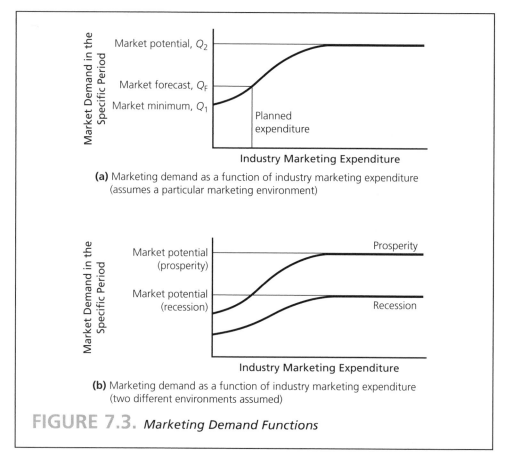

(a) Marketing demand as a function of industry marketing expenditure (assumes a particular marketing environment)

(b) Marketing demand as a function of industry marketing expenditure (two different environments assumed)

FIGURE 7.3. *Marketing Demand Functions*

Source: Kotler and Keller, *A Framework for Marketing Management*, 3rd ed. Upper Saddle River, N.J.: Prentice Hall, 2007.

function—which is determined by the marketing environment—but their marketing spending can influence their location on the function.

Organization Demand and Sales Forecast

Organization demand is the firm's estimated share of market demand at different levels of company marketing effort in a given time period. Ultimately, the company's share of market demand depends on how such factors as its products, services, prices, and communications are perceived relative to its competitors'. If these factors are equal, however, the company's market share depends on the size and effectiveness of its marketing expenditures relative to competitors. Marketing model builders have developed sales-response functions to measure how a company's sales are affected by its marketing expenditures, marketing mix, and marketing effectiveness.[16]

Once marketers have estimated organization demand, they next choose a level of marketing effort to produce an expected level of sales. The *organization sales forecast* is the expected level of organization sales based on a chosen marketing plan and an assumed marketing environment. The organization sales forecast is graphed with company sales on the vertical axis and organization marketing effort on the horizontal axis, as in Figure 7.3. Note that the sales forecast is the result of an assumed marketing expenditure plan.

A *sales quota* is the sales goal set for a product line, corporate division, or sales representative. It is primarily a managerial device for defining and stimulating sales effort. A *sales budget* is a conservative estimate of the expected sales volume and is used primarily for making current purchasing, production, and cash-flow decisions. The sales budget is based on the sales forecast and avoidance of excessive risk, so it is generally set slightly lower than the sales forecast.

Organization sales potential is the sales limit approached by customer demand as the company's marketing effort increases relative to competitors. The absolute limit of company demand is, of course, the total market potential. Even when organization marketing expenditures increase considerably, in most cases organization sales potential is less than the market potential; each competitor has a core of loyal buyers who are not very responsive to other organizations' efforts to woo them.

Estimating Current Demand

In estimating current marketing demand, executives want to examine total market potential, area market potential, and total industry sales and market shares.

Total Market Potential. Total market potential is the maximum number of sales that might be available to all the firms in an industry during a specified period, under a given level of industry marketing effort and environmental conditions. A common way to determine total market potential is to estimate the possible number of buyers and multiply this figure by both the average quantity each purchases and the price of each unit. For example, assume that one hundred million people buy over-the-counter cold medicine each year, the average cold preparation buyer buys three units or boxes a year, and the average price of a box is $7; the total market potential for boxes of cold preparations is $2.1 billion (100 million × 3 × $7).

The most difficult component to estimate is the number of buyers for the specific product or market. Organizations can start with a total population, eliminate groups that obviously would not buy the product, and do research to eliminate groups without interest or money to buy. What remains is a prospective pool of potential buyers that organizations can include in the calculation of total market potential.

Area Market Potential. Because organizations face the problem of selecting the best territories and allocating their marketing budget optimally among them, they need to estimate the market potential of different cities, states, and nations.

Business-to-business marketers primarily use the market-buildup method, whereas consumer marketers primarily use the multiple-factor index method.

The *market-buildup method* calls for identifying all the potential buyers in an area and estimating their potential purchases. This method works well if organizations have a list of all potential buyers and a good estimate of what each will buy—data that can be difficult to gather. An efficient method makes use of the *North American Industry Classification Systems* (NAICS), a six-digit code of classifying industry sectors that provides statistics comparable across the United States, Canada, and Mexico.[17] To use the NAICS, an operating table manufacturer would first determine the six-digit NAICS codes that represent the hospitals, physician practices, and ambulatory surgery centers that are likely to require its products. Then the manufacturer determines an appropriate base for estimating the number of operating tables that will be used, such as customer industry sales. Once the company estimates the rate of operating table ownership relative the customer industry's sales, it can compute the market potential.

Consumer companies also estimate area market potentials; however, because their customers are too numerous to be listed, they often use the *index method*. A drug marketer, for example, might assume that the market potential for drugs is directly related to population size. If Virginia has 2.28 percent of the U.S. population, the company might assume that state will account for 2.28 percent of all drugs sold. In reality, drug sales are also influenced by other factors. Thus, it makes sense to develop a multiple-factor index, with each factor assigned a specific weight. For example, if Virginia has 2.00 percent of the U.S. disposable personal income, 1.96 percent of U.S. retail sales, and 2.28 percent of U.S. population, the respective weights for these factors are 0.5, 0.3, and 0.2. The buying-power index for drugs in Virginia would be

$$0.5(2.00) + 0.3(1.96) + 0.2(2.28) = 2.04$$

In addition to estimating total market potential and area potential, a company needs to know the *actual* industry sales taking place in its market. This information may be available from trade associations and marketing research firms, although not for individual competitors. For example, Nielsen Media Research audits retail sales in various product categories in supermarkets and drugstores and sells this information to interested companies. These audits can give a company valuable information about its total product-category sales as well as brand sales. It can compare its performance to the total industry or any particular competitor to see whether it is gaining or losing share.

It is typically harder for business marketers to estimate industry sales and market share than it is for consumer-good manufacturers. Business marketers have no source equivalent to the Nielsens, and distributors typically will not supply information about how much of competitors' products they are selling. Business-goods marketers therefore operate with less knowledge of their market-share results.

Estimating Future Demand

Forecasting is the art of anticipating what buyers are likely to do under a given set of conditions. Very few products or services lend themselves to easy forecasting of future demand; those that do generally involve a product whose absolute level or trend is fairly constant and for which competition is nonexistent (public utilities) or stable (pure oligopolies). In most markets, total demand and company demand are not stable; the more unstable the demand, the more critical is forecast accuracy and the more elaborate is the forecasting procedure.

Organizations commonly use a three-stage approach to prepare a sales forecast. They first prepare a macroeconomic forecast, which projects such factors as inflation, unemployment, interest rates, consumer spending, business investment, government spending, and payer reimbursement rates. They then prepare an industry forecast and finally an organization-specific sales forecast. Based on these estimates and assumptions that the firm will win a certain market share, marketers issue their final forecast. Methods for sales forecasting are shown in Table 7.4.

TABLE 7.4. Sales Forecast Methods

Forecast Method	Description	Use
Survey of buyers' intentions	Survey consumers or businesses about purchase probability, future finances, and expectations about the economy.	To estimate demand for industrial products, consumer durables, purchases requiring advance planning, and new products.
Composite of sales force opinions	Have sales representatives estimate how many current and prospective customers will buy the company's products.	To gather detailed forecast estimates broken down by product, territory, customer, and sales representative.
Expert opinion	Obtain forecasts from experts such as dealers, distributors, suppliers, consultants, and trade associations; can be purchased from economic forecasting firms.	To gather estimates from knowledgeable specialists who may offer good insights.

(Table 7.4 continued)

Past-sales analysis	Use time-series analysis, exponential smoothing, statistical demand analysis, or econometric analysis to analyze past sales.	To project future demand on the basis of an analysis of past demand.
Market-test method	Conduct a direct market test to understand customer response and estimate future sales.	To better forecast sales of new products or sales in a new area.

Source: Kotler and Keller, *A Framework for Marketing Management,* 3rd ed. Upper Saddle River, N.J.: Prentice Hall, 2007.

SUMMARY

A steady flow of market and competitive information is required for developing effective marketing plans and managing marketing activities. Health care organizations get their information by examining internal records, by applying marketing intelligence scanning, and by conducting marketing research. The information comes in the form of secondary (preexisting) and primary data.

Primary data are drawn from observational research, focus group research, individual in-depth interviews, and well-designed surveys. Surveys supply the final quantitative picture of the market situation. Surveys involve administering a well-tested questionnaire to a sufficient size sample population that is drawn on a probability basis. The data are then turned into findings with the help of statistical analysis and quantitative decision models.

DISCUSSION QUESTIONS

1. Popular marketing metrics such as customer acquisition, satisfaction, and retention can sometimes turn out to be poor indicators of customers' true perceptions and, ultimately, marketing success. Explain how these metrics could mask important marketing problems for hospitals, medical device companies, and health care plans.

2. Senior executives may view marketing research as overly complex, too expensive, or offering no new insights. As a marketing manager, how could you structure a marketing research recommendation to overcome these objections?

3. You are the chief marketing officer of a pharmaceutical company. Your company has received FDA approval for a new prescription-only drug to treat early signs of Alzheimer's disease. How would you measure market demand and develop a sales forecast for this new product?

4. On-line marketing research surveys are becoming more common. What are the pros and cons of using the Web to conduct a focus group? How does the statistical validity and reliability of a quantitative on-line survey compare with the validity and reliability of a telephone survey?

APPENDIX: SECONDARY-DATA SOURCES

A. Internal Sources

Company profit-loss statements, balance sheets, sales figures, sales-call reports, invoices, inventory records, and prior research reports.

B. Government Publications

Statistical Abstract of the United States

County and City Data Book

Industrial Outlook

Marketing Information Guide

Other government publications include the *Annual Survey of Manufacturers*; *Business Statistics*; *Census of Manufacturers*; *Census of Population*; *Census of Retail Trade, Wholesale Trade, and Selected Service Industries*; *Census of Transportation*; *Federal Reserve Bulletin*; *Monthly Labor Review*; *Survey of Current Business*; and *Vital Statistics Report*.

C. Periodicals and Books

Business Periodicals Index

Standard and Poor's Industry

Moody's Manuals

Encyclopedia of Associations

Marketing journals include *Marketing Health Services*, the *Journal of Marketing*, *Journal of Marketing Research*, and *Journal of Consumer Research*.

Useful health care and marketing trade magazines include *HealthLeaders*, *Modern Healthcare*, *B to B*, *Hospitals & Health Networks*, *Advertising Age*, *Chain Store Age*, *Progressive Grocer*, *Sales & Marketing Management*, and *Stores*.

Useful general business periodicals include *Business Week*, *Fortune*, *Forbes*, *The Economist, Inc.*, *Fast Company*, *Wall Street Journal*, *Financial Times*, and *Harvard Business Review*.

D. Commercial Data

Nielsen Company. Ad*Views Media Data, data on products and brands sold through retail outlets (Retail Index Services), supermarket scanner data (Scantrack), data on television audiences (Media Research Services), magazine circulation data (Neodata Services, Inc.), and others.

MRCA Information Services. Data on weekly family purchases of consumer products (National Consumer Panel) and data on home food consumption (National Menu Census).

SAMI/Burke. Reports on warehouse withdrawals to food stores in selected market areas (SAMI reports) and supermarket scanner data (Samscam).

Simmons Market Research Bureau (MRB Group). Annual reports covering television markets, sporting goods, and proprietary drugs, with demographic data by sex, income, age, and brand preferences (selective markets and media reaching them).

Other commercial research houses selling data to subscribers include the Audit Bureau of Circulation; Arbitron, Audits and Surveys; Dun & Bradstreet; National Family Opinion; Standard Rate & Data Service; and Starch.

E. Internet Data—Health Care Industry–Specific Internet Resources

Achoo HeadlineNews. Health care news service covering over 150 news topics, including biotechnology, clinical trials, the pharmaceutical industry, companies, and regulations.

ClinicalTrials. This site helps you find clinical trials in the U.S. and Canada. One can also register for future clinical trials.

Drug InfoNet. Health and medical information as well as links to manufacturer press releases and product approval sites.

eMedicine World Medical Library. Offers resources as dictionary, thesaurus, and translator and gives access to the eMedicine Journal. Also includes a section, "Recalls and Alerts."

Health On the Net Foundation. This site offers online health information, medical articles, dossiers, and a very complete calendar of medical events.

Healthfinder. Links to current and government health news, on-line publications, clearinghouses, databases, and support and self-help groups.

HighWire Press. This site provides a collection of scientific and medical magazines, some full text some indexed. Included are well-known publications such as *Science, Pediatrics*, and the *Proceedings of the National Academy of Sciences*.

Journal of the American Medical Association. Full-text articles available for purchase.

Mayo Clinic. A newsstand with current health news, resources, including information on drugs and diseases.

National Coalition on Health Care. Full-text articles, press releases, reports, and speeches from the U.S. alliance composed of businesses, consumers, and health care providers who want to improve the health care system.

National Library of Medicine. The world's largest biomedical library.

Physicians Online. Physicians on-line site uniting physicians, managed health care organizations, and pharmaceutical companies. Access limited to U.S. physicians and other prescribing health care professionals.

Reuters Health Information. Subscription-based health and medical news. Also includes a news archive and a drug database.

The Lancet. Medical journal from the U.K. Free access to selected articles and pay-per-view option. Also features conferences and discussion groups.

F. Internet Data—General Industry Internet Resources

Lexis Nexis. Contains legal data and nonlegal full text material from 7,100 magazine and newspaper sources (www.lexisnexis.com).

Dun and Bradstreet. Provides Dun and Bradstreet credit information on thousands of companies (www.dnb.com).

Hoovers. Provides detailed profiles on 12,000 corporate firms (www.hoovers.com).

Moody's. Provides credit information and credit ratings of companies (www.moodys.com).

www.marketguide.com. Provides financial information on 10,000 publicly traded companies.

American Marketing Association (www.ama.org).

Commerce Net. Industry association for internet commerce (www.commerce.net).

Gale's Encyclopedia of Associations (www.gale.com).

A Business Researcher's Interests. Provides links to business directories, media sites, marketing-related resources, and much more (www.brint.com).

Bloomberg Personal. Timely news and financial services (www.bloomberg.com).

C/Net. Journalistic coverage of high technology, computers, and the Internet (www.cnet.com).

Company Link. Free basic directory data, press releases, stock prices, and SEC data on 45,000 U.S. firms; more information available to subscribers (www.companylink.com).

EDGAR. Public company financial filings (www.sec.gov/edgarhp.htm).

National Trade Data Bank. Free access to over 18,000 market research reports analyzing trends and competition in scores of industries and for hundreds of products (www.stat-usa.gov).

Public Register's Annual Report Service. Allows searches of 3,200 public companies by company name or industry and offers annual reports via e-mail (www.prars.com/index.html).

Quote.Com. Access to a wide range of business wires, companies' directories, and stock quotes (www.quote.com).

Government Information.

Census Bureau (www.census.gov).

FedWorld. A program of the U.S. Department of Commerce, serves as a clearinghouse for over 100 federal government agencies (www.fedworld.gov).

Thomas. Indexes federal government sites (thomas.loc.gov).

US Business Advisor (www.business.gov)

International Information.

CIA World Factbook. A comprehensive statistical and demographic directory covering 264 countries around the world (www.odic.gov/cia/publications).

The Electronic Embassy (www.embassy.org).

I-Trade. Free and fee-based information services for firms wishing to do business internationally (www.i-trade.com).

The United Nations (www.un.org).

CHAPTER

8

MARKET SEGMENTATION, TARGETING, POSITIONING, AND COMPETITION

LEARNING OBJECTIVES

In this chapter, we will address the following questions:

1. What are the different levels of market segmentation?

2. How can a health care organization divide a market into segments?

3. How can an organization choose the most attractive target markets?

4. How can an organization choose and communicate an effective positioning in the market?

5. How can the organization analyze the competitors' strategies, objectiv
   strengths, and weaknesses?

OPENING EXAMPLE

A Fall Prevention Program for Seniors Succeeds Through Segmentation and Targeting   In Washington State, more people aged sixty-five and older are hospitalized due to falls than people of all other age groups are hospitalized due to motor vehicle accidents. This statistic was at the heart of a comprehensive report prepared by the Washington State Injury Prevention Program, which led to a three-year, $900,000 CDC grant to develop a fall prevention program.

The Washington State Department of Health—believing that a physical fitness program for seniors could decrease the number of falls and, therefore, reduce health care costs—decided to use a marketing approach to test this hypothesis. First, they conducted a market segmentation analysis of the senior population. The analysis divided the senior population by age, fall incidence, and physical fitness level. From the resulting information, the Department found that their target market—people aged seventy to seventy-nine—seemed to have a fall incidence and fitness capacity that could be most easily improved through the physical fitness program.

The Department then selected one county for a test market. Qualitative market research was conducted to understand the target market's perceptions of the fitness program concept. The research asked potential participants about their preferences related to program benefits, barriers to joining, and barriers to regular attendance, and competing programs.

The marketing research conclusions were used to develop the product and a positioning strategy that focused on the particular benefits that were important to the target market. The positioning statement read: "A fitness class for seniors that *works*, as it will improve strength and balance; is *safe*, as it has experienced skilled instructors offering tested exercises; and is *fun*, as it offers an opportunity to meet others and get out of the house. It is an important and worthwhile activity for seniors wanting to stay *independent*, be *active*, and *prevent falls*."

The fitness program was named *S.A.I.L.* (Stay Active and Independent for Life), with a tagline of "A Strength and Balance Fitness Class for Seniors." It consisted of a one-hour strength and balance fitness class that met three times a week with up to twenty participants. A fall prevention booklet was created and distributed that advised seniors how to create an exercise plan, manage health care needs, build a strong foundation for balance, and make a safe home. An optional safety effectiveness assessment was also developed. The research indicated that pricing each S.A.I.L. class at $2.50 would be acceptable. The scheduled meeting times and locations were arranged for the convenience of the prospective participants based on the research respondents' preferences.

Promotional messages built brand awareness, and the media used to deliver the messages were "senior-based" and included senior center newsletter ads and articles, brochures for physicians and senior center staff members, and sandwich board signs at senior centers.

S.A.I.L. has been successful in reducing injuries from falls among Washington State seniors. It has also been adopted by other state health departments throughout the nation.

One important reason for the successful approach used by the Washington State Health Department's S.A.I.L. program was that it employed target marketing. To compete more effectively and reach appropriate customers, many organizations are now embracing this strategy. Instead of scattering their marketing effort using a ''shotgun'' approach, they focus on those consumers they have the greatest chance of satisfying, through a ''rifle'' approach. Target marketing requires that marketers (1) identify and profile distinct groups of buyers who differ in their needs and preferences (market segmentation), (2) select one or more market segments to enter (market targeting), and (3) establish and communicate the distinctive benefits of the organization's market offering (market positioning).

OVERVIEW: MARKET SEGMENTATION

Sellers that use *mass marketing* engage in the mass production, distribution, and promotion of one product for all buyers. Henry Ford epitomized this strategy when he offered the Model-T Ford "in any color, as long as it is black." Coca-Cola also practiced mass marketing when it sold only one kind of Coke, in a 6.5-ounce bottle.

The argument for mass marketing is that it creates the largest potential market, that leads to the lowest costs, that in turn can lead to lower prices or higher margins. Critics note that the increasing splintering of the market and the proliferation of advertising media and distribution channels make it more difficult and increasingly expensive to reach a mass audience. Some claim that mass marketing is dying. Not surprisingly, therefore, many organizations are turning to *micromarketing* at one of four levels: segments, niches, local areas, and individuals.

Segment Marketing

A market segment consists of a group of customers who share a similar set of *needs* and *wants*, such as health insurance customers who want low premiums versus other customers who want generous health care benefits. A *segment* is not a *sector*. "Young, middle-income health insurance buyers" is a sector, not a segment, because these buyers will differ in what they want in a health insurance product. Marketers do not create the segments; their task is to identify different benefit segments and decide which to target.

Because the wants of segment members are similar but not identical, Anderson and Narus urge marketers to present flexible market offerings instead of one standard offering to all of a segment's members.[1] A *flexible market offering* consists of the product and service elements that *all* segment members value, plus *discretionary options*—perhaps for an additional charge—that *some* members value. For example, most health insurance companies offer similar benefits; for an additional charge, customers can obtain vision care benefits that also cover periodic eye examinations and corrective lenses.

Niche Marketing

A *niche* is a more narrowly defined customer group seeking a distinctive mix of benefits. Marketers usually identify niches by dividing a segment into subsegments. For example, LifeInsure.com, a California-based insurance agency, sells life insurance to smokers, charging a high price for coverage to build in profits from this high-risk group. An attractive niche has these characteristics: its customers have a distinct set of needs, they will pay a premium to the firm that best satisfies their needs, the niche is not likely to attract other competitors, the niche company gains certain economies through specialization, and the niche has size, profit, and growth potential.

Segments are fairly large and attract several competitors; niches are fairly small and may attract few rivals. Niche marketers presumably understand and satisfy their customers' needs so well that the customers willingly pay a premium. As marketing efficiency increases, niches that were seemingly too small may become more profitable.[2]

Tom's of Maine, which produces a line of all-natural dental health and other products, often commands a 30 percent premium on its toothpaste because its unique, environmentally friendly products and charitable donation programs appeal to consumers who have been turned off by big businesses.[3] The concept of natural personal care products made without artificial or animal ingredients or chemicals is a market niche that Tom's of Maine has exploited since its founding, in 1970, with a $5,000 loan and a single product. The company is now a leading natural care brand, with nearly two hundred employees and ninety oral and body care products distributed through more than forty thousand retail outlets worldwide. Tom Chappell began with a set of beliefs and values based on a relationship-building model and safe, effective natural products marketed in a socially responsible and environmentally sensitive manner.

The low cost of internet marketing has also led to many small start-ups aimed at niches. The recipe for internet niche-finding success is to choose a hard-to-find product that customers do not need to see and touch. For example, as the cost of pharmaceuticals continues to escalate, there is strong demand for branded drugs at lower prices purchased through the Web. Unfortunately, this demand has led to counterfeiting and illegal channeling of pharmaceuticals from foreign countries. (The problem is so great the FDA has set up a Web site to keep the public informed about this problem: http://www.fda.gov/counterfeit/.)

Local Marketing

Target marketing is tailored to the needs and wants of local customer groups, including trading areas, neighborhoods, and even individual retail outlets. Local hospitals that are owned by national chains provide different mixes of health care services depending on particular market demographics.

FOR EXAMPLE

American Drug, one of the largest U.S. drugstore retailers, had its marketing team assess shopping patterns at hundreds of its Osco and Sav-on Drug Stores on a market-by-market basis. Using scanned data, the company fine-tuned the stores' product mix, revamped store layout, and refocused marketing efforts to more closely align with local consumer demand. Depending on the local demographics, each store unit varies the amount and type of merchandise in such categories as hardware, electrical supplies, automotive products, cookware, over-the-counter drugs, and convenience goods.[4]

Local marketing reflects a growing trend toward grassroots marketing, concentrating on getting as close and personally relevant to individual customers as possible. A large part of local, grassroots marketing is *experiential marketing*, which promotes an offering by connecting it with unique and interesting experiences. One marketing commentator describes experiential marketing this way: "The idea is not to sell something, but to demonstrate how a brand can enrich a customer's life."[5]

Proponents of local marketing see national advertising as wasteful because it fails to address local needs. Opponents argue that local marketing drives up manufacturing and marketing costs by reducing economies of scale. Logistical problems become magnified when organizations try to meet varying local requirements. Also, a brand's overall image might be diluted if the product and message vary in different localities.

Patterns of Market Segmentation

Market segments can be defined in many different ways. One common method is to identify *preference segments*. Suppose buyers are asked to compare how much they value two health care product attributes: ease of use versus low price. Three different patterns can emerge, as shown in Figure 8.1.

1. *Homogeneous preferences.* Figure 8.1(A) shows a market in which all the consumers have roughly the same preferences. The market shows no natural segments. We would predict that health information systems would be similar and cluster around the middle of the scale in both ease of use and price.

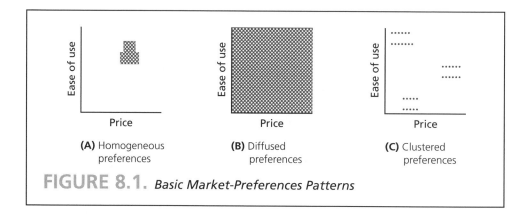

FIGURE 8.1. *Basic Market-Preferences Patterns*

2. *Diffused preferences.* At the other extreme, consumer preferences may be scattered throughout the field of possibilities, as shown in Figure 8.1(B), indicating a high level of variance in consumer preferences. One brand might position in the center to try to appeal to the most people. If several brands are in the market, they are likely to position themselves throughout the field to target consumer preference differences.

3. *Clustered preferences.* An intermediate possibility is the formation of distinct preference clusters called *natural market segments*, as shown in Figure 8.1(C). The first firm in this market might (1) position in the center to appeal to all groups, (2) choose only the largest market segment (*concentrated marketing*), or (3) provide different offerings to different segments that favor ease of use or price. If the first firm to enter chooses one segment, other competitors would enter and introduce different offerings to the other segments.

SEGMENTATION OF CONSUMER MARKETS

Because of the inherent differences between consumer and business markets, marketers cannot use exactly the same variables to segment both. In this section we will discuss segmenting consumer markets; we will present business market segmentation in the following section.

Two broad groups of variables are used to segment consumer markets. Some researchers try to form segments by looking at descriptive characteristics: geographic, demographic, and psychographic. They then examine whether these customer segments exhibit different needs or product responses. Other researchers first try to form segments by looking at behavioral aspects, such as responses to benefits, use occasions, or brands. With the segments formed in this way, the researcher sees whether different characteristics are associated with each consumer-response segment.

Regardless of which type of segmentation scheme is employed, the key is that the marketing program can be profitably adjusted to recognize customer differences. The major segmentation variables—geographic, demographic, psychographic, and behavioral segmentation—are summarized in Table 8.1 and described in the sections that follow.

Geographic Segmentation

Geographic segmentation divides the market into different geographical units such as nations, states, regions, counties, cities, or neighborhoods. A medical supply company

TABLE 8.1. **Major Segmentation Variables for Consumer Markets**

Geographic	■ Nation or country
	■ State or region
	■ City or metro size
	■ Density
	■ Climate
Demographic	■ Age, race, gender
	■ Income, education
	■ Family size
	■ Family life cycle
	■ Occupation
	■ Religion, nationality
	■ Generation
	■ Social class
Psychographic	■ Lifestyle
	—*Activities*
	—*Interests*
	—*Opinions*
	■ Personality
	■ Core values
Behavioral	■ Occasions
	■ Benefits
	■ User status
	■ Usage rate
	■ Loyalty status
	■ Buyer-readiness
	■ Attitude

can operate in one, a few or all geographic areas, but it must pay attention to local variations. Most local community hospitals serve a specific and limited geography called a "service area" (often a radius of only five to ten miles if situated in an urban or suburban locale) and must tailor their offerings to meet the specific needs of their communities. Large hospital groups, such as HCA and Tenet, are capable of either adapting service offerings to local geographic markets or providing the same service configuration across their national spectrum of hospitals.

Regional marketing is capable of drilling down to a specific zip code.[6] Some approaches combine geographic data with demographic data to yield richer descriptions of consumers and neighborhoods. Claritas, Inc. has developed a geoclustering approach called PRIZM (Potential Rating Index by Zip Markets) that classifies over half a million U.S. residential neighborhoods into fifteen distinct groups and sixty-two distinct lifestyle segments called PRIZM Clusters.[7] The groupings take into consideration thirty-nine factors in five broad categories: (1) education and affluence, (2) family life cycle, (3) urbanization, (4) race and ethnicity, and (5) mobility. The clusters have descriptive titles such as *Blue Blood Estates, Winner's Circle, Hometown Retired, Latino America, Shotguns and Pickups*, and *Back Country Folks*. The underlying assumption is that the inhabitants of these clusters tend to lead similar lives, drive similar cars, have similar jobs, and read similar magazines.

Demographic Segmentation

Using this method, the market is divided into groups on the basis of age and other demographic variables. This segmentation method is the most popular because consumer wants, preferences, and usage rates are often associated with demographic variables, and these variables are easy to measure. Even when the target market is described in nondemographic terms such as a personality type, the link to demographic characteristics is needed to estimate the size of the market and the media that can be used to reach it.

The following demographic categories are frequently used to segment markets.

Age and life-cycle stage. Consumer wants, abilities, and health needs change with age. Toothpaste brands such as Crest and Colgate offer three main lines of products to target children, adults, and older consumers. Several medical specialties also focus on different age groups: pediatricians treat children, obstetricians focus on women ages fifteen to fifty, adult cardiologists tend to treat mainly people over age fifty, and, of course, geriatricians treat older adults. Age and life cycle can sometimes be tricky segmentation variables because a product that is intended for a particular age group can actually draw more attention from a completely unexpected group.[8] For example, Viagra and other erectile dysfunction drugs were intended to primarily help men over sixty, but teenagers and young men in their twenties have also adopted these drugs for use with alcohol and other recreational drugs.[9]

Life stage. Persons in the same part of the life cycle may differ in their life stage. Life stage defines a person's major concern, such as their children's school grade levels, marital status and changes, responsibility of caring for an older parent, homeowner status, and so on. These life stages present opportunities for marketers who can help people cope with their major concerns.

Gender. Men and women tend to have different attitudinal and behavioral orientations based partly on genetic makeup and partly on socialization. As an example, women tend to be more communal-minded and men tend to be more self-expressive and goal-directed; women tend to take in more of the data in their immediate environment, whereas men tend to focus on the part of the environment that helps them achieve a goal. Increased sensitivity to women's health care needs and preferences have resulted in health care organizations' seeking more women physicians; investing more resources in women's health concerns related to infertility, menopause, and osteoporosis; and developing better techniques for treating breast cancer.

Disease, organ system, or diagnostic category. Most health care providers first segment their markets according to the disease, organ system, or diagnosis of the patient. Medical subspecialties are organized in this fashion; for example, heart (cardiology), joints (rheumatology), cancers (oncology), hormones (endocrinology), and skin (dermatology). Institutions sometimes specialize along these lines also; for example, some hospitals treat only patients with psychiatric problems, rehabilitation needs, or cancers. Even though many institutions consider themselves to be general hospitals, they will still choose to concentrate their resources in a few select disease categories. Likewise, they may also choose not to provide services in certain health care categories, such as obstetrics.

Payer mix. How patients pay for their care is also an important segmentation variable. Growth in the proportion of the uninsured and Medicaid eligibles relative to commercially insured patients is usually an indicator that financial results will worsen. Most hospitals and physician practices analyze changes in payer mix and reimbursement regulations to ensure that current and new health care services do not jeopardize the financial viability of the organization.

Income. Income segmentation is a long-standing practice in health care. Discretionary services—that is, those elective procedures not covered by insurance— present an opportunity for providers to gain extra revenue. Cosmetic surgery is an example in this category. Providers can also offer extended services for covered benefits, such as private rooms not required for medical reasons. Phillips House is a care center at the Massachusetts General Hospital that caters to international patients and those in the high-end income bracket, as the following description from its Web site explains.

For patients seeking the comfort and elegance characteristic of a fine hotel, the Phillips House is the ideal choice. The Phillips House combines the atmosphere of a luxury hotel with world-class medical and hospital care. A particular market niche for Phillips House is international patients, patients with special needs, and those requiring a high level of personal service. Private rooms have elegant mahogany appointments, customized menus, satellite television with access to foreign channels, business services, and accommodations for guests and members of the entourage.[10]

Increasingly, companies are finding that their markets are "hourglass shaped" as middle market Americans migrate toward more premium products.[11]

Generation. Each generation is profoundly influenced by the times in which it grows up—the music, movies, politics, and defining events of that period. Demographers call these groups *cohorts.* Because cohort members share the same experiences and have similar outlooks and values, effective marketing appeals use the icons and images that are prominent in the targeted cohort's experiences. People born between 1925 and 1945, known as the Silent Generation or as children of the Great Depression, are typically trusting conformists who value stability. These people are often less likely to question medical professionals or to have unrealistic expectations around aging. In contrast, the post–World War II baby boomers grew up questioning authority and strongly attempt to resist the limitations of growing older.

Social class. Social classes are relatively homogeneous and enduring divisions in a society that is hierarchically ordered and whose members share similar values, interests, and behaviors. Social class is distinguished using variables such as income, occupation, education, and type of residence; each class may show distinct health behaviors and health care consumption patterns. For example, certain types of sports injuries, like tennis elbow, are found primarily in the upper and upper middle classes; heroin addiction, on the other hand, is found primarily in the lower classes, as is lead paint poisoning in children.

Psychographic Segmentation

Psychographics is the science of using psychology and demographics to better understand consumers. In *psychographic segmentation*, buyers are divided into different groups on the basis of lifestyle, personality, or values. People within the same demographic group can exhibit very different psychographic profiles.

One of the most popular commercially available classification systems based on psychographic measurements is SRI Consulting Business Intelligence's VALS framework. VALS classifies all U.S. adults into eight primary groups based on personality traits and key demographics. The segmentation system is based on responses to a questionnaire featuring four demographic and thirty-five attitudinal questions. The VALS system is continually updated with new data from more than eighty thousand surveys per year.[12]

The major attributes of the four groups with ample resources are as follows:

1. *Innovators.* Successful, sophisticated, active, "take-charge" people with high self-esteem. Their purchases often reflect cultivated tastes for relatively upscale, niche-oriented products and services.

2. *Thinkers.* Mature, satisfied, and reflective people who are motivated by ideals and value order, knowledge, and responsibility. They favor durability, functionality, and value in products.

3. *Achievers.* Successful career- and work-oriented people who value consensus and stability. They favor established, prestige products that demonstrate success to their peers.

4. *Experiencers.* Young, enthusiastic, impulsive people who seek variety and excitement. They spend a comparatively high proportion of income on fashion, entertainment, and socializing.

The major attributes of the four groups with more limited resources are as follows:

1. *Believers.* Conservative, conventional, and traditional people with concrete beliefs. They favor familiar, American products and are loyal to established brands.

2. *Strivers.* Trendy and fun-loving people who seek approval of others but are resource-constrained. They favor stylish products that emulate the purchases of those with greater material wealth.

3. *Makers.* Practical, self-sufficient, traditional, and family-oriented people who focus on their work and home context. They favor basic products with a practical or functional purpose.

4. *Strugglers.* Elderly, resigned, passive people who are concerned about change. They are loyal to their favorite brands.

You can find out which VALS type you are by going to SRIC-BI's Web site (www.sric-bi.com).

Lifestyle segmentation schemes are by no means universal. The Japanese version of VALS divides society into ten segments on the basis of two key consumer attributes: life orientation (traditional ways, occupations, innovation, and self-expression) and attitudes toward social change (sustaining, pragmatic, adapting, and innovating).

Behavioral Segmentation

In behavioral segmentation, buyers are divided into groups on the basis of their knowledge of, attitude toward, use of, or response to a product. Decision roles are one such variable. People play five roles in a buying decision: *initiator, influencer, decider, payer*, and *user*. Recall our discussion in Chapter Two about the difference between a customer and stakeholder. As another example here, suppose a wife decides to adopt a healthier lifestyle, and she initiates a purchase by requesting a new treadmill for her birthday. The husband may then seek information from many sources, including a friend who has a treadmill and is a key influencer in what models to consider. After presenting the alternative choices to his wife, she chooses the model, he pays for it, and the entire family ends up using it. Different people are playing different roles, but all are crucial in the decision-making process and ultimate consumer satisfaction.

Many marketers believe that behavioral variables—occasions, benefits, user status, usage rate, loyalty status, buyer-readiness stage, and attitude—are the best starting points for constructing market segments.

Occasions. Buyers can be distinguished according to the occasions when they develop a need, purchase a product, or use a product. For example, patients who visit their physician do so when they are feeling ill, when it is time to have a routine physical exam, in preparation for an overseas trip that requires a vaccination, and when they feel a need for medical advice.

Benefits. Buyers can be classified according to the benefits they seek. Some consumers are interested in one particular benefit whereas others want a benefit bundle. The health care market includes four different benefits buyers. The *quality buyer* wants the best product regardless of cost; an example is the patient who chooses a hospital based on the *U.S. News and World Report* annual "Best Hospitals" listing. S*ervice buyers* prefer the best personal treatment; they assume that medical expertise is fairly equal. *Value buyers* are price sensitive; they want the lowest price and highest medical care combination. *Economy buyers* are also price sensitive, but they are concerned much more about price than about care. Consumers largely assume that the health care system can offer the benefits of alleviating pain, providing reassurance and comfort, curing illness, and prolonging life. The responsibility for communicating that these benefits cannot always realistically be provided rests with many stakeholders: employers, payers, providers, government, and media.

User Status. Markets can be segmented into nonusers, ex-users, potential users, first-time users, and regular users of a product. Blood banks cannot rely only on regular donors to supply blood; they must also recruit first-time donors and contact former donors. Each will require a different marketing strategy. Included in the potential user group are consumers who will become users in connection with some life stage or life event. For example, persons who have a loved one who needs blood may start to donate blood regularly after they have seen the need. From the standpoint of company size, market-share leaders focus on attracting potential users, and smaller firms focus on trying to lure users away from the market leader.

Usage Rate. Markets can be segmented into light, medium, and heavy product users. Heavy users are often a small percentage of the market but account for a high percentage of total consumption. For example, physician referrals for hospital admissions often reflect the 80:20 pattern, wherein 80 percent of all hospital admissions come from 20 percent of the total admitting physicians. Since these patterns are critical to financial success, hospitals must ensure that referral data is accurate and comprehensive; they should understand why some physicians refer (and why others do not refer) and develop strategies for further bonding with heavy referrers.

Buyer-Readiness Stage. A market consists of people in different stages of readiness to buy a product. Some are unaware of the product, some are aware, some are informed, some are interested, some desire the product, and some intend to buy. The relative numbers make a big difference in designing the marketing program. Consider an example from India. With the growing consumption of junk foods, obesity and diabetes are becoming more common. In many places, however, people are not aware of what diabetes is. At the start of a health promotion program to combat diabetes, a health agency's effort should therefore focus first on disease awareness-building, advertising using a simple message. Later the advertising should dramatize the benefits of screening tests. The campaign can then move on to a stage that emphasizes the value of treatment.

Loyalty Status. Buyers can be divided into four groups according to brand loyalty status: *hard-core loyals* (who always buy one brand), *split loyals* (who are loyal to two or three brands), *shifting loyals* (who shift loyalty from one brand to another), and *switchers* (who show no loyalty to any brand).[13] A hospital can learn a great deal by analyzing the degrees of consumer brand loyalty. By studying its hard-core loyals, the hospital can identify its products' strengths. By studying its split loyals, the hospital can pinpoint which brands are most competitive with its own. By looking at customers who are shifting away from its brand, the hospital can learn about its marketing weaknesses and attempt to correct them. However, what appear to be brand-loyal purchase patterns may in reality reflect habit, indifference, a low price, easier access, a high switching cost, or the nonavailability of other brands.

Attitude. Five attitude groups can be found in any market: enthusiastic, positive, indifferent, negative, and hostile. For example, hospitals can classify referring physicians into these groups. They thank enthusiastic referrers and suggest that they continue to refer; they reinforce those who are positively disposed; they try to win the referrals of indifferent physicians; they spend no time trying to change the attitudes of negative and hostile physicians.

The Conversion Model has been developed to measure the strength of the psychological commitment to a brand, consumers' openness to change, and the ease with which a consumer can be converted to another choice.[14] The model assesses commitment based on factors such as consumer attitudes toward and satisfaction with current brand choices in a category and the importance of the brand selection decision.[15]

Segmentation of Business Markets

While business markets can be segmented with some of the same variables used in consumer market segmentation—such as geography, benefits sought, and usage rate—marketers must also use other variables. As an example, consider a large hospital attempting to sell its laundry services to smaller hospitals and other health care organizations.

Organization size: Businesses could be segmented by size based on revenue, number of employees, market share, and other variables. The hospital could decide that small hospitals may best fit with its offering.

Geographic location: Geographic divisions could be established as within the same city, within the same county, or within a fifty-mile radius. The hospital may decide to focus on other hospitals that are within a convenient, one-hour radius that can be efficiently served.

Interest profile: The hospital could identify other hospitals, restaurants, nursing homes, or assisted living facilities that have demonstrated an interest in highly sanitary laundry services.

Resource level: Businesses differ in the amount of money that they are willing to invest in particular programs. The hospital would want to segment potential customers by their level of revenue or profit and ability to purchase industrial laundry services.

Buying criteria: Businesses differ in the qualities they prefer in product and service decisions. A business customer that does not value laundry services that place a high priority on sanitation along with a higher price will not be a good prospect for the hospital. For example, uniforms for groundskeepers need to be clean but don't have to be sterile.

Buying process: Businesses differ in how much documentation they require and length of time they take to make a decision. The hospital may want to work with organizations that require less documentation and make decisions quickly.

Sequential Segmentation

Business marketers generally identify segments through a sequential process. Consider a specialty hospital company that first undertook disease-based, macro-segmentation. After considering several markets, it chose to focus on heart disease, and it needed to determine the most attractive mix, within that category, of such products as disease prevention, diagnosis, nonsurgical and surgical treatment, and rehabilitation. Deciding to focus on surgery, it considered the best geographic location, choosing medium-size cities close to major transportation hubs and without competing programs. The second stage consisted of microsegmentation. The company distinguished among customers buying on price, service, or quality. Because the hospital company had a high-service profile, it decided to concentrate on the service-motivated segment.

Business buyers also seek different benefit bundles based on their stage in the purchase decision process:[16]

- *First-time prospects.* Customers who have not yet purchased but want to buy from a vendor who understands their business, who explains things well, and whom they can trust

- *Novices.* Customers who are starting their purchasing relationship and thus want easy-to-read manuals, hotlines, a high level of training, and knowledgeable sales reps

- *Sophisticates.* Established customers who want speed in maintenance and repair, product customization, and good technical support

These segments may also have different channel preferences. First-time prospects prefer to deal with a company sales person rather than a catalog or direct-mail channel, because the latter provide too little information and do not provide a sense of comfort. Sophisticates, on the other hand, may want to conduct more of their buying over electronic channels. By addressing these differences, marketers can successfully start or continue relationships with business customers.

MARKET TARGETING

Once the firm has identified its market segment opportunities, it has to decide how many and which ones to target. Marketers are increasingly combining several variables in an effort to identify smaller, better-defined target groups. Thus a health information systems company may not only identify a group of large health systems, but within that group may distinguish several segments depending on financial ability to buy, age of legacy system, management outlook, and brand preferences. These characteristics have led some market researchers to advocate a *needs-based market segmentation approach*. Roger Best proposed the seven-step approach shown in Table 8.2.

Effective Segmentation Criteria

Not all segmentation schemes are useful. For example, aspirin buyers could be divided into blond and brunette customers, but hair color is undoubtedly irrelevant to the product's purchase. Furthermore, if all aspirin buyers consumed the same number of pills each month, believed all brands are the same, and would pay only one price, this market would be minimally segmentable.

To be useful, market segments must rate favorably on five key attributes:

- *Measurable.* The size, purchasing power, and characteristics of the segments can be measured.
- *Substantial.* The segments are large and profitable enough to serve; each should be the largest possible homogeneous group worth going after with a tailored marketing program.
- *Accessible.* The segments can be effectively reached and served.
- *Differentiable.* The segments are conceptually distinguishable and respond differently to different marketing mix elements and programs. If two segments respond similarly to an offer, they are not separate segments.
- *Actionable.* Effective programs can be formulated for attracting and serving the segments.

Evaluating and Selecting the Market Segments

In evaluating different market segments, the firm must look at two factors: the segment's overall attractiveness and the company's objectives and resources. How

TABLE 8.2. Steps in the Segmentation Process

1. Needs-Based Segmentation	Group customers into segments based on similar needs and benefits sought by customer in solving particular consumption problem.
2. Segment Identification	For each needs-based segment, determine which demographics, lifestyles, and usage behaviors make the segment distinct and identifiable (actionable).
3. Segment Attractiveness	Using predetermined segment attractiveness criteria (such as market growth, competitive intensity, and market access), determine the overall attractiveness of each segment.
4. Segment Profitability	Determine segment profitability.
5. Segment Positioning	For each segment, create a value proposition and the product-price positioning strategy based on that segment's unique customer need and characteristics.
6. Segment "Acid Test"	Create segment storyboards to test the attractiveness of each segment's positioning strategy.
7. Marketing-Mix Strategy	Expand segment positioning strategy to include all aspects of the marketing mix: product, price, promotion, and place.

Source: Best, Market Based Management & Hot Topics & EBIZ PKG, 2nd ed., Copyright 2001. Electronically reproduced by permission of Pearson Education, Inc., Upper Saddle River, New Jersey.

well does a potential segment score on the five key criteria? Does a potential segment have characteristics that make it generally attractive, such as large size, rapid growth, high profitability, substantial scale economies, and low risk? Does investing in the segment make sense given the firm's objectives, competencies, and resources? Some attractive segments may not mesh with the company's long-run objectives, or the company may lack one or more necessary competencies to offer superior value.

Single-Segment Concentration. QHR, formerly Quorum Health Resources, concentrates on the small hospital market for consulting and management services, whereas Ernst & Young focuses on larger hospitals. Through concentrated market-ing, each firm gains a strong knowledge of its target segment's needs and behaviors, thereby achieving a strong market presence. Furthermore, each firm attains operating economies by specializing in the segment's product needs, channels, and promo-tion. Concentrated marketing involves risks, such as a particular market segment's turning sour due to changes in buying patterns or new competition; therefore many companies prefer to operate in more than one segment.

Selective Specialization. Here the firm selects a number of segments, each objec-tively attractive and appropriate. There may be little or no synergy among the segments, but each promises to be a moneymaker. This multisegment strategy has the advantage of diversifying the firm's risk. When Procter & Gamble launched Crest Whitestrips, initial target segments included newly engaged women and brides-to-be, as well as gay males.

Product Specialization. Another approach is to specialize in making a certain prod-uct for several segments. The microscope marketplace is roughly divided into the bio-med, industrial, and geology segments. Although the frames may be the same across markets, the optics and accessory modules change. Each market has its defin-ing uses and sales requirement. The firm makes different microscopes for the different customer groups and builds a strong reputation in the specific product area. The downside risk is that the product may be supplanted by an entirely new technology.

Market Specialization. The firm concentrates on serving many needs of a particular customer group. One health care product example is a firm that sells an assortment of products only to university research laboratories. The firm gains a strong reputation in serving this customer group and becomes a channel for additional products the customer group can use. The downside risk is that the customer group may suffer budget cuts or shrink in size.

Full Market Coverage. Some firms attempt to serve all customer groups with all the products they might need. Large firms can cover a whole market in two broad ways: through undifferentiated marketing or differentiated marketing.

In *undifferentiated marketing*, the firm ignores segment differences and goes after the whole market with one offer. It designs a product and a marketing program that will appeal to the broadest number of buyers and then uses mass distribution backed by mass advertising to create a superior product image. The narrow product line helps hold down the costs of research and development, production, inven-tory, transportation, marketing research, advertising, and product management. The undifferentiated advertising program keeps down advertising costs. Presumably, the company can turn its lower costs into lower prices to win the price-sensitive seg-ment of the market. Lower costs may be accomplished at the expense of customer satisfaction, due to the failure of meeting individual needs; competitors may then have an incentive to reach the neglected segments and to increase market share.

In *differentiated marketing*, the firm operates in several market segments and designs different products for each segment. The best way to manage multiple segments is to appoint segment managers with sufficient authority and responsibility for building the segment's business. At the same time, segment managers should not be so focused as to resist cooperating with other groups in the company.

Consider the following situation: Baxter operated several divisions selling different products and services to hospitals. Each division sent out its own invoices. Some hospitals complained about receiving as many as seven different Baxter invoices each month. Baxter's marketers finally convinced the separate divisions to send the invoices to headquarters so that the company could send one invoice a month to its customers.

Differentiated marketing typically creates more total sales than undifferentiated marketing, but it also increases the costs of product modification, manufacturing, administration, inventory, and promotion. It is difficult to predict how this strategy will affect profitability. Some organizations take differentiated marketing to an extreme, launching more segmented programs than are economically feasible. This strategy can be the result of internal management pressures to keep up with competitors, but narrowing and deepening the product offering based on validated market needs usually results in better financial results. On the other hand, to achieve their missions, many community hospitals try to serve all segments in their service areas, with profitability as a secondary concern.

Additional Considerations

Three other considerations must be taken into account in evaluating and selecting segments: segment-by-segment invasion plans, updating segmentation schemes, and ethical choice of market targets.

Segment-by-Segment Invasion. An organization should enter one segment at a time and avoid letting rivals know which segments will be next. Unfortunately, too many companies fail to develop a long-term segment entry plan, often called an *invasion plan*. When a company's invasion plans are thwarted by blocked markets, the invader must then break into it using a mega-marketing approach. Mega marketing is the strategic coordination of economic, psychological, political, and public-relations skills to gain the cooperation of a number of parties in order to enter or operate in a given market.

Updating Segmentation Schemes. Market segmentation analysis must be done periodically because segments change. One way to discover new segments is to investigate the hierarchy of attributes consumers examine in choosing a brand. This process is called *market partitioning*. Buyers who first decide on price are price dominant; those who first decide on the type of product are product dominant; those who first decide on the brand are brand dominant. Customers also combine their preferences among these features. For example, those who are type/price/brand dominant make up a segment; those who are quality/service/type dominant make up another segment. Each segment may have distinct demographics, psychographics, and mediagraphics.[17]

Ethical Choice of Market Targets. Market targeting sometimes generates public controversy.[18] The public is concerned when marketers take unfair advantage of vulnerable groups (such as children) or disadvantaged groups (such as inner-city poor people) or promote potentially harmful products. The public is concerned when health insurers are unwilling to insure higher-risk patients, even at higher prices. Socially responsible marketing calls for targeting that serves not only the company's interests, but also the interests of those targeted.

MARKET POSITIONING

No organization can succeed if its products and offerings resemble every other product and offering; marketing strategy must be built on **segmentation, targeting,** *and* **positioning (STP).** An organization first discovers different needs and groups in the marketplace. Second, it targets those needs and groups that it can satisfy in a superior way. Then it positions its offering so that the target market recognizes the organization's distinctive offering and image. If an organization does a poor job of positioning, the market will be confused. If an organization does an excellent job of positioning, then it can work out the rest of its marketing planning and differentiation from its positioning strategy.

Positioning is the act of designing the organization's offering and image to occupy a distinctive place in the mind of the target market. The goal is to locate the brand in the minds of consumers to maximize the potential benefit to the organization. A good brand positioning helps guide marketing strategy by clarifying the brand's essence, what goals it helps the consumer achieve, and how it does so in a unique way. The result of positioning is the successful creation of a *customer-focused value proposition*, a cogent reason why the target market should buy the product.

The word *positioning* was popularized by two advertising executives, Al Ries and Jack Trout. They see positioning as a creative exercise done with an existing product: "Positioning starts with a product. A piece of merchandise, a service, a company, an institution, or even a person. . . . But positioning is not what you do to a product. Positioning is what you do to the mind of the prospect. That is, you position the product in the mind of the prospect."[19]

Rather than letting the customer figure out where the product or service exists vis-à-vis its competitors, successful companies position their offerings by pointing out the similarities and differences between brands. Therefore, deciding on a positioning strategy requires that a company determine a competitive frame of reference by identifying the target market, the nature of the competition, and the ideal points-of-parity and points-of-difference in brand associations.

Competitive Frame of Reference

A starting point in defining a competitive frame of reference for a brand positioning is to determine category membership—the products or sets of products with which a brand competes and that function as close substitutes. As discussed later in this chapter, competitive analysis considers a host of factors—including the resources, capabilities, and likely intentions of various other firms—in choosing those markets in which consumers can be profitably serviced.

Target market decisions are often a key determinant of the competitive frame of reference. Determining the proper competitive frame of reference requires understanding consumer behavior and the consideration sets that consumers use in making brand choices. In the United Kingdom, for example, the Automobile Association has positioned itself as the fourth "emergency service"—along with police, fire, and ambulance—to convey greater credibility and urgency.

Points-of-Parity and Points-of-Difference

After a firm defines the customer target market and nature of competition, its marketers can define the appropriate points-of-difference and points-of-parity associations.[20] *Points-of-difference* are attributes or benefits consumers strongly associate with a brand, positively evaluate, and believe that they could not find to the same extent with a competitive brand. Strong, favorable, and unique brand associations that make up points-of-difference may be based on virtually any attribute or benefit.

Points-of-parity, on the other hand, are associations that are not necessarily unique to the brand but may in fact be shared with other brands. Two basic forms are category and competitive points-of-parity. Category points-of-parity are associations consumers view as essential to be a legitimate and credible offering within a certain category, although perhaps not sufficient for brand choice. Consumers might not consider a home health agency to be truly a home health agency unless it is able to send nurses to patient residences, provide advice to improve daily living, and offer various durable medical equipment options. Category points-of-parity may change over time due to technological advances, legal developments, or consumer trends. For example, home health agencies may also need to provide infusion therapies to fit into this category.

Competitive points-of-parity are associations designed to negate competitors' points-of-difference. If a brand can "break even" in those areas where the competitors are trying to find an advantage and can achieve advantages in some other areas, the brand should be in a strong—and perhaps unbeatable—competitive position. To achieve a point-of-parity on a particular attribute or benefit, a sufficient number of consumers must believe that the brand is "good enough" on that dimension. Often, the key to positioning is not so much in achieving a point-of-difference as it is in achieving points-of-parity. This positioning is akin to the integrated, "total solution" strategy we discussed in Chapter Two.

Establishing Category Membership

Target customers are aware that Blue Cross/Blue Shield is a leading health insurance brand, Nexium is a leading heartburn drug brand, and the Mayo Clinic is a leading physician group. Often, however, marketers must inform consumers of a brand's category membership, especially when it is not always apparent; for example, when a new product is introduced. There are also situations in which consumers know a brand's category membership but may not be convinced that the brand is a valid member of the category. For example, physicians may be aware that Agfa produces digital X-ray equipment, but they may not be certain whether Agfa X-ray machines are in the same class with those of Siemens, General Electric, and Kodak. Agfa might find it useful to reinforce category membership.

It is important that consumers understand what the brand stands for and not just what it is *not*. Because brands are sometimes affiliated with categories in which they do not hold membership, they should not be trapped between categories, unless the company is trying to invent a new category. The preferred positioning approach is therefore to inform consumers of a brand's membership *before* stating its point-of-difference; consumers need to know what a product is and what function it serves before deciding whether it dominates the brands against which it competes. There are three main ways to convey a brand's category membership:

- *Announcing category benefits.* To reassure consumers that a brand will deliver on the fundamental reason for using a category, benefits are frequently used to announce category membership. Thus dental tools might claim to have durability and antacids might announce their efficacy in reducing stomach distress.

- *Comparing to exemplars.* Well-known, noteworthy brands in a category can also be used to specify category membership. Using the Agfa X-ray example, Agfa could advertise its market position vis-à-vis its larger competitors to establish itself in the desired category. A corollary technique is for an organization to publicize its affiliations with better-known category leaders. For instance, when Raleigh Community Hospital was a brand without a strong positioning, advertising announced its ownership by Duke Health System, a recognized brand in the category.

- *Relying on the product descriptor.* The product descriptor that follows the brand name is often a very concise means of conveying category origin. For example, Grane Healthcare attaches the descriptor "Pennsylvania's Premier Senior Living Provider" to explain its category.

Choosing Points-of-Parity and Points-of-Difference

Points-of-parity are driven by the needs of category membership (to create category points-of-parity) and the necessity of negating competitors' points-of-difference (to create competitive points-of-parity). In choosing points-of-difference, two important considerations are that consumers find the points-of-difference desirable and that the firm has the capabilities to deliver on the points-of-difference. The three key *consumer desirability criteria* for target customers are that the product must be personally *relevant* and important, *distinctive* and superior, and *believable* and credible.

Additionally, there are three key *deliverability criteria* for points-of-difference: *feasibility*—that is, the organization must be able to actually create the points-of-difference; *communicability*—that is, the brand must substantiate that it can deliver the desired benefit; and s*ustainability*—that is, the positioning must be preemptive, defensible, and difficult to attack.

Creating Points-of-Parity and Points-of-Difference

One common difficulty in creating a strong competitive position is that many of the attributes or benefits that make up the points-of-parity and points-of-difference are negatively correlated. If consumers rate the brand highly on one particular attribute or benefit, they may also rate it poorly on another important attribute. For example, it might be difficult to position a brand as "inexpensive" and at the same time assert that it is "of the highest quality." Moreover, individual attributes and benefits often have positive *and* negative aspects. A health information system is not easily positioned as both "cutting edge" and "a longstanding market leader." A legacy leadership position could be positive and suggest experience, financial stability, and expertise. On the other hand, it could also easily be regarded as negative, as it might imply being rooted in old technology and not innovative.

An expensive but sometimes effective approach to address negatively correlated attributes and benefits is to launch two different marketing campaigns, each one devoted to a different brand attribute or benefit. These campaigns may run concurrently or sequentially. Head & Shoulders shampoo met success in Europe with a dual campaign: one emphasized its dandruff removal efficacy, another highlighted the appearance and beauty of hair after its use. This approach might cause consumers to be less critical when judging the points-of-parity and points-of-difference benefits in isolation.

Linkage with well-known branded ingredients may also lend credibility to a questionable attribute in consumers' minds. Vytorin pairs Merck's Zocor—a highly successful, well-known medication—and Schering-Plough's Zetia. The latter medication was a little-known entity that works synergistically with Zocor to lower cholesterol. The two companies set up a joint venture in 2001 to develop this combination; Vytorin quickly became the world's second-best-selling fixed-combination product ever because it tackles lipid levels convincingly in two entirely different ways. The linkage with a well-known brand helped to establish Zetia's credibility.

Differentiation Strategies

Products must be differentiated to be branded. This differentiation can be based on characteristics of the product or service, but also through attributes of personnel, channels, and images (see Table 8.3).[21]

TABLE 8.3. Differentiation Variables

Product	Services	Personnel	Channel	Image
Form	Ordering ease	Competence	Coverage	Symbols, colors, slogans
Features	Delivery	Courtesy	Expertise	Atmosphere
Conformance	Installation	Credibility	Performance	Events
Durability	Customer training	Reliability		Brand contacts
Reliability	Customer consulting	Responsiveness		
Reparability	Maintenance and repair	Communication		
Style				
Design				
Quality				

Product Differentiation. Physical products vary in their potential for differentiation. At one extreme are health care products that allow little variation, such as scalpels, aspirin, and crutches. Yet even for these, some differentiation is possible. For example, MYCO Medical, a distributor of scalpel blades to physicians, can offer an imported blade at a very low price with extremely responsive sales and account service. At the other end of the spectrum, there are products that can be highly differentiated, such as clinical software and eyeglasses. Products can be differentiated through the following attributes:[22]

- *Form.* This attribute refers to the product's size, shape, or physical structure. For example, aspirin can be differentiated by dosage size, shape, and coating.

- *Features.* The characteristics that supplement the product's basic function are its features. Marketers can identify and select new features by researching needs and calculating *customer value* versus *organization cost* for each potential feature. With a pharmaceutical product, a useful feature can be duration of action; for example, shorter for a sleeping pill and longer for blood pressure medication. Regarding each feature, they should also think about how many customers want it, how much time they should devote to introducing it, and how easily rivals can copy it. Organizations must also think in terms of feature bundles or packages. Health information systems companies often bundle software modules, which lowers product development and packaging costs. As well, pharmaceutical companies manufacture combinations of medications whose branded ingredients would be more costly if purchased separately. Each organization must decide whether to offer feature customization at a higher cost or a few standard packages at a lower cost.

■ *Performance quality.* Most products are established at one of four performance levels: low, average, high, or superior. Performance quality is the level at which the product's primary characteristics operate; for example, how well it does what it claims to do. Firms should not necessarily design the highest performance level possible, but rather the level that is appropriate to the target market and competitors' performance levels. A company must also manage performance quality through time. Continuously improving the product can produce higher returns and market share. Lowering quality in an attempt to cut costs often has dire consequences.

■ *Conformance quality.* Conformance quality reflects the degree to which all of the produced units are identical and consistently meet the promised specifications. The conformance quality of medical devices, such as pacemakers, is easy to evaluate; they are checked often according to preset parameters, and malfunctions have obvious consequences. On the other hand, although the government may monitor manufacturing practices, the consumer may not be able to easily evaluate the potency conformance of medications. The problem with low conformance quality is that the product will disappoint some buyers and may lead to legal repercussions.

■ *Durability.* Durability, a measure of the product's expected operating life under natural or stressful conditions, is a valued attribute for certain products. Buyers will generally pay more for medical devices and equipment that have a reputation for being long lasting. This rule is subject to some qualifications. The additional price must not be excessive, or third-party payers are unlikely to offer reimbursement for it. Furthermore, the product must not be subject to rapid technological obsolescence. Also, as a practical matter, the product must match the life expectancy of the user; an innovative, expensive pacemaker that will last thirty years is not likely to add value when implanted in a ninety-year-old patient.

- *Reliability.* Buyers normally will pay a premium for more reliable products. Reliability is a measure of the probability that a product will not malfunction or fail within a specified time period. Many health care products and services have had reputations for reliability in the past, but such occurrences as internal defibrillator malfunctions have negatively affected company images.

- *Reparability.* Reparability is a measure of the ease of fixing a product when it malfunctions or fails. Ideal reparability would exist if users could fix the product themselves with little cost in money or time. Some products include a diagnostic feature that allows service people to correct a problem over the telephone or advise the user how to correct it.

- *Style.* Style is the product's look and feel to the buyer. Style has the advantage of creating distinctiveness that is difficult to copy. On the negative side, strong style does not always mean high performance. Although health care product manufacturers usually emphasize functionality, style may be used to distinguish a product from its competitors. For example, the advertising campaign for the stomach acid-reducing medication, Nexium, relies on its appearance as "the Purple Pill."

- *Design.* As competition intensifies, design offers a potent way to differentiate and position a company's products and services.[23] Design integrates all of the product qualities. To the organization, a well-designed product is one that is easy to manufacture and distribute. To the consumer, a well-designed product is one that is pleasant to look at and easy to open, install, use, repair, and dispose of after its useful life.

Services Differentiation. When the physical product cannot easily be differentiated, the key to competitive success may lie in adding valued services and improving their quality:

- *Ordering ease.* This benefit refers to how easy it is for the customer to place an order with the company. Baxter Healthcare has eased the ordering process by supplying hospitals with computer terminals that they use to send orders directly to Baxter; UCLA Medical Center and Emory Healthcare now provide access to physician appointments through the hospital Web site.

- *Delivery.* Attributes of how well the offering is delivered include speed, accuracy, and care. Today's customers have grown to expect delivery speed: pizza delivered in half an hour, film developed in one hour, eyeglasses made in one hour, cars lubricated in fifteen minutes. MedScribe, a medical transcription company based in Jacksonville, Florida, uses digital dictation technology to turn around dictated medical records from hospitals across the country in one hour to twenty-four hours, or even less, depending on specific client needs.

■ *Installation.* This feature refers to the work done to make a product operational in its planned location. Differentiating at this point in the consumption chain is particularly important for organizations with complex products. Ease of installation becomes a true selling point, especially when the target market is technology novices. For new hospital customers wishing to convert their legacy health information system to a new McKesson Health product, a specially trained team of McKesson experts is available on-site during the installation period. These McKesson employees have all had direct hospital experience and understand the perspective of the customer.

■ *Customer training.* Training the customer's employees to use products properly and efficiently is a key differentiator. General Electric not only sells and installs sophisticated imaging equipment in hospitals, it also gives extensive training to hospital users of this equipment.

■ *Customer consulting.* Customer needs can go beyond the product purchased. To satisfy total customer requirements, the seller needs to offer other products or services or help customers assess how to best solve their problems. Many customers are willing to pay a premium for these extras because they anticipate improved profitability.[24]

■ *Maintenance and repair.* When something does go wrong, the customer wants to be able to fix it quickly to restore full functioning. Many computer hardware and health care software companies offer technical support over the phone or by fax or e-mail.

A4 Health Systems, a provider of electronic health records, offers on-line technical support or "e-support" for its customers. In the event of a service problem, customers can use various on-line tools to find a solution. Those aware of the specific problem can search an on-line database for fixes; those who are unaware can use diagnostic software that finds the problem and searches the on-line database for an automatic fix. Customers can also seek on-line help from a technician.[25]

Health care service marketers frequently complain that differentiating their services is difficult because they believe that their offering is a commodity. To the extent that customers view a service as fairly homogeneous, they may actually care less about the provider than the price. For example, few patients ask prospective physicians about their training and board certification. One of the more frequent questions in selecting a doctor is whether he or she participates with the consumer's health plan. Although the particular health care service provider is a critical element of service delivery, price is becoming increasingly important to consumers with the growth of high-deductible health plans.

Health care service offerings *can* be effectively differentiated. One approach used by innovative hospitals has been to differentiate as well as improve their product (see sidebar).

HOSPITALS TURN TO BUILDING BETTER HEALING ENVIRONMENTS

There is increasing evidence that well-designed environments that are pleasant, aesthetic, and quiet and naturally lit result in patients healing faster, requiring less medication, and leaving the hospital sooner. Kaiser Permanente noticed that patients in rooms facing the sunniest exposures had shorter hospital stays, used less medicine, and reported higher satisfaction with their hospital experience. Banner Good Samaritan Medical Center in Phoenix developed an outdoor healing garden with desert plants and benches and is able to monitor their patients' conditions via wireless telemetry devices. The St. Francis Medical Center in Peoria, Illinois, developed a third corridor to reduce the noise of passing service and delivery carts. The Montefiore Medical Center in the Bronx, N.Y., introduced a program called "Silent Hospitals Help Healing" by monitoring and discouraging hallway conversations and limiting intercom volumes.

An increasing number of hospitals are rethinking the "hospital experience" from the patient's point of view. No patient is happy walking down the dark halls of a hospital in an open-back blue gown. At Memorial Hermann Healthcare System Hospitals, patients are told they can bring their own pajamas to wear around the hospital.

Two of the Memorial Hermann hospitals are going further. They have added gourmet chefs and room service to replace plain food served only at scheduled times. They are adding healing gardens, more uplifting hospital colors, and soothing music. They are considering adding pet therapy, marble hot tubs, and aromatherapy to replace the smells of rubbing alcohol and disinfectant.

The aim is to change the impersonal character of hospitals to one that "addresses the mental and spiritual aspects of healing." According to Jean Sedita, clinical director of medical-surgical nursing at Memorial Hermann, "It's costly. But when you look at what drives patients to get better, in creating that environment—quiet, stress-free—it helps with the healing process."

Sources: L. Landro, "Hospitals Build a Better 'Healing Environment.'" *Wall Street Journal*, Mar. 21, 2007, p. D9; and "System Looks at the Ins and Outs of Holistic Patient Environment." *Modern Healthcare*, Jan. 8, 2007, p. 36.

Sometimes an organization achieves differentiation through the sheer range of its service offerings and the success of cross-selling its various offerings. The major challenge is that most service offerings and innovations are easily copied. The organization that regularly introduces advances will gain a succession of temporary advantages over competitors and become known as an innovator.

Personnel Differentiation

Service organizations, as well as product companies, can gain a strong competitive advantage through their people. A more satisfied workforce has higher productivity and conveys a better image to its customers. Superior organizations have employees who exhibit *competence* (skill and knowledge), *courtesy* (respect and consideration), *credibility* (trustworthiness), *reliability* (consistent and accurate performance), *responsiveness* (a sense of urgency), and *communication* (desire to understand customers and communicate clearly).[26] Griffin Hospital, in Connecticut, has been successful in differentiating itself as one of the best places in the nation in which to work (see sidebar).

GRIFFEN HOSPITAL USES CUSTOMER FOCUS TO IMPROVE ITS RATING

Griffin Hospital in Derby, Connecticut, was named the fourth best place to work in the nation, according to *Fortune Magazine*'s list of the "Top 100 Companies to Work for 2006"; it was the sixth year in a row it made this list. What is this hospital's secret? Simply stated, it's a relentless focus on patient care with no detail left unattended. This was not always the case with Griffin Hospital.

Located in a working-class, economically depressed region, the hospital's financial situation was poor in the early 1980s. It was losing market share to seven larger health care institutions including nearby Yale–New Haven Medical Center. Griffin's strength was that it was the most affordable hospital in the state. Unfortunately, lower prices also meant less money to invest in new technology and updated facilities. A survey conducted by the hospital in 1982 showed that Griffin was the #1 hospital consumers hoped to *avoid*.

Today, Griffin is giving other hospital executives "benchmarking" tours to show them how to replicate Griffin's success. Outpatient visits have soared 72 percent since 1998, and admissions are up 25 percent since 1999. The consulting firm Total Benchmark Solutions ranked Griffin twelfth among 2,053 hospitals across the nation for the quality of its care.

The Griffin reputation for quality care also attracts like-minded employees and doctors. Although Griffin employees are paid 5 to 7 percent *less* in a fiercely competitive field with chronic labor shortages, the hospital had more than 5,100 applicants in 2005 for only 160 jobs. Focusing on patient care and customer service is attractive to doctors and nurses whose job satisfaction is directly related to the level of care they are able to offer. For example, decentralized nursing stations, or pods, allow nurses to have easier access to patient rooms. The Griffin patient-to-nurse ratios are among the highest nationally. Each nurse cares for only four patients during day shifts, while the norm in other hospitals is usually seven to ten patients. Overhead paging in the patient care areas is limited to just ten to twelve pages each day so patients can get more rest and get better faster.

To make sure that employees and doctors clearly understand the importance of patient-centered care, each new member of the team meets with Griffin CEO Patrick Charmel and two other top executives on their first day of work. "We know clearly from the orientation session that Pat and I do that the clinicians are coming to Griffin because of the approach to patient care. It's the reason they went into their professions [in the first place back] when they were in school," according to William Powanda, a Griffin Hospital vice president.

Source: R. Kalra, "2 State Employers on Fortune's List." *Hartford Courant*, Jan. 11, 2006.

Channel Differentiation

Organizations can achieve competitive advantage through the way they design their distribution channel *coverage*, *expertise*, and *performance*. Drug wholesalers achieve a competitive advantage through channel performance. Biomet, in the orthopedic implant product segment, has also distinguished itself by developing and managing high-quality direct-marketing channels.

Image Differentiation

Buyers respond differently to company and brand images. *Identity* is the way in which an organization aims to help customers recognize its products or position itself. *Image* is the way the public perceives the company or its products. An effective image establishes the offering's character and value proposition, conveys its character in a distinctive way, and delivers emotional power beyond a mental image. To be effective, both identity and image need to be consistently conveyed through every communication vehicle and brand contact, including symbols, colors, slogans, atmosphere, media, and special events.

COMPETITIVE FORCES AND COMPETITORS

It would seem a simple task for an organization to identify its competitors. Stryker knows that Synthes is a major orthopedic implant competitor; Pfizer knows that its statin drug Lipitor competes with AstraZeneca's Crestor. However, the range of an organization's actual and potential competitors is actually much broader than it may first appear. An organization is more likely to be hurt by emerging competitors or new technologies than by current competitors. Rapid health care service market changes in China illustrate this point (see sidebar).

CHINA BECOMES AN ACTIVE HEALTH CARE MARKET

Local Chinese hospitals, which are mostly state-owned, now have several new global competitors that they probably did not anticipate. Leading international health care providers are speeding up efforts to market Western-style medical services to China's elite. The competitive moves are targeting high-income Chinese who have traditionally used their local hospitals but who are now considering other options due to rising personal income levels.

For example, Chindex International, a U.S.-based health care company that targets the Chinese market, has joined with Fesco Insurance Brokerage, the Chinese state-run human resources group, to introduce a new insurance plan aimed mainly at upper-income Chinese. Wealthy Chinese who frequently travel abroad now want the same health care and payment options as foreigners. Chindex has two hospitals operating under the brand United Family Hospitals & Clinics (UFHC) in Beijing and Shanghai, and it expects to open two more. While more Chinese can now afford UFHC services, the new insurance product will assist buyers in planning for their health care needs.

HCA, the largest hospital chain in the U.S., is also considering offering a new patient referral service for wealthy Chinese, to assist them in visiting Western hospitals for various medical procedures. Cedars-Sinai Medical Center, the Los Angeles hospital that caters to the Hollywood Set, is also attempting to develop patient referrals from China. The Medical Center has employees who speak fluent Mandarin.

Source: Financial Times Limited, Oct. 24, 2006.

Industry Concept of Competition

An *industry* is a group of firms that offers a product or class of products that are close substitutes for each other. Industries are classified according to number of sellers; degree of product differentiation; presence or absence of entry, mobility, and exit barriers; cost structure; degree of vertical integration; and degree of globalization. In the following section, we pick up from the discussion of strategy in Chapter Five.

Number of Sellers and Degree of Differentiation. The starting point for describing an industry is to specify the number of sellers and determine whether the product is homogeneous or highly differentiated. These characteristics give rise to four industry structure types. In a *pure monopoly*, only one firm provides a certain offering in a specific area (such as a regional power company). An unregulated monopolist might charge a high price, do little or no advertising, and offer minimal service. If partial substitutes are available and there is some danger of competition, the monopolist might invest in more service and technology. A regulated monopolist is required to charge a lower price and provide more service as a matter of public interest.

In an *oligopoly*, a small number of usually large firms produce offerings that range from highly differentiated to standardized. In *pure oligopoly*, a few organizations produce essentially the same commodity (such as gasoline), so all have difficulty charging more than the going price. If competitors match services, the only way to gain a competitive advantage is through lower costs; however, as noted previously, price wars are destructive for all industry members. In *differentiated oligopoly*, a few organizations (such as hospitals) put forward offerings partially differentiated by quality, features, styling, or services. Each competitor may seek leadership in one attribute, attract customers seeking that attribute, and charge a premium for its special expertise or product.

Monopolistic competition means that many competitors are able to differentiate their offers in whole or in part. An example is assisted living facilities. Competitors focus on market segments in which they can better meet customer needs and charge more. In *pure competition*, many competitors offer the same product and service, so without differentiation all prices will be the same. No competitor will advertise unless advertising can create psychological differentiation (such as in health insurance), in which case the industry is in actuality monopolistically competitive.

An industry's competitive structure can change over time; this is often due to events in other parts of its sector. For example, in the 1980s the traditional health insurance market changed from being composed overwhelmingly of traditional indemnity plans to predominantly managed-care products. As these plans became more competitive, they offered pharmaceutical benefits. When costs for this benefit rose, pharmaceutical benefit management (PBM) firms were created, altering the supply chain and industry structure for wholesalers.

Degree of Vertical Integration. Many organizations benefit from *vertical integration*—integrating backward or forward to offer a total solution that advantageously positions its services and products vis-à-vis competitors. An example is the internationally known Aravind Eye Care System in Madurai, India. This eye-care hospital not only provides quality and affordable eye care to all, but also conducts research, provides training for specialists. and manufactures intra-ocular lenses, pharmaceuticals, and sutures for use in cataract surgery.

Vertical integration often lowers costs, and firms gain a larger share of the value-added stream. Also, a vertically integrated firm can manage prices and costs in different parts of the value chain to earn profits where taxes are lowest. On the other hand, vertical integration may raise costs in certain parts of the value chain and restrict a firm's strategic flexibility, which is why organizations outsource activities that specialists can handle better and more cheaply.

Market Concept of Competition

Using the market approach, competitors are organizations that satisfy the same customer need. For example, a customer who buys a flu vaccination wants disease prevention—a need that can be satisfied by a personal physician, a "minute clinic" in a drug store, an urgent care center, a hospital emergency room, or a county health department. The market concept of competition reveals a broader set of actual and potential competitors. Rayport and Jaworski suggest profiling a company's direct and indirect competitors by mapping the buyer's steps in obtaining and using the product. They suggest a *competitor map* composed of three concentric domains, with the center listing consumer buying activities; the first outer ring listing direct competitors with respect to each consumer activity; and the second outer ring listing indirect competitors that may increasingly become direct competitors (see Figure 8.2). This type of analysis highlights both the opportunities and the challenges a company faces.[27]

Analyzing Competitors

Once an organization identifies its primary competitors, it must ascertain their strategies, objectives, strengths, and weaknesses.

Strategies. A group of firms following the same strategy in a given target market is called a *strategic group*.[28] For example, suppose an organization wants to enter the surgical supplies industry. What is its strategic group? It discovers a *range* of possibilities that can be characterized by the dimensions of product quality and level of vertical integration. For example, analysis of this group would find that Group A (narrow product line, high cost, high quality, and low vertical integration) has one competitor (Teleflex Medical), while group B (full product line, moderately priced, lower quality, and the same vertical integration) has three (Davis & Geck, Chengbiao Medical

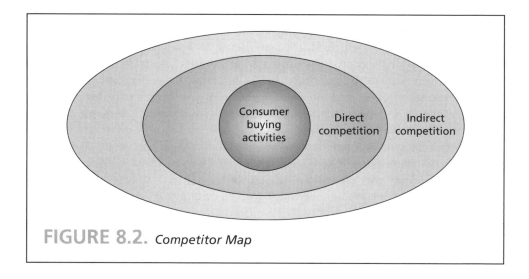

FIGURE 8.2. *Competitor Map*

Supplies, and Johnson & Johnson). Important insights emerge from this analysis. First, the height of the entry barriers differs for each group. Second, if the company successfully enters a group, the members of that group become its key competitors.

Objectives. Once a company has identified its main competitors and their strategies, it must ask, What is each competitor seeking in the marketplace? What drives each competitor's behavior? Many factors shape a competitor's objectives, including size, history, current management, and financial situation. If the competitor is a division of a larger company, it is important to know whether the parent company is running it for growth or profits or is milking it.[29]

Note that companies differ in the emphasis they put on short-term versus long-term profits. Many U.S. firms have been criticized for operating on a short-run model, largely because current performance is judged by stockholders who might lose confidence, sell their stock, and cause the company's cost of capital to rise. Japanese firms operate largely on a market-share-maximization model. They receive much of their funds from banks at a lower interest rate and in the past have readily accepted lower profits. An alternative assumption is that each competitor pursues some mix of objectives: current profitability, market-share growth, cash flow, technological leadership, or service leadership. Finally, an organization must monitor competitors' expansion plans.

Strengths and Weaknesses. When analyzing competitors, an organization should monitor three variables:

1. *Share of market.* The competitor's share of the target market

2. *Share of mind.* The percentage of customers who named the competitor in response to the statement "Name the first company that comes to mind in this industry"

3. *Share of heart.* The percentage of customers who named the competitor in response to the statement "Name the company from which you would prefer to buy the product"

Companies that make steady gains in mind share and heart share will inevitably make gains in market share and profitability. To improve market share, many companies benchmark their most successful competitors, as well as world-class performers.

Selecting Competitors. After the company has conducted customer value analysis and examined competitors carefully, it can focus its attack on one of the following classes of competitors: strong versus weak, close versus distant, and "good" versus "bad."

- *Strong versus weak.* Most organizations aim at weak competitors because this tactic requires fewer resources per share point gained. The organization should also compete with strong competitors to keep up with the best. Even strong competitors have some weaknesses.

- *Close versus distant.* Most organizations compete with competitors who resemble them the most, yet companies should also recognize distant competitors, as they can offer substitutes for the organization's products or services. For example, an orthopedic clinic that offers rehabilitation services competes not only with local sports medicine programs but also with on-line instructional resources.

- *"Good" versus "bad."* Every industry includes "good" and "bad" competitors.[30] An organization should support its good competitors and attack its bad competitors. Good competitors play by the industry's rules; they make realistic assumptions about the industry's growth potential; they set prices in reasonable relation to costs; they favor a healthy industry; they limit themselves to a portion or segment of the industry; they motivate others to lower costs or improve differentiation; and they accept the general level of their share and profits. Bad competitors try to buy share rather than earn it; they take large risks; they invest in overcapacity; and they upset industrial equilibrium.

Competitive Strategy

An organization can gain further insight into its competitive position by classifying its competitors and itself according to the roles each plays as market leader, market challenger, market follower, or market nicher. On the basis of this classification, the company can take specific actions in line with its current and desired roles.

Market-leader strategies. Many industries contain a very small number of firms that are the acknowledged market leaders. Such leaders may have one or more of the following characteristics: having the largest market share; leading the other firms in price changes, new product introductions, distribution coverage, and promotional intensity; and being opinion or thought leaders. Ries and Trout argue that well-known products generally hold a distinctive position in consumers' minds. Nevertheless, unless a dominant firm enjoys a legal monopoly, it must be sure not to miss key developments. A product innovation may affect the leader, such as when a relatively unknown firm (Fonar) developed the first open and first stand-up MRI scanners. Another risk is that the dominant firm might look old-fashioned compared with newer, energetic rivals; some customers may want to "buy futures" in dealing preferentially with these innovative firms.

Enduring as market leader calls for action on three fronts: expanding total market demand, protecting its current market share through good defensive and offensive actions, and trying to increase its market share, even if market size remains constant.

Expanding the total market. The dominant firm normally gains the most when the total market expands. If Americans increase their purchases of health insurance, UnitedHealth Group stands to gain because it sells the largest share of the nation's health insurance. It can attract buyers who are unaware of the product or who are resisting it because of price or the lack of certain features. An organization can search for new buyers who might use the product (market-penetration strategy), those who have never used the product category (new-market segment strategy), or those who live elsewhere (geographical-expansion strategy).

To increase usage, marketers can boost the *level* or *quantity* of consumption or increase the *frequency* of consumption. Consumption can sometimes be increased through packaging or product design. Increasing frequency of use involves identifying additional opportunities to use the brand in the same basic way or finding completely new and different ways to use it. Product development can also spur new uses. Chewing gum manufacturers are exploring ways to make "nutraceutical" products as a cheap, effective delivery mechanism for medicine. The majority of Adam's chewing gums (ranked number two in the world) claim health benefits. Aquafresh and Arm & Hammer are two dental gums that have also achieved some success.[31]

Defending market share. While trying to expand total market size, dominant organizations must also defend current business against domestic and foreign rivals. The most constructive response is *continuous innovation* in new offerings, customer services, distribution effectiveness, and cost cutting. Additionally, leaders must consider which segments to defend, even at a loss, and which to surrender. The aim of defensive strategy is to reduce the probability of attack, divert attacks to less threatening areas, and lessen their intensity. A dominant firm can choose from six defensive strategies.

1. *Position defense.* This action involves occupying the most desirable market space in the minds of the consumer and making the brand virtually impregnable. Market leaders often own key category benefits that play a crucial role in consumer choice; for example, Johns Hopkins has held the number one spot in the *U.S. News & World Report*'s annual "Best Hospitals" list for sixteen years in a row.

2. *Flank defense.* Although position defense is important, the market leader should also erect outposts to protect a weak front or possibly serve as an invasion base for counterattack. For example, an academic medical center could build primary care practices in areas that it wants to penetrate for increased referrals for tertiary services.

3. *Preemptive defense.* A more aggressive maneuver is to attack before the competitor starts its offense. An organization can launch a preemptive defense in several ways. It can wage guerrilla action across the market—hitting one competitor here, another there—and keep everyone off balance, or it can try to achieve a grand market envelopment. Another approach is to send out market signals and dissuade competitors from attacking.[32] A firm can also introduce a stream of new products supported by preannouncements—deliberate communications regarding future actions.[33] For example, McKesson, a leader in health information systems, could announce the release of a new and improved version of its software months before it is actually offered. Of course, it must launch when it says it will be ready. Past failures in this tactic have caused stock prices to plummet in sectors ranging from pharmaceuticals to information technology.

4. *Counteroffensive defense.* When attacked, most market leaders will respond with a counterattack. In a counteroffensive, as in actual battle, the leader can meet

the attacker frontally, hit its flank, or launch a pincer movement. An effective counterattack is to invade the attacker's main territory so that it will have to pull back to defend the territory. Another common form of counteroffensive is the exercise of economic or political clout. The leader may try to crush a competitor by subsidizing lower prices for the vulnerable product with revenue from its more profitable products—being careful to avoid legal repercussions of predatory pricing. As mentioned above, the leader may also prematurely announce that a product upgrade will be available, to cause customers to hesitate before buying the competitor's product.

5. *Mobile defense.* Here, the leader stretches its domain over new territories that can serve as future centers for defense and offense through market broadening and market diversification. With market broadening, the organization focuses on the underlying generic need, not the current product, and gets involved in R&D across the whole range of technology associated with that need. Thus hospitals have been known to recast themselves into "systems" that enter into arrangements with physician practices, educational services, urgent care, diagnostic services, clinical research, and other medical areas. Market diversification involves shifting into unrelated industries. When U.S. tobacco companies like Reynolds and Philip Morris finally acknowledged the health hazards associated with cigarette smoking, they were not content with position defense or even with looking for cigarette substitutes. Instead they quickly moved into new industries, such as beer, liquor, soft drinks, and frozen foods.

6. *Contraction defense.* Large companies sometimes recognize that they can no longer defend all of their territory. The best course of action then appears to be planned contraction (also called strategic withdrawal), giving up weaker territories, and reassigning resources to stronger territories. Coastal Physician Services, best known for staffing hospital emergency departments, decided to enter the managed care business in 1994. Several years later, after significant financial losses, Coastal sold its unprofitable health plan subsidiary.

Expanding market share. Market leaders can improve profitability by increasing their market share. In many markets, one share point is worth tens of millions of dollars. Because the cost of buying higher market share may far exceed its revenue value, a company should consider four factors before pursuing increased market share:

- *The first factor* is the possibility of provoking antitrust action. Jealous competitors are likely to cry "monopoly" if a dominant firm makes further inroads.

- *The second factor* is economic cost. Profitability may fall, not rise, with further market share gains beyond a certain level. "Holdout" customers may dislike the company, be loyal to competitive suppliers, have unique needs, or prefer dealing with smaller suppliers. Also, the cost of legal work, public relations, and lobbying rises with market share. Pushing for higher market share is less justified when there are few scale or experience economies, unattractive market segments exist, buyers want multiple supply sources, and exit barriers are high.

Some leaders have even increased profitability by selectively decreasing market share in weaker areas.[34] This strategy was particularly successful in the managed care industry when companies such as Aetna shifted from a market share maximization strategy to one that better managed a smaller book of business, thus returning to it profitability.

- *The third factor* is pursuing the wrong marketing-mix strategy. Companies that successfully gain share typically outperform competitors in three areas: new-product activity, relative product quality, and marketing expenditures.[35] As mentioned previously, companies that cut prices more deeply than competitors typically do not achieve significant gains, as enough rivals meet the price cuts and others offer other values so that buyers do not switch.

- *The fourth factor* is the effect of increased market share on actual and perceived quality.[36]

Other Competitive Strategies. Firms that are not market leaders in an industry are often called *runner-up* or *trailing* firms, even though they may be quite large in their own right. These firms can adopt one of two postures. They can attack the leader and other competitors in an aggressive bid for further market share (market challengers), or they can take a self-protective stance (market followers).

Market-challenger strategies. A market challenger must first define its strategic objective. If it decides to increase market share, the challenger must decide who to attack. Attacking the market leader can potentially result in a high payoff if that leader is not serving the market well. The risk with this strategy is that this action may get the attention of the market leader, which may then acquire the competitor. Such a scenario developed when, in 2006, United Health Group bought Nevada-based Sierra Health Services, Inc. The challenger can also attack firms of its own size that are underperforming, underfinanced, have aging products, charge excessive prices, or are not satisfying customers in other ways. A third choice is to attack small local and regional firms.

Given clear opponents and objectives, there are five general market challenger options:

- *Frontal attack.* Match the opponent's product, advertising, price, and distribution. The side with the greater resources will win. If the competitor can convince the market that its offering is equal to that of the leader's—and if the market leader does not retaliate—a modified frontal attack can be effective.

- *Flank attack.* A flanking strategy is another term for identifying shifts in market segments that are causing gaps to develop, then filling the gaps and developing them into strong segments. Because they use fewer resources, flank attacks are particularly attractive to a small challenger and are much more likely to succeed than a frontal attack.

  In a geographical flank attack, the challenger spots areas in which a rival is underperforming. The other flanking strategy is to serve uncovered market needs, as minute clinics inside drug stores did when they increased immediate access to very basic primary care without an appointment or prolonged waiting.

■ *Encirclement attack.* The encirclement maneuver is used to capture a wide slice of the opponent's territory through a "blitz." It involves launching a grand offensive on several fronts. Encirclement makes sense when the challenger commands superior resources in a particular niche and believes a swift encirclement will break the opponent's will.

■ *Bypass attack.* The most indirect assault strategy involves bypassing the opponent and attacking easier markets to broaden one's resource base. Three lines of approach are diversifying into unrelated products, diversifying into new geographical markets, and leapfrogging into new technologies to supplant existing products. *Technological leapfrogging* is a bypass strategy practiced in high-tech industries.

■ *Guerrilla warfare.* This strategy consists of small, intermittent attacks intended to harass and demoralize the opponent, eventually securing permanent footholds. The guerrilla challenger uses both conventional and unconventional means of attack, such as selective price cuts and intense promotional campaigns. Normally, guerrilla warfare is practiced by a smaller entity against a larger one. It *can* be costly, but it is usually less expensive than a frontal, encirclement, or flank attack. If the challenger hopes to beat the opponent, the guerrilla warfare must be backed by a stronger attack, based on more specific strategies such as product innovation, improved services, distribution innovation, manufacturing cost reduction, or intensive advertising promotion. A challenger's success depends on combining several strategies to improve its position over time.

Market-follower strategies. Theodore Levitt has argued that a strategy of *product imitation* might be as profitable as a strategy of *product innovation.*[37] The innovator bears the expense of developing the new product, getting it into distribution, and educating the market about its useful features. The reward for all this work and risk is normally market leadership, even though another firm can then copy or improve on the new product. Although it probably will not overtake the leader, the follower can achieve high profits because it did not bear any of the innovation expense.

Many companies prefer to follow rather than challenge the market leader. Patterns of "conscious parallelism" are common in capital-intensive, homogeneous-product industries in which the opportunities for product differentiation and image differentiation are low, service quality is often comparable, and price sensitivity is high. Short-term grabs for market share provoke retaliation, so most firms present similar offers to buyers, usually by copying the leader. This dynamic keeps market shares highly stable.

This situation does not mean that market followers lack strategies. A market follower must know how to hold current customers and win a fair share of new customers. Each follower tries to bring distinctive advantages to its target market—location, services, or financing. Because the follower is often itself a major target of attack by challengers, it must keep its manufacturing costs low and its product quality and services high. It must also enter new markets as they emerge. The follower has to define a growth path, but one that does not invite competitive retaliation. Normally a follower earns less than the leader. No wonder Jack Welch, former CEO of GE, told his business units that each must reach either the number one or two position in its market—or else.

Market nicher strategies. An alternative to being a follower in a large market is to be a leader in a small market or niche. Smaller firms normally avoid competing with larger firms by targeting small markets of little or no interest to the larger firms. Firms with low shares of the total market can be highly profitable through smart niching (see sidebar).

The main reason market nichers can be highly profitable is that they know the target customers so well that they can meet their needs better than other firms

MEETING A BASIC AND ESSENTIAL NEED FOR HOME CARE

Mark Terry had spent his entire career as an information technology staffing manager; but in 2000, he suspected that the IT industry was due for a downturn. Terry decided that he would use his staffing experience to make a change. He recognized that there was a strong need for senior home care when his own family experienced problems finding quality care. One of his most striking "aha" moments was learning that there are quality alternatives to Medicare and nursing homes that can allow anyone to remain independent.

Terry decided to open Right At Home Senior Care and also a RAH Staffing franchise in Colorado Springs, Colorado, to meet the need for non-medical, continuing senior care. Right at Home Senior Care can provide respite care to a senior when his or her regular caregiver is unavailable, sick, or on vacation. Other services include driving senior clients to doctor's appointments, helping with light housekeeping, or even cooking dinner. While these services may seem mundane, they are becoming increasingly important as our population ages and families live further apart. This niche service generates most of its referrals from hospitals, nursing homes, assisted-living facilities, hospices, and home health agencies that need follow-up care for their patients and clients.

Terry's other complementary company, RAH Staffing, recruits and contracts with caregivers to deliver services for Right at Home. RAH Staffing sources registered nurses, licensed practical nurses, and certified nurse assistants not only to support the needs of Right at Home, but also to provide staff for nearby hospitals and physician offices.
Source: Adapted from B. Hurley, "Company Finds Welcome Niche, Rewards in Home Care." *Colorado Springs Business Journal*, Jan. 9, 2004.

selling to this niche. As a result, the nicher can charge a substantial premium over costs. The nicher achieves a *high margin*, whereas the mass-marketer achieves *high volume*.

Nichers have three tasks: creating niches, expanding niches, and protecting niches. This strategy carries a major risk in that the market niche might dry up or be attacked. The company is then stuck with highly specialized resources that may not have high-value alternative uses. The key idea in nichemanship is specialization, such as in the following categories:

- *End-user specialist:* The firm specializes in serving one *type* of end-user customer. For example, a *value-added reseller (VAR)* customizes the computer hardware and software for specific customer segments and earns a price premium in the process.[38]

- *Vertical-level specialist:* The firm specializes at some vertical level of the production-distribution value chain.

- *Customer-size specialist:* The firm concentrates on selling to either small, medium-sized, or large customers. Many nichers specialize in serving small customers who are neglected by large firms.

- *Specific-customer specialist:* The firm limits its selling to one customer or just a few. Many firms sell their entire output to a single company.

- *Geographic specialist:* The firm sells only in a certain locality, region, or area of the world.

- *Product or product-line specialist:* The firm carries or produces only one product line or product; for example, a firm may produce only lenses for microscopes, or a retailer may carry only health supplements.

- *Product-feature specialist:* The firm specializes in producing a certain type of product feature. A hyperbaric oxygen chamber company manufactures only multiplace chambers for groups of patients treated together and not monoplace chambers that are designed to treat patients individually.

- *Job-shop specialist:* The firm customizes its products for individual customers.

- *Quality-price specialist:* The firm operates at either the low-quality or the high-quality end of the market.

- *Service specialist:* The firm offers one or more services not available from other firms.

- *Channel specialist:* The firm specializes in serving only one channel of distribution.

Because niches can weaken, the firm must continually create new ones. The firm should "stick to its niching" but not necessarily to its niche. *Multiple niching* is preferable to *single niching* because, by developing strength in two or more niches, the company increases its chances for survival.

Balancing Customer and Competitor Orientations

We have stressed the importance of an organization's positioning itself competitively as a market leader, challenger, follower, or nicher. Yet a company must not spend *all* its time focusing on competitors. A competitor-centered firm looks at what competitors are doing, such as increasing distribution, cutting prices, and introducing new services. It then formulates reactions, including increasing advertising expenses, meeting price cuts, and increasing the sales promotion budget. This kind of planning has advantages and disadvantages. On the positive side, the organization develops a fighter orientation, training its marketers to be alert for weaknesses in its competitors' and its own position. On the negative side, the organization is too reactive. Rather than formulating and executing a consistent customer-oriented strategy, it determines its moves based on its competitors' moves rather than its own goals.

A *customer-centered company* focuses more on customer developments in formulating its strategies. Its marketers might learn, for example, that the total market is growing at five percent annually, while the quality-sensitive segment is growing at nine percent annually. They may also find that the deal-prone customer segment is growing fast, but these customers do not stay with any one supplier for very long. Additionally, they may find that more customers are asking for a twenty-four-hour hotline that no else offers. In response, this company could put more effort into reaching and satisfying the quality segment, avoid cutting prices, and research the possibility of installing a hotline.

Clearly, the customer-centered company is in a better position to identify new opportunities and set a strategy toward long-run profits. By monitoring customer needs, it can decide which customer groups and emerging needs are the most important to serve, given its resources and objectives.

SUMMARY

Health care organizations and providers will be most successful when they choose to serve a part of the market well rather than the whole market poorly. They need skills in market segmentation, targeting, positioning, differentiation, and competitive analysis.

A market can be viewed at four levels: the mass market, a segment market, a niche market, or a local market. The consumer market can be segmented geographically, demographically, psychographically, and behaviorally.

The health care organization must decide on which and how many segments to target. The choices are single segmentation, selective specialization, product specialization, market specialization, and full market coverage. The firm should prepare a segment-by-segment invasion plan and periodically update the segmentation basis, while following ethical principles in its choices of target markets.

For each target market, the organization has to develop a positioning using points-of-parity and points-of-difference. Differentiation can be based on product, service, personnel, channels, or image.

Much of the health organization's strategy must be derived from analyzing who the competitors are and identifying their objectives, strategies, strengths, and weaknesses. The dominant firm will aim to maintain leadership by expanding the total market, defending its market share, and expanding its market share. Other competitors will decide to either challenge the leader, follow the leader, or enter a narrow niche.

Although the firm must continuously monitor its competitors' moves, it must remember to maintain an even stronger focus on its target customers' current and changing needs.

DISCUSSION QUESTIONS

1. The CEO of your medical transcription service company feels that the company sells a commodity. He believes that the only point of differentiation from competitors is price. How would you design a segmentation analysis to reveal different groups of buyers of medical transcription services? Can you propose what segments might exist?

2. Clinipace, a small clinical software company, wants to choose a major pharmaceutical company to sell its software. What criteria might Clinipace use to choose a Fortune 500 company to initially approach?

3. All six hospitals in a major market use the benefit of "high-quality care" as the basis of their positioning strategy. As a new marketing consultant to one of these hospitals, what other positionings can you advise your client to consider?

4. A group of community-based physicians competes with an academic medical center (AMC) in the same market to offer endoscopy services. The physician group charges patients and third-party payers lower fees than the AMC. A regional health plan has contracted with the AMC but refuses to contract with the physicians. The physicians suspect that the AMC has used its bargaining power to influence the health plan. Is this unfair competition? What marketing strategies could the physicians use to secure a contract with the health plan?

PART

3

APPLYING THE MARKETING MIX

CHAPTER

9

SHAPING AND MANAGING PRODUCT AND SERVICE OFFERINGS

LEARNING OBJECTIVES

In this chapter, we will address the following questions:

1. What are the differentiating characteristics of products and services?

2. How can a health care organization build and manage its product mix and product lines?

3. What are the major tools for distinguishing your product offerings from competitor offerings?

4. How can a health care organization differentiate and market its service offerings?

OPENING EXAMPLE

Three Organizations Cooperate to Redesign The Wellness Community   A remarkable health care service product concept emerged from a Labor Day pool party in Sarasota, Florida, in 2005. Johnette Isham, then the vice president of academic affairs at the Ringling College of Art and Design, was visiting her friend "Charlie" Ann Syprett, a board member of The Wellness Community of Southwest Florida. The Wellness Community of Southwest Florida is part of the international Wellness Community, a network of nonprofit organizations dedicated to providing psychosocial support, education, and hope for all people affected by cancer—at no cost to the patients and their loved ones. The Ringling College, also in Sarasota, is a private, not-for-profit, undergraduate college that offers a range of art and design degrees, including a Continuing Studies certificate in "Art and Healing." Out of the pool party came a health care product idea that will both improve cancer patient outcomes and possibly reduce health care costs.

The Wellness Community and the Ringling College decided to work together to recreate The Wellness Community facility using evidence-based design. This market-driven, interdisciplinary approach integrates space planning, human factors, social psychology, sustainability factors, and esthetics to provide a facility that is more responsive to user needs. The partnership provided the initial team of artists, designers, students, and health care professionals in consultation with staff, cancer patients, and caregivers to create an optimal healing environment. This design strategy was guided by The Wellness Community mission and its "Patient Active" concept that states: "People with cancer who participate in their fight for recovery from cancer will improve the quality of their life and may enhance the possibility of their recovery."

A growing body of evidence indicates that improving the design of medical and therapeutic settings supports the healing process. London's Guy's and St. Thomas's hospitals used a co-design approach in 2003 to engage patients and health care professionals in the redesign of their maternity facilities. A key result was that this quality designed facility had a positive effect on the emotional experience of patients, as well as on employee's morale and staff retention. Also, patient volume increased by 15 percent and midwifery vacancies dropped. Another study at Pittsburgh's Montefiore Hospital showed that drug costs were 21 percent lower for surgery patients in better designed, better-lit rooms than for patients in traditional rooms with less natural lighting. Additional results were less use of pain medication and earlier discharges—both leading to lower health care costs.

The Wellness Community also established a partnership with Florida State University's College of Medicine in Sarasota. The purpose was to assess the impact of the new optimal healing environment on patient outcomes and satisfaction. These types of partnerships will enable The Wellness Community to help more cancer patients in Southwest Florida;

add to the body of knowledge surrounding integrating design, green architecture, and healing; and become a model for the twenty-six other Wellness Communities worldwide.

The Wellness Community's Building Hope campus has acquired a five-acre lot that is surrounded by a 300-acre nature preserve. It is working with an expanded list of over twenty community partners, and it has designed a LEED-certified facility and a garden to amplify the power of place in healing.

Source: Interview with Johnette Isham, Building Hope Project Director of The Wellness Community and organizational placemaking consultant.

Marketing planning begins with designing an offering to meet target customers' needs or wants. The customer will judge the offering by four basic elements: product features, quality, services mix, and price. In this chapter, we examine the product—the first, and most necessary, component of the "4 Ps" (product, price, place, and promotion).

OVERVIEW: DISTINGUISHING PRODUCT TYPES AND LEVELS

Many people usually think of a product as a tangible offering, but a product can be much more. A *product* is anything that can be offered to a market to satisfy a want or need; thus it includes *physical goods, services, experiences, events, places, properties, organizations, information*, and *ideas*.

Product Levels: The Customer Value Hierarchy

In planning its market offering, the health care organization needs to address five product levels (see Figure 9.1).[1] The fundamental level is the *core benefit* that the customer is really seeking. A patient visiting a hospital to deliver a baby wants a safe, healthy birth. The purchaser of aspirin is buying headache relief. Marketers, therefore, must see themselves as benefit providers.

At the second level, the marketer has to turn the core benefit into a *basic product*. Thus a patient hospital room in a maternity department includes a bed that also serves as a delivery table, a scale, and a recliner, and it supports high-intensity lights and an ultrasound machine.

At the third level, the marketer prepares an *expected product:* a set of attributes and conditions buyers normally expect when they purchase this product. Expectant mothers can expect a clean gown, fresh bedding, working lamps, acceptable food, and a relative degree of quiet.

At the fourth level, the marketer may offer an *augmented product* that exceeds customer expectations. For hospitals in developed countries, these augmented

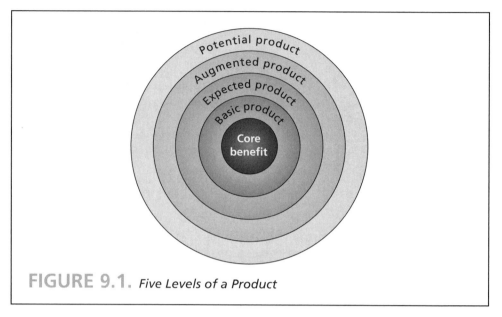

FIGURE 9.1. *Five Levels of a Product*

Source: Kotler and Keller, 2006, p. 372.

products often include the following features: access to care, coordination of care, information and education, physical comfort, continuity and transition to home, emotional support, involvement of family and friends, and respect for patient preferences.[2] This augmented offering arises from the intense competition for patients in these markets. In developing countries and emerging markets such as China and India, however, competition occurs mostly at the expected product level.

Differentiation takes place mainly at the level of product augmentation and leads the marketer to look at the user's total *consumption system:* the way the user performs the tasks of getting and using products and related services.[3] However, we offer a few cautionary notes about implementing a product-augmentation strategy. First, each augmentation adds cost. Second, augmented benefits soon become expected benefits and necessary competitive points-of-parity. Today's hospital "guests" not only expect cable or satellite television with a remote control but many also demand high-speed internet access. Third, as companies raise the price of their augmented product, some competitors may offer a stripped-down version at a much lower price. Examples include simpler medication administration pumps and glucose monitoring devices.

At the fifth level is the *potential product*, which encompasses all the possible augmentations and transformations the product or offering might undergo in the future. Here is where companies search for new ways to delight customers and distinguish their offering. For example, addressing the preferences of women's families was the driving forces throughout all of the design process of the new Birth Place at Gaston Memorial Hospital; it is expected that as family preferences evolve, so will the Birth Place (see example box).

FOR EXAMPLE

The Birth Place at Gaston Memorial Hospital—Innovative Service Product Benefits

The Birth Place at Gaston Memorial Hospital in Gastonia, North Carolina, is a fifty-two-suite family birthing center that allows mothers to stay in one room for their entire stay, from delivery to checkout. Each suite has a full-size sofa bed, refrigerator, internet access, TV, VCR/DVD/CD player, and a whirlpool bathtub. The ambiance includes reflecting pools, flowing water, trees, plants, and restful, soothing art and sculpture. Family spaces include a media room, dining room, and children's play room. Parents and their family have access to the Resource Center, which includes a health education library with internet access, children's library, consultation room, and classroom. Comprehensive integrated electronic security for newborn, patient, family, and provider safety is built in. Because of its unique design, the Birth Place is getting the attention of nurses, doctors, and architects nationwide.

Product Characteristics

One way in which marketers classify health care products is on the basis of durability, tangibility, and service. For each combination of these features there is an appropriate marketing-mix strategy.[4]

Health care products can be classified into three groups, according to their durability and tangibility (or lack thereof):

- *Nondurable goods* are tangible goods normally consumed in one or a few uses, like aspirins and bandages. Because these goods are consumed quickly and purchased frequently, the appropriate strategy is to make them available in many locations, such as pharmacies, food stores, and mass merchandisers. Most nondurable goods makers charge only a small markup and advertise heavily to encourage trial and build preference, achieving profitability on volume sales. However, nondurable health care goods have lower levels of advertising and higher markups than their nonhealth care counterparts, such as soft drinks and toiletries. Pharmaceuticals are an exception in this category, since they may be one-time use products with large markups and are heavily promoted. Of course, medications for chronic illness may fit more into the traditional pattern of this category.

- *Durable goods* are tangible products that normally survive many uses, such as imaging equipment, operating tables, hospital beds, and wheelchairs. They can also be internal implants such as pacemakers and artificial joints. Durable products normally require more personal selling and service, command a higher margin, and require more seller guarantees.

- *Services* are nondurable and intangible goods. In the next section we discuss the features of services that distinguish them from tangible products.

Combinations of these three groups occur frequently. For example, a cardiologist may (1) find a blockage in any artery in the heart while performing an angiogram, (2) open the blockage with a balloon-tipped catheter (angioplasty), and (3) insert a metal mesh (stent) in the artery to keep it open. The cardiologist's procedures are *services* that use *nondurable goods* (catheters) and *durable goods* (stent).

THE NATURE OF SERVICES

Health care has led the way in job growth in this country: from 2001 to 2006, 1.7 million new jobs were added to this sector, while in the rest of the economy employment outside was flat. During the same period, information technology companies lost 1.1 million positions. The Bureau of Labor Statistics reports that the service-producing sector will continue to be the dominant employment generator in the economy, adding 20.5 million jobs by 2010. Employment in the service-producing sector is expected to increase by 19 percent during the 2000–2010 period, whereas manufacturing employment is expected to increase by only 3 percent.[5] This growth has led to an increasing interest in the special problems and opportunities of the marketing of services.[6]

Distinctive Characteristics of Services

Health care services have four distinctive characteristics that greatly affect the design of marketing programs for them: *intangibility, inseparability, variability*, and *perishability*.

Intangibility. Unlike physical products, services cannot be seen, tasted, felt, heard, or smelled before they are bought. The person getting a face-lift cannot see the results before the purchase, and the patient in the psychiatrist's office cannot know the exact outcome.

To reduce uncertainty, buyers look for evidence of quality by drawing inferences from the place, people, equipment, communication material, symbols, and price that they observe. Health care service companies can thus try to demonstrate their service quality through *physical evidence* and *presentation*.[7] The service provider's task is to "manage the evidence," to "tangibilize the intangible."[8] Whereas product marketers are challenged to add abstract ideas, service marketers are challenged to add physical evidence and imagery to abstract offers.

For example, a hospital can develop a look and style of dealing with patients, family members, physicians, and visitors that reflects its intended customer value proposition. Unlike airlines, hotels, or banks, health care service companies rarely seem to strategically position themselves in this manner. An exception is the Lasky Skin Center (see Field Note 9.1).

FIELD NOTE 9.1.

The Lasky Skin Center   A dermatology and plastic surgery physician practice in Beverly Hills, California that caters to Hollywood celebrities, the Lasky Skin Center has made its service message tangible through a number of marketing tools:

1. *Place:* The exterior and interior have clean lines. The layout of the reception area, the exam and procedure rooms, and the traffic flow are planned carefully. An elegant home-like atmosphere, including a fireplace, has been designed. Waiting times are not noticeably long.

2. *People:* Personnel are busy, but not too busy to be attentive to patients, and they are cross-trained to increase efficiency. Staff morale and customer service orientation are a top priority. The rule is that "the patient is always right—even if he or she really isn't."

3. *Equipment:* Computers, lasers, cameras, and furniture not only appear to be state-of-the-art but actually are. Most important, the treatment offerings must be state-of-the-art as well.

4. *Communication material:* Printed materials—text and photos—suggest quality and refinement. Patient information sheets reflect the product image and clearly communicate the clinic's positioning through graphic treatments and content.

5. *Symbols:* The name and symbol suggest stability and excellence in service.

6. *Price:* Charges are judged to be average for the services provided in this upscale demographic market. Prices are adjusted, however, if patients are significantly inconvenienced by an unusually long waiting time or need to reschedule their appointments.

Source: Interview with Mark G. Rubin, M.D., owner of the Lasky Skin Center.

Service marketers must also be able to transform intangible services into concrete benefits—a process for which Carbone and Haeckel propose a set of concepts under the term *customer experience engineering*.[9] Companies must first develop a clear picture of what they want the customer's perception of an experience to be and then design a consistent set of *performance* and *context clues* to support that experience. In the case of a hospital, a good surgical outcome is a performance clue; a context clue is whether the surgeon and nurses act in a professional manner. The context clues in a hospital are delivered by people (*humanics*) and things (*mechanics*). The hospital assembles the clues in an *experiential blueprint*, a pictorial representation of the various clues. This technique is often used in training simulations.

Inseparability. Services are typically produced and consumed simultaneously. In contrast, tangible goods are frequently manufactured, put into inventory, distributed through multiple resellers, and consumed later. If a person renders the service, then the provider is part of the service. Because the consumer is also present as the service is produced, provider-client interaction is a special feature of services marketing. With advances in technology, however, presence need not require physical proximity. For example, physicians may monitor patients in the intensive care unit by electronic surveillance. Furthermore, medical specialists may render opinions and advice from a distance, thanks to advances in telecommunications ("telemedicine").

In the case of health care services, buyers are becoming increasingly sensitive to service delivery. For example, a patient in a "consumer-driven health plan" with high out-of-pocket requirements may be dissatisfied when presented with a bill for physician services if she "only sees the nurse." In traditional markets, when many customers have the same strong provider preferences, price is raised to ration the preferred provider's limited time. In health care, however, prices (provider charges) are usually fixed by contract (as with an insurance company) or law (as with government-sponsored health care programs in the United States and other countries). The physician provider market has reacted to this constraint by offering "concierge service" for an additional fee. In this model, primary care physicians charge $500 to $1,500 per person per year and offer prompt access and longer appointment times; the extra charge enables these doctors to have many fewer patients in their panel.

Non-price strategies also exist for getting around this limitation. The service provider can learn to work with *larger* groups. For example, some psychotherapy services and diet counseling for diabetes and obesity can be performed well on a group basis. Individual sessions can then augment treatment as necessary.

Variability. Services are highly variable because they depend on who provides them and when and where they are provided. To address quality concerns, service providers try to standardize their products; however, because the circumstances that require each delivery are unique, the service is never *exactly* the same each time it is rendered.

Unfortunately, service variability can lead to medical errors. Filling the wrong prescription, injecting the wrong medication, operating on the wrong limb—such errors kill thousands of people each year. Patients are becoming more aware of this variability and are increasingly seeking sources of information before receiving care. To increase quality, service firms often take three steps:

1. *Invest in good hiring and training procedures.* Because most services are provided by people, recruiting the right employees at all skill levels and providing them with excellent training is crucial. Ideally, employees should exhibit competence, a caring attitude, responsiveness, initiative, problem-solving ability, and goodwill. They must also be empowered to solve customer problems as soon as they occur.

2. *Standardize the service-performance process throughout the organization.* Standardization can be helped by preparing medical *service blueprints* that depict events and processes in a flowchart, with the objective of recognizing potential safety failures. For example, Evanston Northwestern Healthcare is training its doctors and nurses to follow the safety checks that airline pilots use, and the Great Ormond Street Hospital for Children in London is adopting some of the techniques of race-car pit crews to minimize errors in transferring patients postoperatively.[10]

3. *Monitor customer satisfaction.* Firms can employ formalized suggestion and complaint systems, customer surveys, and comparison shopping. They can also develop customer information databases and systems to permit more customized service.

Perishability. You cannot store services; you can only build capacity to perform them when they are needed. The perishability of services is not a problem when demand is predictable and the firm has excess capacity. Unfortunately, ensuring that capacity is always present in health care is very expensive. For example, hospitals may need to hire more expensive temporary nurses to meet seasonal demand.

There are several strategies for producing a better match between demand and supply in many service businesses; but as health care needs can be a matter of life and death and can be very time-sensitive, only a few can be used.[11] For example, operations research says that maximal efficiency comes from seeing the shortest visits first (similar to the express checkout lane at the supermarket). In emergency rooms, this principle is used by employing parallel "fast track" programs, which see the least complex health problems that will take the shortest time to treat.

On the supply side, part-time employees can be hired to serve peak demand. Peak-time efficiency routines can also be introduced; for example, stipulating that only certain laboratory tests or X-rays will be performed during certain hours (unless an emergency requires otherwise). Sharing services with other providers, such as use of high-tech medical equipment, can also help reduce the strain of peak demands. For any growing business, a major challenge is deciding when to add permanent excess capacity in anticipation of growth.

Efficient use of scarce personnel is a related important concern, particularly regarding hospital nursing (see Field Note 9.2). Trained nurses are in short supply,

FIELD NOTE 9.2.

The Nurse Shortage Will Only Get Worse   The service performance of hospitals, clinics, nursing homes, and other health care institutions critically depends on having a sufficient number of registered nurses on staff. Yet U.S. health care facilities are facing a serious shortage. In 2000, this national nursing shortage approached 6 percent, with demand exceeding supply by 110,000. Looking ahead to 2020, nurse demand will increase by 40 percent, but nurse supply will increase by only 6 percent, resulting in a 29 percent nurse shortage by 2020.

The nurse shortage directly affects the quality of health care. A decreased number of nurse staffed hospital beds causes increased crowding in hospital emergency rooms. Reduced staff also results in an increased incidence of urinary tract infections and bleeding.

What are the contributing factors to this nurse shortage? Fifty-one percent of the nursing workforce is over forty-five years of age, and their retirement rate may not be filled by enough newly trained nurses. Women who consider nursing as a career are facing greater alternative career opportunities. The pay is low, the working conditions in hospitals and nursing homes are stressful, and there are insufficient part-time work opportunities for those nurses who do not want to work full time. Some nurses now prefer to work in less stressful environments such as in the home health sector or the doctor's office.

Normally one would expect the states and federal government to address this problem, but their tight budgets have been used to meet other pressing demands. Seeing limited public involvement, Blue Cross and Blue Shield of Florida (BCBSF) decided to use its expertise and resources in the following undertaking:

- To provide incentives for students to go into the field of nursing

- To provide incentives for colleges and universities to pool their resources and work together as teams to offer additional opportunities for students to study nursing

- To increase the pool of groups (such as Hispanics and African Americans) who are underrepresented among those entering the field

- To increase the pool of nursing educators available to teach in the field

- To involve health care facilities directly as partners to help solve their nursing shortages

As a catalyst, BCFSF has provided $5.6 million in the past two years to support nursing, prenursing, and allied health professional education in Florida. It has leveraged state matching grants and partnered with non-profit foundations, colleges, physician groups, and hospitals to improve the nurse supply.

Source: S. Ullmann, P. Martin, C. Kelly, and J. Homer, "Strategic Giving and the Nursing Shortage," *International Journal of Nonprofit and Voluntary Sector Marketing*, Feb. 2006, pp. 3–11. Copyright John Wiley & Sons Limited. Reproduced with permission.

partly because of the hard work involved and the low level of pay. Using staffing ratio guidelines (such as intensive care: one nurse per two patients; medical/surgical: one nurse per four to six patients) can help hospitals staff the appropriate number of nurses in different departments.[12]

VIEWING THE PRODUCT MIX

A *product system* (or *product line*) is a group of diverse but related items that function in a compatible manner. For example, a hospital might have a cancer product line consisting of diagnostic imaging and lab services, chemotherapy, radiation therapy, and counseling (independent services that are coordinated and scheduled to treat cancer patients). A *product mix* (also called a *product assortment*) is the set of all products and items a particular seller offers for sale. A product mix consists of various product systems and independent services. Hospitals that use product-line management offer a comprehensive range of clinical services, but they set priorities for specific clinical product specialties. For example, at Vanderbilt University Medical Center, there are managers for each of six product lines: cancer, children's services, heart, emergency services, orthopedics, and imaging.

A company's product mix has width, length, depth, and consistency.

- The *width* of a product mix refers to how many different product lines the company carries. Vanderbilt has a stated product-mix width of six lines. (In fact, Vanderbilt has many additional product lines that it ranks as lower priorities and does not actively market.)

- The *length* of a product mix refers to the total number of items in the mix. Health care service product-mix length assessments are complex. At Vanderbilt, the number of items in the mix is many hundreds, with numerous overlaps. The children's services product line alone is drawn from all of the services offered by the department of pediatrics, clinic programs and services, surgical services, primary care practices, off-site specialty practices, and many more.

- The *depth* of a product mix refers to how many variants of each product in the line are offered. The Vanderbilt cancer product line may have a depth of three if the cancer product is distinctly managed for adults, children, and specialty care for women.

- The *consistency* of the product mix refers to how closely related the various product lines are in such features as end use, production requirements, or distribution channels. The Vanderbilt product lines are consistent insofar as they are health care services that go through the same distribution channels. The lines are less consistent insofar as they perform different functions for patients.

These product-mix dimensions permit the organization to expand its business in four ways. It can add new product lines and widen its product mix; lengthen each product line; add more product variants to each product and deepen its product mix; and pursue more product-line consistency. To make these product and brand decisions, it is useful to conduct a product-line analysis.

MANAGING PRODUCT LINES

In large hospitals like Vanderbilt University Medical Center and health care companies such as GlaxoSmithKline Pharmaceuticals, the product mix consists of a variety of product lines. In offering a product line, the company normally develops a basic platform and modules that can be expanded to meet different customer requirements.

Product-Line Analysis

Product-line managers need to know the purpose and the sales and profits of each item in their line to determine which items to build, maintain, harvest, or divest.[13] They also need to understand each product line's market profile.

Purpose. While many product lines are calculated to be offered at a profit, some are introduced to support the organization's mission of providing care for a community. The purpose and role of the product line must therefore be understood before considering sales and profits.

Sales and Profits. Marketers should develop a sales and profit analysis report for their product lines. A simple approach would measure the sales revenue and profit margin for each product in the line. Suppose that in a five-product line the first item accounts for 50 percent of total sales and 30 percent of total profits and the first two items account for 80 percent of total sales and 60 percent of total profits. If sales of these two items were suddenly hurt by a competitor, the line's sales and profitability could collapse; therefore, sales of these items must be carefully monitored and protected. At the other extreme, suppose the fifth item delivers only 5 percent of the product line's sales and profits. The product-line manager may consider dropping this item unless it has strong growth potential or is a necessary part of a profitable portfolio package.

A classic example of the importance of a least profitable item is maternity services in general hospitals. Traditionally, this product line has lost money, but hospitals offer these services for at least two reasons. First, it is part of their community service mission. From a marketing standpoint, the second reason is more important: women are the household decision makers. If a woman has a good experience in childbirth, the family is more likely to use the hospital for other (more profitable) services.

Market Profile. In reviewing how a line is positioned against competitors' lines, the marketing manager can use product mapping to compare competitive offerings. Individual products are plotted on a graph with two or more dimensions that represent the product attributes most important for buyers. For a pharmaceutical product, the dimensions could be efficacy, the likelihood of side effects, potential for interaction

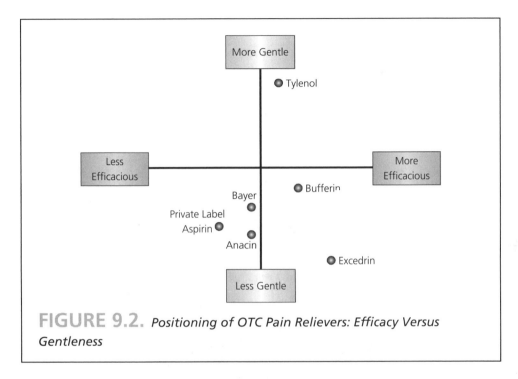

FIGURE 9.2. *Positioning of OTC Pain Relievers: Efficacy Versus Gentleness*

Note: Positioning is for illustrative purposes only.

with other medications, cost and compliance. The product map in Figure 9.2 shows how a product compares to competitors' offerings using the first two dimensions. The map also reveals possible locations for new items. If a company can forecast strong unmet demand and can produce and price this product at low cost, it could consider adding this item to the line. Another benefit of product mapping is that it identifies market segments.

Application: Hospital Product-Line Analysis

Copland has developed a product-line analysis that helps hospitals determine where to invest resources to increase market share for selected product lines.[14] The steps are as follows:

1. *Calculate costs, revenue, and margin by DRG.* Diagnosis related groups (DRGs) have been developed by the Centers for Medicare and Medicaid Services (CMS) to reimburse hospitals for inpatient stays through the Medicare program. Each inpatient admission is assigned a primary DRG, based on the reason for the admission. Using this assigned category, CMS pays the hospital a fixed amount; therefore, whether the hospital loses money or makes a profit depends on its costs. The cost data can be used to measure profitability by DRG, as shown in Table 9.1.

TABLE 9.1. Hospital DRG Array

Description	Actual Payment	Variable Costs	Operating Revenue	Surplus/ Deficit Funds	Operation Revenue/ Discharge	Number Discharge to Break Even
Total Trauma (s)	$211,357	$41,319	$170,038	$75,007	$9,447	0
Total Cardiac Care (s)	$657,088	$243,466	$413,622	($29,022)	$7,131	4
Total General Surgery	$3,517,430	$1,125,706	$2,391,724	$75,422	$5,461	0
Total Other Surgery	$1,697,890	$727,201	$970,689	($434,088)	$5,333	81
Total Cancer Care (s)	$541,597	$174,914	$366,683	$5,397	$5,238	0
Total Cancer Care (m)	$2,234,351	$664,074	$1,570,277	$254,709	$4,969	0
Total Orthopedics (m)	$753,810	$208,405	$545,405	($241,388)	$4,622	52
Total Orthopedics (s)	$3,533,240	$1,193,734	$2,339,506	($423,114)	$4,215	100
Total Renal/Urology (s)	$786,281	$258,922	$527,359	($21,148)	$3,906	5

Total Neuro (s)	$473,611	$144,128	$329,483	$20,029	$3,876	0
Total Women's Health	$850,362	$239,908	$610,454	$82,206	$2,677	0
Total Respiratory	$3,529,933	$1,180,382	$2,349,551	($178,858)	$2,619	68
Total Neuro (m)	$1,434,127	$438,188	$995,939	($75,193)	$2,534	28
Total Dental	$35,693	$15,547	$20,146	($9,291)	$2,518	4
Total Psychiatry	$1,938,377	$556,597	$1,391,740	($647,268)	$2,425	267
Total Cardiac Care (m)	$3,646,299	$1,207,841	$2,438,458	($41,865)	$2,377	18
Total Medicine	$4,327,546	$1,391,665	$2,935,881	($298,182)	$2,312	129
Total Trauma (m)	$119,567	$36,219	$83,348	($5,939)	$1,984	3
Total Renal Urology (m)	$389,414	$156,900	$232,514	($107,848)	$1,970	55

(Table 9.1 continued)

Description	Actual Payment	Variable Costs	Operating Revenue	Surplus/ Deficit Funds	Operation Revenue/ Discharge	Number Discharge to Break Even
Total Obstetrics	$878,054	$312,715	$565,339	($172,470)	$1,343	128
Total Ophthalmology	$13,061	$8,347	$4,714	($5,508)	$786	7
Total Substance Abuse	$67,097	$38,776	$28,321	($75,303)	$405	186
Total Newborn	$260,810	$143,423	$117,387	($216,536)	$302	718
Totals	$31,896,995	$10,508,377	$21,398,578	($2,470,251)	$78,450	1,853

Note: (s) = surgical; (m) = medical

Source: A. Copland, "Talking to Your Boss In His/Her Language: The Marketing/Finance Interface," presentation made at UNC-Chapel Hill School of Public Health, Chapel Hill, N.C., Aug. 2001.

2. *Group DRGs by product-line and measure margins.* The data will show the degree of profit or loss for each hospital product. As mentioned earlier, profitability is not the only reason for marketing a given product; there are many other humanitarian and strategic reasons. Nevertheless, hospitals should at least be aware of which products have negative margins and which have positive ones. The product-line analysis should be considered in the context of the hospital strategic plan, the expected changes in payer mix, and reimbursement levels for the various product lines.

3. *Make effective marketing management decisions.* Product line analysis can tell management where to find surplus revenue, focus process improvements, look for new services, and identify services to discontinue—ideally within the strategic framework of the organization.

4. *Analyze market share.* Environmental data from primary and secondary data sources should be used to augment institutional data. The state hospital association is the best initial source; it can furnish statistics on admissions and discharges by product line for the relevant market.

    Table 9.2 shows a breakout by service line of market share for a rural hospital. The first column on the left is hospital market share by service line, subtracted from 100 percent to estimate competitors' share. The next column reduces this amount by 15 percent—the amount this hospital estimates will always use a nearby tertiary hospital. The data indicate how many total discharges there were for each service line in the primary market. The potential capture share percentage is multiplied by the total number of discharges to calculate the number of potential discharges that could be captured. This number is then multiplied by the average charges by product-line to calculate potential incremental revenue gained.

5. *Calculate costs of increasing market share.* Following calculation of potential operating revenue available, the fixed and variable costs to add market share can be estimated. Once these results are quantified, product-line investments and projected rates of return on invested capital can also be forecast.

6. *Replicate product-line analysis for other products.* Profitability updates per service line, market share analyses, and a detailed analysis of where patients can be acquired by zip code or census block can be added. From this detailed geographic data, strategic marketing plans can be aimed at specifically targeted groups.

7. *Measure marketing return on investment.* By measuring the results of the marketing efforts to increase market share, a marketing ROI can be calculated. A sample calculation is shown in Table 9.3.

TABLE 9.2. Market Share Capture Potentials

Primary Service Area Service Lines	Percentage Lost Volume[a]	Potential Percentage Capture[b]	Adjusted[c] Potential Discharge Capture	Potential Revenue[d]
Cancer Care (m)	48	33	107	$ 918,121
Cancer Care (s)	65	50	12	$ 132,302
General Surgery	50	35	30	$ 499,290
Medicine	38	23	242	$2,020,942
Neurological (m)	42	27	20	$ 211,120
Neurological (s)	100	85	82	$ 504,136
Ophthalmology	100	85		
Orthopedics (s)	52	37	10	$ 166,462
Renal/Urology (s)	62	47	14	$ 118,000
Women's Health	38	23	8	$ 67,300
Total			525	$4,637,673

Notes:
(m) = medical; (s) = surgical
[a]Based on market share by service line, which provides a basis for estimating capture potential.
[b]Subtracts 15 percent of cases going to tertiary competitor from previous column.
[c]The figures in this column represent the previous column's percentage converted into discharges. The discharges are then arbitrarily divided in half to reflect an understated potential capture.
[d]The revenue projections are based on the data for "Average Charges/Discharge" by Service Line.
Conclusions: A conservative capture of 525 additional discharges would increase market share from 62 percent to 68 percent. This percentage increase is equivalent to approximately $773,000 per percentage point. It is reasonable to expect a 3-percent additional market share.
Source: Copland, 2001.

TABLE 9.3. **Hospital Product-Line Marketing Return on Investment**

Incremental Discharges	100
Net revenue from discharges (net patient revenue less all patient costs)	$100,000
Marketing costs to increase discharges	$70,000
Return on investment	$30,000 or 42.9%

SUMMARY

Every health care organization has to define its products and services. A product can be viewed on five levels: core benefit, basic product, expected product, augmented product, and potential product. We can distinguish among nondurable products, durable products, and services. Services have four characteristics: intangibility, inseparability, variability, and perishability.

The health care organization can describe its product mix in terms of its width, length, depth, and consistency. These dimensions will change as the organization decides to add, enlarge, reduce, and terminate different products and services based on doing a hospital product line analysis.

DISCUSSION QUESTIONS

1. Marketers who specialize in health care services often consider service marketing to be fundamentally different from product marketing. Marketers who specialize in health care products take exception to this claim; they believe that the fundamentals of marketing are largely applicable to both services and products. Analyze both sides of this argument and then select and support a position.

2. The basic, expected, augmented, and potential product levels revolve around a core product benefit. You are advising a family medicine physician on making his practice market-driven. Develop a chart that explains the five product levels and how they apply to this solo physician's practice.

3. When drug maker GlaxoSmithKline PLC launched Requip for restless-legs syndrome, few consumers had heard of the problem, and some physicians

were skeptical that it even existed. Despite these problems, the drug is now very successful. Should the marketing of a health care product that is not immediately recognized as responding to a health care need (a) have more government oversight and control or (b) be left to allow market forces to decide its value?

4. Research studies show that surgery patients in rooms with much natural light require less pain medication and have drug costs 21 percent less than for equally ill patients assigned to darker rooms. How could a hospital use this study to enhance its product design and to market its inpatient surgery services to patients, physicians, and payers?

CHAPTER

10

DEVELOPING AND BRANDING NEW OFFERINGS

LEARNING OBJECTIVES

In this chapter, we will address the following questions:

1. Why is it important to develop new health care products in spite of the risks?

2. What are the nine steps in effectively developing and launching a new product?

3. How can a company build a strong brand around its offering?

4. What are the main stages of the product life cycle and how do they help management understand the behavior of health care products and services over time?

OPENING EXAMPLE

Blue Cross Blue Shield of North Carolina Successfully Launches A New Individual Health Care Insurance Product In 1996, Blue Cross Blue Shield of North Carolina (BCBSNC) launched a new individual health care insurance product called "Blue Advantage." This offering, an extension of the nationally licensed Blue Cross Blue Shield brand, introduced new product features and successfully leveraged the brand.

Compared to the group insurance, the market for individual health insurance has traditionally been much riskier for insurers. Despite underwriting, pools of individuals have always generated higher overall levels of medical costs and insurance claims compared with large groups that had less risk and medical cost variability. Two reasons for this disparity are that (1) individuals have more and better information about their own health status than insurance companies do, and (2) the sickest individuals will seek insurance products with the best benefits. Because of this high insurance risk, many companies in the individual market exclude preexisting conditions from coverage.

BCBSNC product research showed that existing individual insurance products differed from those of large groups by having (1) fewer benefits, (2) lower lifetime maximum coverage amounts, (3) higher deductibles, and (4) higher out-of-pocket maximum amounts. It was no surprise, then, when their research indicated that individual insurance customers were dissatisfied with these product characteristics; they preferred to have the richer benefits common among group insurance products.

BCBSNC decided to stimulate sales of its renamed individual product, Blue Advantage, by changing three features. First, the plan replaced a high deductible with a $30 co-payment for doctor visits. Consumers benefited from this innovation because the cost to visit a physician was now predictable. Also, both patients and BCBSNC benefited because plan members were now more likely to seek medical care before an illness or injury became more serious and required more costly care.

The second innovation was a waiver for preexisting conditions. Because medical problems can be wide-ranging, consumers are never really confident that a specific problem will be covered; the insurer could potentially decide that this problem was somehow related to an excluded preexisting condition and deny payment. Blue Advantage eliminated this risk.

Finally, BCBSNC used a different technique to reach prospective Blue Advantage customers. By using television ads, direct mail, and the BCBSNC website, which consumers could use to obtain a policy quote, the plan lowered its administrative costs by 80 percent compared with the traditional broker channel. Consumers also benefited from this approach. By their applying for coverage on-line, the average individual policy underwriting time was reduced from an average of forty days to just thirteen days. Thirty-eight percent of applicants applying on-line were approved for coverage instantly.

The results of this campaign were striking. The plan's percentage of business-to-consumer revenue increased from 20 percent to 45 percent. Cost savings were passed along to consumers through lower premiums. Eventually, three of the major BCBSNC competitors marketing individual insurance products were forced to withdraw from the market because of falling market shares.

By conducting appropriate marketing research, this health plan was able to enter a market segment that was previously ill-served and overpriced. It not only used its marketing information to penetrate this sector, but relied on its strong brand (Blue Cross Blue Shield) to quickly dominate it.

OVERVIEW: THE NEW OFFERING DEVELOPMENT PROCESS

Health care organizations need to grow their revenue over time by developing new products and expanding into new markets. Pharmaceutical companies must research and develop new, more effective, and safer drugs. Medical equipment companies must bring out new products that perform better at a lower cost. Surgeons must acquire new skills to deliver safer and more effective care. In addition to providing high-quality medical care, hospitals must also offer new services and procedures that make patients more comfortable in their surroundings.

Some health care organizations put product innovation at the forefront of all they do. The Brigham and Women's Hospital in Boston, one of the most innovative academic medical centers, clusters related services to form disease-oriented strategic business units. These strategic units—such as cancer, cardiovascular, orthopedics and arthritis, and women's health—are managed using a matrix structure that promotes collaboration and crosses departmental boundaries. The product development process is driven by scientific discoveries, translational research, and clinical trials and is supported by market demand measurement and forecasting. For example, heart surgeons and interventional cardiologists work together at Brigham and Women's Hospital to develop hybrid therapies that involve catheterization and drug-eluting stents (drug-coated or medicated stents) as well as percutaneous valve repair procedures. At many other academic medical centers that are not focused on innovation and integration, doctors often compete rather than collaborate with each other.

Marketers play a key role in the new-product development process by identifying opportunities, measuring the size of the opportunity, suggesting needed features, and working with R&D and others in every stage of development.

Challenges in New Product Development

A health care company can add new products to its portfolio through acquisition, development, or cooperative venture with another organization. The acquisition route can take three forms: The company can buy other companies, acquire patents, or buy a license or franchise.

In developing new products, the company can either create them itself or contract with independent researchers or new-product-development firms. Six categories of new products can be identified:[1]

■ *New-to-the-world products:* New products that create an entirely new market. When they were first introduced, devices such as implantable defibrillators and quinolone antibiotics were in this category.

■ *New product lines:* New products that allow a company to enter an established market for the first time (see Field Note 10.1).

FIELD NOTE 10.1.

Can Success in Health Insurance Translate to Success in Banking? The Blue Cross and Blue Shield Association and several other health care insurers are diversifying into the health care banking business. The new Blue Healthcare Bank, owned by thirty-three Blue Cross and Blue Shield companies, received a federal savings bank charter in February 2007.

The Blues are hoping to take advantage of a market opportunity. Its marketing research shows that demand for health care banking services is increasing because:

1. Consumers are accepting higher insurance deductibles in order to have more moderate monthly premiums.

2. Providers are beginning to see an increase in bad debt and the number of days in accounts receivable.

3. Hospitals and physicians are attempting to collect their fees in advance for services rendered.

4. The number of health plan members eligible to have Health Savings Accounts (HSAs) is estimated to grow from forty million to forty-five million people by 2010. HSAs allow members with qualifying health plans to deposit a percentage of their earnings in special accounts and withdraw the funds to pay their insurance deductibles and other specified medical expenses. Members do not pay taxes on these funds.

Blue Healthcare Bank will allow customers to manage and direct health care spending via debit cards linked to their HSAs, flexible spending accounts, and employer-financed health reimbursement accounts. An estimated twelve to fifteen Blue Cross and Blue Shield companies are expected to begin offering the new banking services to their consumer-driven health plan members in 2007. By 2010, Blue Healthcare Bank is projected to have health savings account deposits in excess of $500 million.

Blue Cross and Blue Shield, which serves about 98 million members or nearly one in three Americans, joins UnitedHealth Group and Humana in the health care banking business. Time will tell whether these insurers will be as proficient in banking as they are in managing claims.

Source: R. Roberts, "Blue Cross Association Enters Health Care Banking," *Kansas City Business Journal*, Feb.13, 2007.

- *Additions to existing product lines:* New products that supplement a company's established product lines. Medtronic is known, among other items, for its pacemakers and cardiac catheters. To augment its existing product line, it developed a device (the ablation catheter) to detect and destroy areas of the heart that cause abnormal heart rhythms.

- *Improvements and revisions of existing products:* New products that provide improved performance or greater perceived value and replace existing products. Pharmaceutical companies often seek drug delivery systems that will enable patients to take medications once a day rather than in multiple doses.

- *Repositioning:* Targeting of existing products to new markets or market segments. Angiotensin converting enzyme (ACE) inhibitors were originally developed to lower high blood pressure. Subsequent research showed they are also effective in treating heart failure and preventing kidney disease in diabetics.

- *Cost reductions:* New products that provide similar performance at lower cost. Generic pharmaceuticals are the most obvious example in this class.

In developing these new products, firms can also engage in cooperative ventures, which can take a variety of forms, including the following:

Joint product development. Alexian Brothers Hospital, in Elk Gove Village, Illinois, teamed up with rival Northwest Community Hospital in Arlington Heights to develop and run a free community clinic. This venture helps both institutions fulfill their missions of community service while helping to reduce costly emergency room visits.

Joint venture. TAP Pharmaceuticals is a stand-alone company with its own products. It is co-owned by Japan's Takeda Pharmaceuticals and Chicago's Abbott Laboratories.

Comarketing. To expand the breadth and depth of sales force efforts, companies that own certain products will enlist other firms for help. The other companies may even be competitors for other products. In 2006 Novartis Pharmaceuticals signed a copromotion agreement with TAP for the antiviral drug Famvir. The reason for this alliance was TAP's strength in the OB/GYN sector.

Provision of complementary expertise. It is common for small biotechnology or medical product firms to contract with larger companies to provide a variety of services, such as conducting large clinical trials, helping file for drug or device approval, and furnishing a sales force and other marketing functions.

Fewer than 10 percent of all new products are truly innovative and new; for example, a new chemical entity in the pharmaceutical sector or an innovative device to treat a previously incurable condition. These types of products involve the greatest cost and risk because they are new to both the company and the market place.

Most new health care product activity is devoted to improving existing products.[2] There are several product marketing strategies for current products:

- *Expanding use in the product category.* The clinical guidelines for treating conditions evolve as new research findings become available. For example, new standards that promote increasingly lower levels of cholesterol and blood pressure create opportunities for pharmaceutical companies to reach new customers and augment sales to existing ones.

- *Implementing new uses for the same product.* Sildenafil citrate (Viagra) was originally approved for use to treat erectile dysfunction. It is now approved for primary pulmonary hypertension (high pressure in the blood vessels of the lung).

- *Improving the same product.* Modifications of the same product may make it more convenient or suitable for customers. For example, a smaller version of an existing catheter may help a cardiologist more easily perform certain procedures.

- *Expanding the market for eligible consumers.* One frequent tactic that pharmaceutical companies employ is conducting testing of an existing drug in the pediatric market shortly before patent expiration. This activity not only serves to expand the potential size of the market but, due to certain laws, extends the patent life. Although this strategy is legal, we must note that initial delaying of research in this manner raises important ethical questions.

- *Combining an existing product with a new and innovative product.* Companies can enhance sales of an existing product by pairing it with a new and innovative one. For example, as mentioned previously, Merck combined its established, cholesterol-lowering drug, simvistatin (Zocor) with Schering-Plough's newer and innovative medication, ezetimibe (Zetia) into one pill they comarket as Vytorin. Vytorin lowers cholesterol much better than either drug alone. Another example is the creation of drug-eluting stents to keep blocked coronary arteries open after angioplasty. This product combined existing stent technology with new drugs. The category rapidly went from nonexistent to about 85 percent of market share in the United States.

Of course, several of the described tactics can be employed simultaneously and have different purposes for different companies. For example, Exubera is an inhaled form of insulin that was comarketed by Pfizer and Sanofi Aventis. Pfizer contributed its extensive, effective sales force and used this new offering to augment its product line (its other diabetic product is the pill Glucotrol XL). Sanofi Aventis already had an insulin product (injectable Lantus) and looked to Exubera to extend its category offering with this new delivery method. (Unfortunately, after Pfizer bought the drug from Sanofi Aventis in 2006, sales were far lower than expected. Pfizer announced in October 2007 that it was pulling Exubera from the market.)

Facing the Risks

Although successful companies must constantly innovate, new products fail at a disturbing rate. Recent studies put the failure rate of new consumer products at 95 percent in the United States and 90 percent in Europe.[3] Several factors hinder new-product development:

- *Shortage of important opportunities in certain areas.* There are few ways left to improve some basic products (such as latex gloves).

- *Fragmented markets.* Companies may have to aim their new offerings at smaller market segments, which can mean lower sales and profits for each product. (Sometimes this fragmentation is financially beneficial. For example, some pharmaceutical companies reap large margins and special patent protection from introducing orphan drugs—products that are used to treat rare diseases.)

- *Social and governmental constraints.* New products have to satisfy consumer safety and environmental concerns. In many countries in which the central government strongly controls health care practice and innovation, product cost is a major consideration in their adoption and diffusion.

- *Cost of development.* A company typically has to generate many ideas to find just one worthy of development, and it often faces high R&D, manufacturing, and marketing costs. A challenge companies constantly face is where to allocate finite R&D funds to ensure the biggest return.

- *Capital shortages.* Many startup companies with good ideas often have problems raising the funds needed to research and launch them.

- *Faster required development time.* Companies must learn how to compress development time by using new techniques, strategic partners, early concept tests, and advanced marketing planning. The time of patent exclusivity is as valuable a resource as the product itself.

- *Shorter product life cycles.* When a new product is successful, rivals are quick to copy its features and benefits.

  New products can fail for many reasons:

- Negative market research findings are ignored or misinterpreted.

- The idea is good, but the market size is overestimated.

- The product is not well designed.

- The product is incorrectly positioned in the market, not advertised effectively, or overpriced.

- The product fails to gain sufficient distribution coverage or support.

- Development costs are higher than anticipated.

- Competitor response is stronger than expected.

What can a company do to develop successful new products? Cooper and Kleinschmidt found that the number one success factor is a unique, superior product.[4] Such products succeed 98 percent of the time, compared with products with a moderate advantage (58 percent success) or minimal advantage (18 percent success). Another key success factor is a well-defined product concept prior to development. The company carefully defines and assesses the target market, product requirements, the competition, and product benefits before proceeding. Other success factors are technological and marketing synergy, quality of execution in all stages, and market attractiveness. Health care marketing managers also need to consider third-party payers, regulations, and multiple decision makers that may be very different from one another.

Steps in the New Product Development Process

This section covers the eight main stages involved in new product development: idea generation, concept development, concept testing, market strategy development, business analysis, product development, market testing, and commercialization.

Idea Generation.   Some marketing experts believe that the greatest opportunities and highest leverage with new products are found in the "fuzzy front end"—uncovering the best possible set of unmet needs or technological innovation by talking with customers.[5] Griffin and Hauser suggest that conducting ten to twenty in-depth experiential interviews per market segment often elicits the vast majority of customer needs.[6]

Technical companies can learn a great deal by studying those "lead customers" who make the most advanced use of the company's products and who recognize the need for improvements before other customers do.[7] Medtronic, a medical device company, has salespeople and market researchers regularly observe spine surgeons who use their own and competitive products, to learn how they can be improved. Other employees throughout the company can also be a source of ideas for improving production, products, and services.

Ideas for new products can come from other sources, such as top management, scientists, competitors, suppliers, distributors, inventors, patent attorneys, university and commercial laboratories, industrial consultants, advertising agencies, marketing research firms, and industrial publications. Although ideas can come from anywhere, their chances of receiving serious attention often depend on someone in the organization becoming a *product champion*. The constant challenge for a firm is to ensure that organizational structure and culture facilitate a free flow of ideas.

Idea screening. Since product development costs rise substantially with each successive development stage, an effective idea-screening process can be critical. Most companies require new product ideas to be described on a standard form that can be reviewed by a new product committee. The description states the product idea, the target market, competition, market size estimate, price, development time and costs, manufacturing costs, and rate of return. With respect to this last feature, in view of finite resources, the company must simultaneously consider all new ideas, to gauge which have the best chance of success vis-à-vis the others.

The new product committee then reviews each idea against a set of criteria; for example:

- Does the product meet a need? If so, how well?
- Would it offer superior value?
- Can it be distinctively advertised?
- Does the company have the necessary know-how and capital to develop, produce, and launch it?
- Will the new product deliver the expected sales volume, sales growth, and profit?

Concept Development. Attractive ideas must be refined into testable product concepts. A *product idea* is a possible tangible offering or specific service the company might introduce to the market. A *product concept* is an elaborated version of the idea expressed in meaningful consumer terms. Consumers do not buy product ideas; they buy product concepts.

A product idea can be turned into several concepts by answering questions such as, Who will use this product? What primary benefit should this product provide? When (under what circumstance) will people consume this product?

Suppose that an academic medical center (AMC) has some space that it wants to use to offer a new medical service. It can develop several concepts for the space:

- *Concept 1:* An outpatient orthopedic clinic for postoperative patients needing rehabilitation
- *Concept 2:* Sports medicine clinics open until 9 PM on weekdays and on Saturdays to cater to local athletes
- *Concept 3:* An occupational health center that targets employers with large volumes of workers' compensation cases

Each concept represents a *category concept* that also defines the product's potential competition. An outpatient orthopedic clinic would compete against independent orthopedic physician practices and other hospital rehab centers. A sports medicine clinic would compete against urgent care centers and primary care physicians. The academic medical center could prepare a *product-positioning map* to show where each alternative space use would compete with others on such product attributes as convenience and price.

Next, the chosen product concept has to be turned into a *brand concept* using a *brand-positioning map* to reflect the positioning of the specific competitors. The gaps in the map based on the most important brand attributes would indicate opportunities for the AMC. The AMC would not want to position the product next to an existing brand, unless that brand is weak or inferior.

Concept Testing. Concept testing involves presenting the product concept to appropriate target consumers and getting their reactions. The concepts can be presented symbolically or physically. The more the tested concepts resemble the final product or experience, the more dependable concept testing is.

Today firms can use computerized *rapid prototyping* to design products (for example, medical devices) and then produce models of each. Potential consumers can then view these models and give their reactions.[8] Companies are also using *virtual reality* to test product concepts, including services. Virtual reality programs use computers and sensory devices (such as gloves or goggles) to simulate a reality equivalent of the new product or service.

After gathering this information, researchers measure the product concept's viability by having consumers respond to the following questions:

1. *Communicability and believability:* Are the benefits clear to you and believable?

   If the scores are low, the concept must be refined or revised.

2. *Need level:* Do you see this product solving a problem or filling a need for you?

   The stronger the need, the higher the expected consumer interest.

3. *Gap level:* Do other products currently meet this need and satisfy you?

   The greater the gap, the higher the expected consumer interest. The need level can be multiplied by the gap level to produce a *need-gap score*. A high need-gap score means that the consumer sees the product as filling a strong need that is not satisfied by available alternatives.

4. *Perceived value:* Is the price reasonable in relation to the value?

   The higher the perceived value, the higher the expected consumer interest.

5. *Purchase intention:* Would you (definitely, probably, probably not, definitely not) buy the product?

   A high score would come from consumers who answered the previous three questions positively. When the consumer is not the principal payer, the consumer's desire to use the product must take into account whether the payer will include some of the expense as a covered benefit. For example, Germans highly value spa care; however, this traditional benefit has been eliminated by health plans as part of other strategies to curb rapidly rising health care costs in that country.

6. *User targets, purchase occasions, purchasing frequency:* Who would use this product, under what circumstances, and how often?

The respondents' answers indicate whether the concept has a broad and strong consumer appeal, identify the products this new product competes against, and highlight which consumers are the best targets. The need-gap levels and purchase-intention levels can be checked against norms for the product category to gauge whether the concept will be a winner, a long shot, or a loser.

Conjoint analysis. Consumer preferences for alternative product concepts can be measured through conjoint analysis, a method for deriving the utility values that consumers attach to varying levels of a product's attributes.[9] Using conjoint analysis, researchers collect responses from presenting the data two attributes at a time. For example, respondents may be shown a table with three price levels and three package types and asked which of the nine combinations they would like most, followed by which one they would prefer next, and so on. They are then shown a further table consisting of trade-offs between two other variables. The trade-off approach may be easier to use when there are many variables and possible offers. The drawback is that respondents are focusing on only two variables at a time, whereas at the time they choose a product, multiple factors may simultaneously come into play (see Field Note 10.2 for an example of how conjoint analysis is applied).

FIELD NOTE 10.2.

Conjoint Analysis Maps Consumer Preferences to Product Design Choosing the particular attributes to include in a successful product or service offering need not be based on luck, convenience, or engineering suggestions. Conjoint analysis is a marketing research tool that can be used to find out from consumers which product attributes have the greatest utility for them in a situation in which there must be trade-offs.

Ratcliffe used conjoint analysis to quantitatively examine patients' preferences for liver transplantation services. He started by assessing the relative importance of six attributes: (1) the chance of successful liver transplant or health outcome, versus these process characteristics of the service: (2) waiting time, (3) continuity of contact with the same medical staff, (4) amount of information received about the transplant, (5) follow-up support received, and (6) distance of the transplantation center from home.

Following a pilot study of forty patients, to identify and confirm the six product elements, a sample of patients who had received a liver transplant (n = 213) were surveyed. Interestingly, the results of this conjoint study indicated that even in the extreme case of a life-saving intervention the majority of respondents would exchange a reduction in health outcome for an improvement in the process characteristics of the liver transplantation service.

Where cost is included as an attribute, conjoint analysis has been used to estimate the willingness of consumers to pay for treatments and or services for which decisions must be made concerning the allocation of scarce health care resources. San Miguel applied conjoint analysis to consider women's preferences for two surgical procedures in the treatment of menorrhagia (excessive menstrual bleeding): hysterectomy and conservative surgery. The results indicated that conservative surgery was preferred to hysterectomy as indicated by higher utility scores and a marginal willingness to pay to have conservative surgery rather than hysterectomy.

A health insurer may want to trade off preventive against curative benefits when defining its benefit package, and estimates of willingness to pay can assist in determining whether the user values a product enough to actually use it. Telser used a conjoint approach with elderly individuals to measure demand for a new medical device that had not yet been developed. The study was sponsored by the Swiss government to decide if this device should be a mandated health insurance benefit. The device was a hypothetical hip protector that lowered the risk of hip fracture by different amounts.

The conjoint study included the elements of marginal willingness to pay, level of reduction of the risk of fracture, ease of handling, wearing comfort, and out-of-pocket cost. The target market was surveyed by conducting five hundred personal interviews. The results suggested that although individuals are interested in reducing the risk of a hip fracture, they are not willing to wear an uncomfortable, bulky protector. The overall willingness to pay for the product was negative, and as a result, the product was not included as a mandatory health insurance benefit.[10]

Conjoint analysis has become one of the most popular concept development and testing tools, particularly for pharmaceutical companies. In using it for drug design, marketers ask physicians what features they prefer in certain treatment categories, including effectiveness, side effects, cost to patient, need to use with other medications to achieve the desired effect, and manufacturer's reputation.

Although preference data can be used to estimate market share, the company may not launch the product even if these numbers are favorable. Given the results of the conjoint analysis, the firm may find that, considering the features consumers want, the product cannot furnish a sufficient profit to justify its launch.

Marketing Strategy Development. Following a successful concept test, the new-product manager will develop a preliminary marketing-strategy plan for introducing the new product into the market. The plan consists of three parts. The first part describes the target market's size, structure, and behavior; the planned product positioning; and the sales, market share, and profit goals sought in the first few years. The second part outlines the planned price, distribution strategy, and marketing budget for the first year. The third part describes the long-run sales and profit goals and marketing-mix strategy.

Business Analysis. After management develops the product concept and marketing strategy, it can evaluate the proposal's business attractiveness. Management needs to prepare sales, cost, and profit projections to determine whether they satisfy company objectives. If they do, the concept can move to the development stage. As new information is gathered, the business analysis will undergo revision and expansion.

Estimating total sales. Total estimated sales are the sum of estimated first-time sales, replacement sales, and repeat sales. Although the firm has determined potential market size in a previous step, here analysis of the pattern of sales is introduced. This pattern depends on whether the product is a one-time purchase (an assisted living home), an infrequently purchased product (a colonoscopy to screen for cancer or a PET scanner), or a frequently purchased product (medication for a chronic illness). For one-time purchased products, the rate of sales growth rises at the beginning, peaks, and later approaches zero, as the number of units or potential buyers attains a steady state that is determined solely by new entrants into the market.

Infrequently purchased products exhibit replacement cycles dictated by physical wearing out or by obsolescence associated with changing styles, features, and performance. Sales forecasting for tangible products in this category calls for estimating first-time sales and replacement sales separately.

For frequently purchased products, the number of first-time buyers initially increases and then decreases as fewer buyers are left (assuming a fixed population). Repeat purchases occur soon, providing that the product satisfies its customers. The sales curve eventually plateaus, representing a level of steady repeat-purchase volume and a fixed percentage of new customers who enter the market. (See the section below on product life cycles.)

Estimating costs and profits. Cost estimates and projections come from a variety of company sources; for example, R&D, manufacturing, marketing, and accounting departments. One of the great challenges of determining product cost is how to allocate the indirect expense component. This allocation problem is especially daunting for products, such as pharmaceuticals or devices, that have been developed over a number of years. Although generally accepted accounting principles (GAAP) can provide some guidance, the company must choose a consistent method that meets its needs.

Health care organizations use the same methods as other industries to evaluate the financial success of their ventures. The simplest is *break-even analysis*, in which management estimates how many units of the product the company needs to sell to cover its fixed and variable costs. Some firms use price and cost data to estimate the time it would take to recoup investment and manufacturing costs. Another method is net present value (NPV) analysis, which uses discounted cash flows to determine whether an investment meets targeted rates of return.

Another, more complex method of estimating profit is *risk analysis* simulations, which employ estimates—for example, optimistic, pessimistic, and most likely—for each uncertain variable that might affect profitability. The simulation generates probability distributions of possible outcomes and computes an expected rate of return.[11]

The place the product occupies in the business's portfolio can determine which of these tools it will use to evaluate profitability. For example, if a nonprofit hospital offers a service that fulfills an unmet community need, it will pay more attention to total budgeted costs rather than financial profitability measures. A pharmaceutical company that seeks benefit only from augmenting its product line may be concerned with break-even calculations for its new offering.

Product Development. If the product concept passes the business analysis test, it is developed into a prototype that (1) embodies the key attributes described in the product-concept statement, (2) performs safely under normal use and conditions, and (3) can be produced within the budgeted manufacturing costs. By designing and testing products through simulation, companies achieve the flexibility to respond to new information and to resolve uncertainties by quickly exploring alternatives. Because this step involves a significant increase in investment of money and other resources, it is critical for the company to decide whether it will proceed.

The task of translating target customer requirements into a working prototype is helped by a set of methods known as *quality function deployment* (QFD). The methodology takes the list of desired *customer attributes* (CAs) generated by market research and turns them into a list of *engineering attributes* (EAs) that the engineers can use. For example, customers of a proposed laboratory centrifuge may want a certain acceleration rate (which is a CA). Engineers can turn this need into the required horsepower and other engineering equivalents (which are EAs). The methodology permits measuring the trade-offs and costs of providing the customer requirements. A major contribution of QFD is that it improves communication among marketers, engineers, and the manufacturing employees.[12]

Lab scientists must not only design the product's functional characteristics but also communicate its psychological aspects through physical cues. How will consumers react to different colors, sizes, and weights? In the case of a mouthwash, a yellow color supports an "antiseptic" claim (Listerine), a red color supports a "refreshing" claim (Lavoris), and a green or blue color supports a "cool" claim (Scope). Marketers need to supply development people with information on what attributes consumers seek and how consumers judge whether these attributes are present. The design process must also consider cross-cultural differences in preference for such attributes as color, product formulation, and taste.

Market Testing. Consumer testing can take several forms, from bringing consumers into a laboratory to giving them samples to use in their homes. In-home placement tests are common with products consumers can use themselves, like glucometers for diabetics.

After management is satisfied with functional and psychological performance, the product is ready for a brand name, packaging, and a market test. The new product is introduced into an authentic setting to enable the makers to learn how large the market is and how patients, physicians, hospital personnel, and others react to handling, using, and repurchasing the product.

Health care consumer-goods market testing. In testing consumer products, the company seeks to estimate four usage variables: trial, first repeat, adoption, and purchase frequency.

In each of these categories there are four major methods of market testing, which we list here from the least to the most costly. These methods are particularly helpful to pharmaceutical companies moving from a prescription-only drug to over-the-counter (OTC) status.

1. *Sales-wave research.* In sales-wave research, consumers who initially try the offering at no cost are reoffered the product, or a competitor's product, at slightly reduced prices. The consumers are reoffered this product as many as three to five times (sales waves), while the company notes how many selected that product again, along with their reported level of satisfaction.

2. *Simulated test marketing.* Simulated test marketing calls for finding thirty to forty qualified shoppers and questioning them about brand familiarity and preferences in a specific product category. These people are then invited to a brief screening of both well-known and new commercials and print ads. Consumers then receive a small amount of money and are invited into a store, where they may buy any items in the relevant product class. The company notes how many consumers buy the new brand and competing brands. This process provides a measure of the ad's relative effectiveness against competing ads in stimulating trial use. Consumers are asked the reasons for their purchases or their lack of purchases. Those who did not buy the new brand are given a free sample. Some weeks later, they are interviewed again by phone to determine their opinions about product attitudes, usage, satisfaction, and repurchase intention and are offered an opportunity to repurchase any products.

3. *Controlled test marketing.* In this method, a research firm manages a panel of stores that will carry new products for a fee. The company with the new product specifies the number of stores and geographic locations it wants to test. The research firm delivers the product to the participating stores and controls shelf position, number of facings, displays, point-of-purchase promotions, and pricing. Sales results can be measured through electronic scanners at checkout. The company can also evaluate the impact of local advertising and promotions during the test.

4. *Test markets.* The ultimate way to test a new consumer product is to fully introduce it into test markets. The company conducts a full advertising and promotion campaign in these markets similar to the one that it would use in a national marketing campaign. This method permits assessing the impact of

alternative marketing plans by varying the approaches in different cities: a full-scale test can cost over $1 million, depending on the number of test cities, the test duration, and the amount of data the company wants to collect.

In spite of its benefits, many companies today are skipping full test marketing programs and relying on faster and more economical methods, such as smaller test areas and shorter test periods.

Business-goods market testing. Business goods can also benefit from market testing. Expensive medical equipment such as CT scanners will normally undergo both alpha testing (within the company) and beta testing (with outside customers such as hospitals). During beta testing, the vendor's technical people observe how test customers use the product; this practice often exposes unanticipated problems and alerts the vendor to customer training and servicing requirements. The vendor can also observe how much value the equipment adds to the customer's operation, which can inform subsequent pricing.

Another common test method for business goods is to introduce the new product at trade shows. The vendor can observe how much interest buyers show in the new product, how they react to various features and terms, and how many express purchase intentions or place orders.

Commercialization. If the company proceeds with commercialization, it will face its largest costs to date. For example, this step requires gearing up for large-scale manufacturing and launch of a full marketing campaign. To introduce a major new drug into the national market, the company may have to spend between $25 million and $100 million in advertising, promotion, and other communications in the first year.

BUILDING THE BRAND

One of the most important skill sets a marketer can have is the ability to create, enhance, maintain, and protect brands. Strategic brand management involves the design and implementation of marketing activities and programs to build, measure, and manage brands to maximize their value. Most large tangible product companies are aware of the strategic need to craft and manage brand identity. Unfortunately, at many health care service organizations, branding is not strategic but only tactical and frequently is limited to controlling the use of the corporate identity.

The American Marketing Association defines a brand as a name, term, sign, symbol, or design, or a combination of these, intended to identify the goods or services of one seller or group of sellers and to differentiate them from those of competitors.

A brand identifies attributes of the seller or maker. Whether it is a name, trademark, logo, or another symbol, a brand is a seller's promise to consistently deliver a specific set of features, benefits, and services. The best brands convey a sense of trust.[13] Brands have up to six levels of meaning (see Table 10.1).

TABLE 10.1. **Levels of Brand Meaning**

Meaning	Description	Example
Attributes	A brand brings to mind certain attributes.	Mayo Clinic suggests "patients first," treatment of last resort, collaborative doctors.
Benefits	Attributes must be translated into functional and emotional benefits.	The attribute "patients first" could translate into the functional benefit of "I feel less tension and stress as a patient."
Culture	The brand may represent a certain culture.	Mayo represents a tradition based on founder William Mayo's 1910 vision that medicine is a "cooperative science."
Personality	The brand can project a certain personality.	Mayo may suggest an intelligent, wise, and caring doctor or a peaceful healing oasis (place).
User	The brand suggests the kind of customer who buys or uses the product.	Mayo services are purchased by a diverse group ranging from international royalty to people living near one of its more than sixty primary care clinics or twenty-one owned or managed hospitals.

Source: Adapted from a chart in P. Kotler, *A Framework for Marketing Management,* 2nd ed. Upper Saddle River, N.J.: Prentice-Hall, 2003, p. 217.

Promoting a brand based on only one category of meaning can be risky. A new, competitive brand may more effectively deliver the underlying benefit, or the benefit of your product may become less important to buyers. Effective brands strive to engage customers on a deeper level by satisfying multiple needs and fostering a relationship with the product.

Most consumer health care products carry a brand name. A few might be labeled with just a generic name, such as aspirin or iodine. In that case, they may carry a lower price because the product has lower-quality ingredients, low-cost commodity ingredients, lower-cost labeling and packaging, or minimal advertising. (Lower quality is less true of generic and over-the-counter pharmaceuticals, because the FDA regulates the chemical composition of generic drugs.)

Health service organizations do not often pay the same attention to branding as do product firms. For example, although all physicians and hospitals have names, they may not have the status of brands. However some physicians may have achieved widespread recognition and preference, whether simply due to their quality work or through further leveraging by some personal marketing (see Field Note 10.3).

FIELD NOTE 10.3.

Physicians Become Brands It is almost unavoidable that certain physicians will become well-known brands, even if they never undertake any marketing or public relations efforts to become well known. The fact is that people needing a physician almost always ask others "Who are the best physicians?" A physician's reputation is built through their patients' satisfaction and word of mouth. And physicians who invent new medical procedures become known nationally and internationally, such as Dr. Michael DeBakey (world-famous heart surgeon), Dr. Jonas Salk (inventor of the Salk vaccine against infantile paralysis), and Dr. Kenneth Cooper (developer of aerobics).

But even in large cities, there are "star" physicians by specialty.

Consider Dr. Lowell Scott Weil. Dr. Weil is a celebrity podiatrist. He is the team podiatrist for the Chicago Bears and the Chicago White Sox, and a podiatry consultant to the Chicago Bulls. He was also team podiatrist for the U.S. Gymnastics Olympic Team. It is not surprising that he numbers among his patients some star athletes, ballerinas, and others prone to foot injuries.

Part of his early fame came from his contributions in the area of foot surgery implants. He codeveloped surgical implants with Dow Corning, Richards Manufacturing, and Collagen Corporation. Some are no longer in use, he says, because "things change so quickly . . . and each invention stimulates others in the field to develop even better versions of the device."

He worked with Dr. Steve Smith to develop one of the most famous podiatric surgical residency programs, Northlake Hospital, in a suburb north of Chicago. The Northlake program serves over one hundred patients a week because of its excellent teaching staff. "Back then, it was known as the 'Mayo Clinic of the feet,'" said Dr. Weil.

Podiatrists have experienced some tensions with orthopedic doctors. Weil says that orthopedists will take foot cases but often aren't as up to date with the latest methods and after-surgery procedures as podiatrists. He would be much happier getting the foot cases and recommending ankle and knee work to orthopedists.

Dr. Weil is an established brand, partly because of his training and surgical contributions, and partly because he often hangs out with Mike Ditka, Michael Jordan, and other athletes at the ball games or in his offices.

Source: M. Gorman, "Podiatrist to the Bears, Bulls, and White Sox," *Podiatry Today*, April 1991.

Sellers of health care products and services who are successful at branding find that the cost and effort can provide the following benefits:

- Making it easier for the seller and buyer to process orders
- Legally protecting unique product features (particularly when a trademark is registered)
- Allowing the seller to attract loyal, profitable customers
- Permitting the organization to charge more because the brand has higher perceived quality
- Helping the seller segment markets by offering different brands with different features for different benefit-seeking segments
- Allowing the firm to more easily launch extensions because the brand has high credibility
- Helping build the corporate image, easing the way for new brands and wider acceptance by distributors and customers
- Reducing marketing costs because of high brand awareness and loyalty
- Giving an organization more leverage in negotiating with its channel partners
- Offering some defense against price competition
- Helping customers distinguish quality differences and shop more efficiently

The strategic brand management process involves three main stages:

1. Developing the brand
2. Measuring brand equity
3. Repositioning the brand

We will discuss each of these processes in the following section.

Developing the Brand

The health care organization must start by choosing a brand name. Desirable qualities for a brand name include the following:

- It should suggest something about the product's benefits. Example: Hemopure, a human blood substitute from Biopure, a company that manufactures artificial blood.

- It should suggest product qualities. Example: HealthStream Express, an online training solution designed to meet the needs of smaller health care organizations.

- It should be easy to pronounce, recognize, and remember. Example: BluePerks, the health service discount program from Blue Cross Blue Shield of Tennessee.

- It should be distinctive. Example: Aircast, a manufacturer of orthopedic support supplies.

Although creating a brand identity certainly involves choosing a name, logo, colors, tagline, and symbol, the process goes beyond these visual cues. Branding offers a contract to the customer regarding how the brand will perform—and the contract must be honest. Consider the following example:

FOR EXAMPLE

Several years after it purchased a community hospital in an adjacent community, an academic medical center (AMC) in the Southeast wanted to change its name in order to leverage the AMC brand and increase market share.

Focus group research was conducted with members of the target market in the nearby area to learn which specific names would be most appealing and why. The research showed that if the community hospital were branded with the name of the AMC, the market would expect the same physicians and level of quality as the AMC. They would also expect a quick and easy transfer from the hospital to the AMC if specialty care was needed. Unfortunately, the AMC did not follow the preferences of the market; it simply changed the signage on the community hospital to reflect the new ownership. The mediocre financial performance of the community hospital did not improve.

Brand strategy varies according to whether the brand is a functional brand, an image brand, or an experiential brand. Consumers purchase a *functional brand* to satisfy a functional need, such as urgent care for a minor illness or injury or a bandage for a wound. Functional brands rely heavily on "product" or "price" features. *Image brands* have features that consumers differentiate from other choices based on such attributes as quality. Image brands also convey a statement about the user—typically something positive. An example of selecting a health care image brand could be a patient choosing to visit a hospital just because it has been highly ranked in the *U.S. News & World Report*. As the image brand says something about the person who uses it, reliance on external sources for brand choice is logical. *Experiential brands* involve the consumer beyond simply acquiring the product. The consumer encounters "people" and "place" with these brands, as happens when a patient visits a medical resort at Vail, Colorado, for an elective plastic surgery procedure combined with a family vacation.

Over time, each type of brand can be developed further. A company can introduce line extensions whereby an existing brand name is extended to new variations in the product category, as in the following example:

FOR EXAMPLE

Hospital Corporation of America (HCA) made the line extension decision in the mid-1980s when it started to use its Nashville-based flagship hospital's brand name on every hospital that it owned or managed nationwide. This extension was intended to achieve marketing communication economies of scale and foster consumer and physician belief that the HCA hospital in their local community would represent high-quality care. The company placed the brand name "HCA" as prefix in all of its hospitals' signage and marketing communications. Unfortunately, the quality of hospital services delivered by the different HCA hospitals varied widely, and the brand integrity was degraded. When HCA merged with Columbia Health care, the names of all the hospitals changed again: the "HCA" brand name was replaced with the "Columbia" brand name. Not long after the merger, Columbia was prosecuted by the federal government for billing irregularities and other alleged wrongdoing. It took several years, but eventually the Columbia brand name was removed and the local hospitals once again returned to the names in use before the HCA branding campaign started.

An organization can also extend its brand name into new product categories; introduce several brands in the same product category; introduce new brands with new brand names in a new product category; and cobrand with another well-known name.

An excellent example of cobranding is the adult oncology collaboration among Dana-Farber Cancer Institute and two Partners HealthCare hospitals, Massachusetts General Hospital and Brigham and Women's Hospital in Boston. Each year, the three hospitals that comprise Dana-Farber/Partners Cancer Care provide comprehensive, multidisciplinary services to more than twelve thousand new cancer patients. Patients come from around the world for access to treatments that offer the greatest promise and clinicians who are renowned for their excellence and compassion.

Increasing brand awareness will create name recognition, brand knowledge, and possibly some brand preference, but it does not create brand bonding. Brand bonding occurs when customers experience the organization delivering on its benefit promise.

Heidi and Don Schultz recommend a six-step brand development process for marketing managers:[14]

1. Organizational values should be used to support the brand.

2. All employees need to live the value proposition.

3. Organizations need to create positive customer experiences at every contact point.

4. Organizations should define the brand's basic essence to be delivered in every market.

5. Firms must use the brand-value proposition to drive their strategy, operations, and product development.

6. Organizations need to measure brand-building results according to measures such as customer retention and customer advocacy.

Measuring Brand Equity

Brands vary by the power and value they have in the marketplace. At one end of the spectrum are brands that are unknown. At the opposite end are brands with a high level of *brand awareness*. For example, if you ask the average person to name a brand of health insurance, chances are the answer will be "Blue Cross." Brands with high awareness are further segmented by the value of their *brand acceptability* and *brand preference*. The ultimate brand goal is to have a high level of *brand loyalty*. Aaker has identified five levels of customer attitude toward brands in general:[15]

1. Customer will change brands, especially for price reasons. No brand loyalty.

2. Customer is satisfied. No reason to change the brand.

3. Customer is satisfied and would incur costs by changing brand.

4. Customer values the brand and sees it as a friend.

5. Customer is devoted to the brand.

Brand equity in this framework is highly related to how many customers are in classes 3, 4, and 5. When patients feel very positive about their physician, hospital, or medicine brand, we say that the brand equity of these respective entities is high.

Marketing managers can maximize their brand's equity by understanding the associations consumers make among the brand's chief perceived attributes as well the strength of these connections. Often these links are graphically displayed in *brand concept maps.* For example, the Mayo Clinic brand has associations including "leader in medical research," "best doctors in the world," and "known world-wide"; these associations relate to product attributes and brand character as well as consumer emotions. The individual maps are then aggregated into consensus maps and can be segmented by consumer type (such as expert, novice, and nonusers). Brand concept maps provide managers with a clear image of a brand's strengths and possible weaknesses.

Brand equity is usually tracked with a set of metrics such as awareness, acceptability, preference, market share, and relative price compared to competitors. *Brand valuation*, on the other hand, refers to estimating the total financial value of the brand. This value has important implications for stock pricing and the financial terms of mergers and acquisitions.

Companies need to periodically audit their brands' strengths and weaknesses. One tool, Kevin Keller's brand report card, is designed to assess whether a brand has the ten characteristics of a strong brand:[16]

1. It excels at delivering the benefits customers truly desire.
2. It stays relevant to customers over time.
3. Pricing truly reflects consumers' perceptions of value.
4. It is properly positioned.
5. It stays consistent.
6. Subbrands relate to one another in an orderly way within a portfolio of brands.
7. A full range of marketing tools is employed to build brand equity.
8. The brand's managers understand what the brand means to customers.
9. The organization gives the brand proper support and sustains it over the long term.
10. The organization consistently measures sources of brand equity.

By developing metrics to grade a brand according to how well it addresses each characteristic, managers can come up with a comprehensive brand report card. They should apply the same scorecard to their competitors' brands to understand their relative strengths and weaknesses.

Repositioning the Brand

An organization will occasionally discover that it may have to reposition a brand because of new competitors or changing customer preferences. Several situations might warrant repositioning moves. A well-known hospital such as the Mayo Clinic may decide to open in new locations and build a reputation as a national or international hospital system. An over-the-counter brand may face a new challenge and want to reposition itself, as happened in 1982 when McNeil's Tylenol brand was the target of random retail poisonings in the Chicago market. McNeil immediately withdrew its product from the market, repackaged it to prevent tampering, and repositioned its brand to make safety, as well as effectiveness, its major selling points.

Repositioning is usually called for when hospitals are merged. Consider the merger of the New York Hospital and the Presbyterian Hospital in 1998 under the new name NewYork-Presbyterian Healthcare System:[17]

FOR EXAMPLE

Because these rival institutions were direct competitors, they duplicated many of the same services. Further, although each of these teaching hospitals had a distinguished history, both were ailing because of changing economic and social conditions. For example, Presbyterian's neighborhood began to change after World War II with an influx of poorer residents and exodus of the more affluent patients to other hospitals. The merger was undertaken to cut costs and build a stronger single hospital system. Fortunately, the hospital hired Dr. Herbert Pardes, the nation's first psychiatrist to run a major medical center. Although he merged all of the hospitals' administrative functions and moved to consolidate many medical units, in order to satisfy local interests he preserved separate clinical areas in psychiatry, neurosurgery, and pediatrics, in spite of redundancies He implemented a patient-centered ethic in the hospital by such actions as personally visiting patients' bedsides, requiring nurses to memorize all the patients' and family members' names, and having the rooms and lobbies repainted in soothing pastel hues—all of which won plaudits from patients, doctors, and nurses. Through the hospitals' combining a large dose of human compassion with effective management, the repositioned brand image of a caring hospital earned NewYork-Presbyterian *U.S. News and World Report*'s ranking of top medical institutions for six years in a row, and in 2005 *New York* magazine ranked it as the overall leader in its "Best Hospitals" survey. The brand repositioning also translated into a successful fundraising campaign—nearly $1 billion in seven years.

MANAGING THE STAGES OF THE PRODUCT LIFE CYCLE

In an environment as dynamic as health care, an organization's marketing strategy must change as the product, market, and competitors change over time. In this section we describe the concept of the *product life cycle* (PLC) and the changes that organizations make as the product passes through each stage of the life cycle.

To say that a product has a life cycle is to assert four things:

- Products have a limited life.
- Product sales pass through distinct stages, each posing different challenges, opportunities, and problems to the seller.

- Profits rise and fall at different stages of the product life cycle.

- Products require different marketing, financial, manufacturing, purchasing, and human resource strategies in each life-cycle stage.

Product Life Cycles

The PLC concept can be used to analyze a product category (pharmaceuticals), a product form (drug tablets), a product (statin drugs), or a brand (Lipitor). Most product life-cycle curves are divided into four stages: introduction, growth, maturity, and decline. The shapes of these curves will depend on the nature of the product and the environment in which it is used. The units on both axes also vary with the product. Sales can range from hundreds of thousands to billions of dollars. Likewise the time can vary, from weeks to centuries (consider aspirin use).

1. *Introduction:* A period of sales growth as the product is introduced in the market. Profit margins are frequently nonexistent because of the heavy expenses of product introduction. Because of this large allocation of development costs at this point, sales volume is used to measure success.

2. *Growth:* A period of rapid market acceptance and substantial profit improvement. Sales volumes as well as rate of increase in that volume are measures of success; for example, new prescriptions in the case of a pharmaceutical launch.

3. *Maturity:* A slowdown in sales growth because the product has achieved acceptance by most potential buyers. Profits stabilize or decline because of increased competition. Actual profitability figures are now used to gauge product success.

4. *Decline:* Sales show a downward drift and profits erode.

Three common PLC patterns are shown in Figure 10.1.

The first pattern is characteristic of products that become rapidly popular but for which enthusiasm dies rather quickly. In consumer goods, these products would

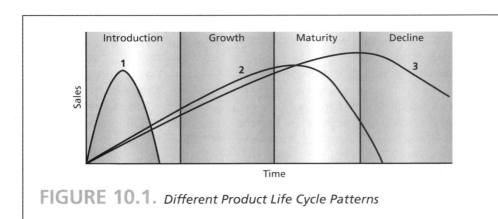

FIGURE 10.1. *Different Product Life Cycle Patterns*

be considered fads. In health care, fads may play a role in alternative medical products or practices; for example, the Grapefruit Diet. Another reason for this pattern, however, is the emergence of unanticipated safety concerns shortly after product launch. Further, this pattern may be normal for some products; for example, different influenza vaccines are produced annually to cover anticipated strains; the vaccine is administered in the United States over several months and then ceases to be used.

The second pattern is more typical of most products and services. After introduction, a steady growth pattern develops into the product's maturity. At that time, the need (demand) for the product declines, or competitors offer substitutes that may have enhanced value, or both may occur. Successful product revisions, such as new features or uses, can result in additional peaks, resulting in a scalloped pattern (not shown in the figure).

The third pattern is for products that have long-established needs and for which competition is minimal. An example in this category is smallpox vaccines. Vaccination started in earnest in the United States during the Revolutionary War and gained in popularity and use over the next two centuries. The vaccine use declined as incidence of the disease waned worldwide and then ceased when the WHO finally declared it eradicated in 1980.

Services also have identifiable life cycles. For a quarter of a century, treating coronary artery disease through surgical and catheter-based intervention has been a highly profitable business for hospitals. Coronary artery bypass grafts, or CABGs, are high-margin surgeries (surgeries with a high profit margin) that circumvent blocked arteries in the heart using vascular tissue frequently taken from veins in the patient's leg. CABG volumes started to slow down a couple years after the introduction of stents in the mid-1990s. Then CABG volumes slowed down further with the advent of the more "efficacious" drug-eluting stents (see Figure 10.2).

We will now discuss each phase of the product life cycle patterns in more depth.

Introduction Stage and the Pioneer Advantage

The introduction stage takes place when the new product or service is first made available to the marketplace. Introduction into one or more markets takes time, and sales growth is apt to be slow. Sales of new health care products and services are slowed by such additional factors as product complexity, regulatory approval, and establishing channel partners, such as physicians and third-party payers.

In the introduction stage, costs are high because of low adoption and heavy production, distribution, and promotion expenses. Promotion costs-to-sales ratios are at their highest because of the need to build awareness, secure distribution channels, and generate trial purchases. Profits are negative or low in the introduction stage. Firms focus on those potential customers who are the readiest or most able to buy. In the consumer goods sector, these customers usually come from higher-income groups; in the health care field, the greatest potential is in the group with comprehensive health insurance benefits. In developing countries, where government resources are

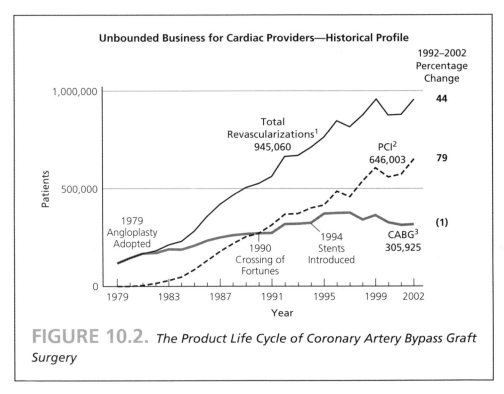

FIGURE 10.2. *The Product Life Cycle of Coronary Artery Bypass Graft Surgery*

Notes:
[1]ICD-9-CM codes 36.00-02, .05, .06, .10–17, .19; individual patients.
[2]ICD-9-CM codes 36.00-02, .05, .06; individual patients.
[3]ICD-9-CM codes 36.10-17, .19; individual patients.
Source: Innovations Center Futures Database, the Advisory Board Company, Washington, D.C., 2006.

scant and private insurance companies are rare, firms focus on those with the greatest disposable incomes.

In addition to all the new product characteristics previously mentioned, companies must also decide *when* to enter the market. To be first can be rewarding, but also risky and expensive. To come in later makes sense if the firm can bring superior technology, quality, or brand strength. For example, by being the first drug introduced in the U.S. market for erectile dysfunction, Pfizer's Viagra has retained sales leadership over rivals Cialis (Eli Lilly) and Levitra (copromoted by Bayer, GlaxoSmithKline, and Schering Plough). On the other hand, American Home Products (now part of Wyeth) was first in the market to produce fenfluramine, which dieters combined with phentermine to lose weight. When the combination was subsequently found to cause heart valve problems, the former medication was pulled from the market and resulted in a multibillion-dollar legal settlement.

In an age in which the rate of technology development is increasing, companies must also reduce cycle time for their products. This process spans drug discovery, small and large clinical trials, patent application, and launch of drug into the market. One study found that products that came out six months late—but on budget—earned an average of 33 percent less profit in their first five years; products that came out on time but 50 percent over budget cut their profits by only 4 percent.[18]

Growth Stage

If all goes well and the new product satisfies market needs, sales will start climbing. Early adopters like the product, and additional consumers start buying it. New competitors enter, introduce new product features, and expand distribution.

Prices remain where they are or fall slightly, depending on how fast demand increases. It should be noted that price competition is not typically a feature of noncommodity products, like branded pharmaceuticals. Companies frequently maintain their promotional expenditures at the same or at a slightly increased level to meet competition and to continue to educate the market. Sales rise much faster than promotional expenditures, causing a welcome decline in the promotion cost-to-sales ratio. Profits increase during this stage as promotion costs are spread over a larger volume and unit manufacturing costs fall. During this stage, firms must watch for a change from an accelerating to a decelerating rate of growth; the firm can use several strategies to sustain rapid market increases:

- Improve product quality, add new product features, and improve styling.
- Add new models and flanker products (for example, products of different sizes, flavors, and so forth that protect the main product).
- Enter new market segments.
- Increase distribution coverage and enter new distribution channels.
- Shift from product-awareness advertising to product-preference advertising.
- Lower prices to attract the next layer of price-sensitive buyers.

These market expansion strategies strengthen the firm's competitive position. A firm in the growth stage faces a trade-off between high market share and high current profit. By spending money on current product improvement, promotion, and distribution, it can capture a dominant position, forgoing maximum current profit in the hope of garnering even greater future returns.

Maturity Stage

At some point, the rate of sales growth will slow, and the product will enter a stage of relative maturity. This stage normally lasts longer than the previous stages and poses big challenges to marketing management. *Most current products are in the maturity stage of the life cycle, and most marketing managers cope with problems of the mature product.*

This stage divides into three further phases: growth, stable, and decaying maturity. In the first phase, the sales growth *rate* starts to decline. There are no new distribution channels to fill. In the second phase, sales flatten on a per capita basis because of market saturation. Most potential consumers have tried the product, and future sales are governed by population growth and replacement demand. In the third phase, decaying maturity, the *absolute level* of sales starts to decline, and customers begin switching to other products.

The sales slowdown creates overcapacity in the industry, which leads to intensified competition. Competitors scramble to find niches, engage in frequent markdowns, and increase advertising and consumer promotion. In commercial markets, they may also increase R&D budgets to develop product improvements and line extensions and make deals to supply private brands. A shakeout begins, and weaker competitors withdraw. The industry eventually consists of well-entrenched competitors whose basic drive is to gain or maintain market share.

Surrounding these dominant organizations is a multitude of competitors that occupy highly specialized market niches, including market specialists, product specialists, and customizing firms. A firm can dominate a market niche by becoming a quality leader, service leader, or cost leader. The issue facing a firm in a mature market is where to place itself among these competing companies.

Market Modification. The company might try to expand the market for its mature brand by working with the two factors that make up sales volume:

$$\text{Volume} = \text{number of brand users} \times \text{usage rate per user}$$

It can try to expand the number of brand users by these methods:

- *Converting nonusers.* The key to the growth of LASIK eye surgery is the constant search for new users to whom ophthalmologists can demonstrate the benefits of not using eyeglasses or contact lenses.

- *Entering new market segments.* When Mayo Clinic decided to establish primary care clinics and alliances with hospitals in Jacksonville, Florida, and Phoenix, Arizona, it boosted market share and expanded its referral network.

- *Winning competitors' customers.* GlaxoSmithKline's Flonase brand nasal spray is continually battling against branded and generic nasal sprays offered by other companies.

Product Modification. Managers also try to stimulate sales by modifying the product's characteristics through quality improvement, feature improvement, or style improvement.

Quality improvement aims at increasing the product's functional performance. A manufacturer can often overtake its competition by launching a "new and improved" product. This strategy is effective to the extent that the quality is improved, buyers accept the claim of improved quality, and a sufficient number of buyers will pay for higher quality. For example, Marion Merrill Dow (now part of Sanofi-Aventis) was a product innovator with its cardiovascular drug Cardizem (diltiazem). Because of its relatively short half-life, patients needed to take this medication every six to eight hours. When generic competition threatened market share, the company launched Cardizem SR, which could be taken every twelve hours. When generics subsequently challenged *that* medication, the company introduced once-a-day Cardizem CD. Because the delivery and form of the longer-lasting formulations were new, the company did well for years by extending its patents.

Feature improvement aims at adding new features (for example, size, weight, materials, additives, accessories) that expand the product's versatility, safety, or convenience. We presented the example of Vytorin (Zocor and Zetia) earlier. This strategy has several advantages. New features build the company's image as an innovator, win the loyalty of market segments that value these features, provide an opportunity for free publicity, and generate sales force and distributor enthusiasm. The chief disadvantage is that feature improvements are easily imitated, unless they include unique components or they can derive a market share gain from being first of its kind.

Style improvement aims at increasing the product's esthetic appeal. The periodic introduction of new car models is largely about style competition, as is the introduction of new packaging for consumer products. Before Northwestern Memorial Hospital built its new facility, the organization conducted extensive market research to understand what its potential patients desired in facility appearance. The consistent reply was: "We want a hospital that doesn't look like a hospital." Using this feedback, the design resulted in a building that looks more like an upscale hotel than a health care institution. In this case, starting anew using marketing research was not only possible but desirable. Companies can run risks, however, if style changes interfere with or confuse the public's positive perception of the brand. Imagine if, in the example that began this chapter, Blue Cross Blue Shield not only designed a new product but also modified its logo. Tampering with that trusted brand identity could have doomed the new product launch.

Marketing Program Modification. Product managers may also try to stimulate sales by modifying other marketing program elements. They should ask the following questions:

- *Prices:* Would a price cut attract new buyers? If so, should the list price be lowered, or should prices be lowered through price specials, volume or early-purchase discounts, or easier credit terms? Alternatively, would it be better to raise the price to signal higher quality?

- *Distribution:* Can the organization obtain more product support through its existing outlets and referral channels, or should it introduce the product into new distribution channels?

- *Advertising:* Should advertising expenditures be increased? Should the message or copy be changed? Should the media mix be changed? Should the timing, frequency, or size of ads be changed?

- *Personal selling:* Should the number or quality of salespeople be increased? Should the basis for sales force specialization be changed? Should sales territories be revised? Should sales force incentives be revised? Can sales-call planning be improved?

- *Services:* Can the company speed up delivery? Can it extend more technical assistance to customers? Can it extend more credit?

Marketers often debate which tools are most effective in the mature stage. For example, would the company gain more by increasing its advertising or its sales-promotion budget? Sales promotion has more impact at this stage because consumers have reached equilibrium in their buying habits and preferences, and psychological persuasion (advertising) is not as effective as financial persuasion (sales-promotion deals). Many consumer-packaged-goods companies now spend over 60 percent of their total promotion budget on sales promotion to support mature products. Other marketers argue that brands should be managed as capital assets and supported by advertising. Brand managers often use sales promotion because its effects are quicker and more visible to their superiors, but excessive sales-promotion activity can hurt the brand's image and long-run profit performance.

Decline Stage

Sales eventually decline for a number of reasons, including technological advances, shifts in consumer tastes, and increased domestic and foreign competition. All lead to overcapacity, increased price cutting, and profit erosion. The decline might be slow, as in the case of X-ray film or paper-based medical records, or rapid, as in the case of laparoscopic surgery replacing certain procedures. Sales may plunge to zero, or they may petrify at a low level.

As sales and profits decline, some firms withdraw from the market. Those remaining may reduce the number of products they offer, withdraw from smaller market segments and weaker trade channels, cut their promotion budgets, or reduce prices further, or a combination of these actions. Unfortunately, many companies have not developed a policy for handling aging products.

With declining drug R&D productivity and maturing product portfolios, it is especially important for pharmaceutical companies to maximize revenues through lifecycle management. A classic example of rapid decline is when a patent expires for a pharmaceutical and generics enter the market. Upon patent expiration, companies risk losing up to 80 percent of brand sales, highlighting the importance of implementing successful strategies for brand protection and market expansion. Pharmaceutical companies need to maximize revenue at all stages of the product lifecycle and minimize the impact of generic competition on their brands. Examples of possible strategies to address the loss of market share to generics include the following: obtaining rapid approval for over-the-counter branded versions—for example, Claritin; indication expansion—for example, expanding approved use to a new population, like children, or new illness categories; and reformulation, as mentioned in the earlier example of Cardizem.

Unless there are strong reasons for retention, such as complementing a product line, carrying a weak product is very costly to the firm. It absorbs a disproportionate share of uncovered overhead and management's time, while requiring frequent price and inventory adjustments, short production runs, and both advertising and sales force attention that might be better used to make healthy products more profitable. Outmoded products can also cast a shadow on the company's image. The biggest cost might well lie in the future; failure to eliminate weak products may delay an aggressive search for more innovative replacement products.

In handling aging products, a company faces a number of tasks and decisions. The first task is to establish a system for identifying weak products. Many companies appoint a product-review committee, with representatives from marketing, R&D, operations, and finance. The controller, marketing, and strategic planning departments usually supply data and analysis for each product, showing trends in market size, market share, prices, costs, and profits. The managers responsible for questionable products complete rating forms showing where they think sales and profits will go, with and without any changes in marketing strategy. The product-review committee then makes a recommendation for each product—leave it alone, modify its marketing strategy, or drop it.[19]

Although some companies abandon aging products, others look for opportunities. A prime example is Ovation Pharmaceuticals. According to founder Jeffrey Aronin:[20]

With the consolidation of big pharma, it became clear that bigger pharma companies needed to focus on much-larger products to get the growth they wanted. This meant a marginal drug for a company would no longer meet the financial threshold and would no longer receive commercial or clinical dollars.

We recognized that we could acquire these products and add value through lifecycle management—new product improvements and new indications—as well as commercial efforts. This is not a completely new concept, but what I saw that was different and important for our business to concentrate on is the high-need drugs with a focused specialty physician group. We have stayed true to this with five central nervous system (CNS) drugs and three rare disease drugs [www.ovationpharma.com].

BUILDING, MAINTAINING, AND TERMINATING A BRAND

The presence and extent of industry exit barriers can significantly influence when a firm abandons declining markets.[21] Such exit barriers include legal or moral obligations, contracts with joint venture partners, lack of alternative opportunities, and government restrictions. In studying declining industries, we see that five strategies are available to a firm:[22]

- Increase the firm's investment (to dominate the market or strengthen its competitive position).

- Maintain the firm's investment level until the uncertainties about the industry are resolved.

- Decrease the firm's investment level selectively, by dropping unprofitable customer groups, while simultaneously strengthening the firm's investment in lucrative niches.

- Harvest ("milk") the firm's investment to recover cash quickly.

- Divest the business quickly by selling or disposing of its assets as advantageously as possible.

An example is a commercial health care insurer that may decide to drop a product that may involve a whole customer segment, like small businesses. If the product has strong distribution and residual goodwill, the company can probably sell it to another firm. If the company can't find any buyers, it must decide whether to liquidate the brand quickly or slowly. In either case, it must decide how and how long to serve existing customers while exiting the market. As well, it must consider the consequences for its reputation in terms of its more profitable lines. Hospitals that cease to provide certain services face similar issues. For example, the University of Chicago Hospitals (among other institutions in the city and around the country) pulled out of the regional trauma care network in late 1980s, citing significant financial losses. Communities were outraged when they learned that victims of gunshot wounds and auto accidents would need to travel miles for emergency care.

The attractiveness of the sector and the company's competitive strength in it can also influence withdrawal decisions. For example, a company that is in an unattractive industry but possesses competitive strength can consider shrinking selectively. A company that is in an attractive industry and has competitive strength should consider strengthening its investment.

The Product Life Cycle (PLC) Concept: A Critique

Although the PLC concept helps marketers interpret product and market dynamics and can be used for planning and control, it is less useful as a forecasting tool. The theory has its share of critics, and Dhalla and Yuspeh assert that the PLC is difficult to validate.[23] Their research shows that some product classes (such as anti-inflammatory medications) have maturity stages that last for centuries, assuming that they satisfy some basic need. Product forms (such as aspirin) tend to exhibit less stability than product class. They assert that the PLC applied to brands (such as Bayer aspirin) has even less validity, claiming that life-cycle patterns are too variable in shape and duration. Critics also allege that marketers can seldom identify the correct stage of the product. For example, it may appear to be mature when actually it has reached a plateau prior to another upsurge. They also charge that the PLC pattern is the *result* of marketing strategies rather than an inevitable course that sales must follow. Consider the following scenario:

FOR EXAMPLE

Suppose a brand is acceptable to consumers but has a few bad years because of such factors as poor advertising, delisting by a major chain, or entry of a "me-too" competitive product backed by massive sampling. Instead of thinking in terms of corrective measures, management begins to feel that its brand has entered a declining stage. It therefore withdraws funds from the promotion budget to finance R&D on new items. Because of these actions, the following year the brand does even worse. The PLC is a dependent variable that is determined by marketing measures; it is not an independent variable to which companies should adapt their marketing programs.[24]

Because the PLC focuses on what is happening to a particular product or brand, rather than on what is happening to the overall market, it yields a product-oriented picture rather than a market-oriented picture. Firms need to visualize a market's evolutionary path as it is affected by new needs, competitors, technology, channels, and other developments. In the course of a product's or brand's existence, its positioning must change to keep pace with market developments.

SUMMARY

Every health care organization must be skilled in developing new products and services to meet the changing market demands. The risks of new product development are many, but it is even more risky to not change with the times.

The challenge is to master the eight steps of new product development: idea generation and screening, concept development, concept testing, market strategy development, business analysis, product development, market testing, and commercialization.

Each new product or service needs a branding strategy that includes naming the product and developing a logo, tagline, color, and symbols. Success in branding will be reflected in rising brand equity.

The branded product will pass through four stages of a product life cycle: introduction, growth, maturity, and decline. A different set of marketing strategies is required in each stage. For example, in the mature stage, strategies of market modification, product modification, and marketing program modification can extend the product's profitable life. At the same time, marketers should recognize that there is nothing inevitable about the product's life cycle.

DISCUSSION QUESTIONS

1. A hospital introduced an annual health testing service geared to executives. How can the hospital marketer identify the four PLC stages for this product line as it evolves? What would be the signs of this service entering the decline stage and what strategies can be used to resurrect it if it enters this stage?

2. Health information systems companies have earned a reputation for marketing new products that do not always perform as promised. Would you classify this perception as new product failure? Why or why not?

3. Brands can clearly indicate to their target markets that they are in a particular category. Explain three ways in which they accomplish this goal and provide examples for a business-to-consumer (B2C) health care product or service and a business-to-business (B2B) health care product or service.

4. You are working in the marketing department of a health plan that seeks to increase penetration in the Hispanic market segment. You need to decide if it would be better to market a new line under a new brand name or use the existing brand name under a line extension strategy. List the advantages and disadvantages of each strategy and present your recommendation.

CHAPTER

PRICING STRATEGIES AND DECISIONS IN HEALTH CARE

LEARNING OBJECTIVES

In this chapter, we will address the following questions:

1. How do health care consumers, providers, and companies process and evaluate prices?

2. What are the different methods and seven steps for setting an initial price for a product or service?

3. How should prices be adapted to meet varying circumstances and opportunities?

4. When should an organization initiate a price change?

5. How should an organization respond to a competitor's price change?

6. What influence do government and private payers have on pricing decisions?

OPENING EXAMPLE

How Johnson & Johnson Tried to Reduce the Price of Its Stents to Save Its Market Share If a medical device company lowers its product prices, does its rival need to respond in kind? Consider the following example.

Boston Scientific introduced its drug-eluting Taxus cardiac stent in 2004. Stents are used to prop open narrowed arteries after they have been opened through a procedure known as angioplasty. The drug-eluting coatings reduce the buildup of scar tissue that can lead to the need for repeat procedures. After its introduction, Taxus immediately captured two-thirds of the market from Johnson & Johnson's coated stent, Cypher, which had received FDA approval almost one year before. These stents were the only drug-eluting versions in the market at the time.

Within the year, Johnson & Johnson dropped the price of Cypher by 19 percent, from $2,900 to $2,350; however, its market share did not significantly change. Boston Scientific lowered the Taxus price by only 4 percent, from $2,675 to $2,575, also maintaining its market share.

Few physicians choose stents based simply on price. Instead, they rely on scientific data about effectiveness, ease of use, ready availability, and product service. To this customer segment, a higher-priced product can be a better value than the lower-priced one. Although Boston Scientific changed positions with Johnson & Johnson as the premium-priced brand, it maintained the leading market share.

The price cut was a competitive move made by Johnson & Johnson after it had struggled with manufacturing and supply problems. Cardiologist Joe Kozina at Mercy General Hospital in Sacramento said that he was offered the lower-priced Cypher stent, but continued to use the Taxus because he finds it is easier to place in blood vessels. "Pricing makes no difference if I can't get the stent into the patient," Kozina said.

Other physicians who experience fewer clinical differences are more price sensitive; they see Boston Scientific following the market and lowering its prices.

Source: Kerber, R., "Price Fight Is Looming Over Stents," *Boston Globe*, Jan. 31, 2005.

OVERVIEW: UNDERSTANDING PRICING

Every nonprofit and for-profit health care organization sets prices on its services and products. The concept of price is the same whether it is termed a co-payment (for a doctor's visit or pharmaceutical purchase), a deductible (for a hospital admission), a per diem (a hospital price to an insurer), tuition (for medical school education), or a room-and-board fee (for a nursing home stay).

Price is the single marketing element that results in revenue; the others all result in costs. Price is also more easily and quickly changed than product features, channel structure, and promotional strategies and tactics. Price can also communicate to the market the company's value and positioning of its product or brand. A well-designed and marketed product can command a price premium and reap big profits for its products—as some of the leading drug companies have found. Many marketers, however, neglect their pricing strategies—one survey found that managers spent less than 10 percent of their time on pricing.[1] As Johnson & Johnson realized in the opening example, pricing decisions and repercussions are very complex—especially in the rapidly changing health care environment. Health care marketers need to remember that a price decision will impact the organization and its marketing strategy, target markets, and brand positionings. It will also affect its customers and competitors as well as the marketing environment.

Because of the presence of health insurance, until recently consumers have been shielded from price concerns. However, consumers are now more engaged in price-seeking due to their increased out-of-pocket expenses. Further, new software applications are allowing buyers to compare prices instantaneously through on-line robotic shoppers or "shopbots." For example, the relatively high price of pharmaceuticals has encouraged consumers to use the Web to shop for drugs sold in the United States and internationally. At the same time, computer technology makes it easier for *sellers* to use software that monitors customers' movements over the Web and allows them to customize offers and prices.

Current Issues

The public often views pricing in the health care sector as inconsistent and mysterious. For example, consumers often ask, Why is it that one pill costs pennies and another that apparently does the same thing costs a hundred times as much? Service prices also can vary widely, as the examples in Field Note 11.1 illustrate. This problem is often compounded by providers who are unsure of their charges. For example, the California HealthCare Foundation hired a mystery-shopping firm to send mock low-income patients to sixty-four hospitals to get prices on different procedures. They didn't succeed; the hospitals were not set up to put price tags on services.[2]

FIELD NOTE 11.1.

Prices Vary Enormously for the Same Medical Service Patrick Fontana received a $900 bill for the cost of diagnostic imaging after he twisted his left knee on the golf course. Because he had a high-deductible health plan, he was responsible for the whole bill. Because of this expense, he decided to forward the bill to a claims adjuster, My Medical Control, a web-based company that reviews bills from doctors and hospitals. A representative from My Medical Control contacted the imaging facility and succeeded in saving Patrick Fontana $200—less a 35 percent fee for collection. The varying reimbursement schedules negotiated between the nation's 850,000 providers and more than 6,000 health plans are not public, and even insurers do not know what other health plans are paying.

For example, the Wills Eye Hospital in Philadelphia estimates that a cornea transplant would cost $15,000, but the reimbursement rate negotiated by local insurers puts it closer to $4,700. The average national rate is estimated to be $3,900.

Source: Michael Mason, "Bargaining Down That CT Scan Is Suddenly Possible," *New York Times*, Feb. 27, 2007, p. D5.

The term *transparency* is applied to a situation in which prices are readily available to consumers *before* the service is rendered. As a result of price inconsistencies and lack of such transparency, local and state governments have become involved, particularly in how hospital pricing affects patients. For example, state attorneys general have sued hospitals for allegedly price gouging the poor and uninsured. Also, some thirty-two states now require that hospitals provide pricing information to the public on request. Some hospitals are providing this information themselves through their state associations. For instance, the Georgia Hospital Association runs a Web site that lists fees for common medical procedures at 141 acute care hospitals in that state.

Private insurance companies have also become involved in transparency issues. For example, Aetna has made available on-line the prices that it has negotiated with Cincinnati-area doctors for hundreds of medical procedures and tests.

Having described some of the public's concerns over health care costs, we now explore approaches that organizations can use to set their prices. When reading the sections that follow, keep in mind that pricing methods depend on a combination of who the *payer* is, what the *product* (or service) is, and the *location* where it is used. We will focus on three types of payers (consumers, government, and private parties) and discuss the pricing decisions that are important to each of them.

CONSUMER PAYERS

When insurance is *not* involved in payment, the pricing situation is relatively straightforward. In this case, the seller has more leeway to price the product using all the traditional tools of market analysis. Although we include the following pricing principles in this consumer section, many can be applied to pricing for other payers.

Consumer Psychology and Pricing

With respect to health care services and products, consumers have traditionally been *price takers;* that is, they accept prices at face value or as given. With the growth of consumer-directed health plans, whereby individuals are responsible for more out-of-pocket expenses, this situation is changing. Consumers are more actively processing price information in terms of their knowledge from prior purchases, formal communications (advertising, sales calls, and brochures), informal communications (friends, colleagues, or family members), and point-of-purchase or on-line resources.[3] To understand how consumers arrive at their perceptions of prices, we consider three key features—*reference prices, price-quality inferences*, and *price cues*.

Although consumers of many non–health care goods and services have a fairly good knowledge of price, surprisingly few can accurately recall specific prices of products or services.[4] To help themselves, they often employ a *reference price*, comparing a product's stated price to an internal reference price (pricing information from memory) or an external frame of reference (such as a posted "regular retail price").[5]

Sellers often attempt to manipulate reference prices. For example, a seller can situate its product among expensive products to imply that it belongs in the same class. Reference price thinking is also encouraged by setting a high suggested charge (indicating that the product was priced much higher originally) or pointing to a competitor's high price.[6] Clever marketers also try to frame the price to signal the best value possible. For example, a relatively more expensive item can be seen as less expensive by breaking the price down into smaller units; a $500 annual health club membership fee may be perceived as more expensive than one priced at "under $50 a month."[7] Because consumers price health care services relatively infrequently, reference pricing is less of a factor in that sector. Health care consumer products more often fall into this category.

Many consumers use price as an indicator of quality when other information is not available. *Price-quality inferences* are especially effective with ego-sensitive products for which consumers pay with disposable income. In the luxury markets, such products include perfumes, champagne, and expensive cars; health care examples primarily involve cosmetic products and procedures. When alternative information about quality is available, price may become a less significant indicator of quality. For example, health care consumers have a wide range of scales and ratings available for evaluating and selecting a high-quality hospital with a national reputation (see Field Note 11.2).

FIELD NOTE 11.2.

Using the Web to Price-Shop for Health Care Services   The average consumer has difficulty gauging the price of health care services. According to a 2006 Harris Interactive on-line consumer survey, sponsored by employee benefits provider Great-West Healthcare, respondents thought that the average price for a four-day hospital stay was $7,762. The actual cost was $20,000. The cost for a routine doctor's office visit was thought to be $95. The average price of a physician visit was, in reality, $200. The respondents estimated $680 for an emergency department visit, but the true cost was actually lower—$400.

Traditionally, consumers paid less attention to health care prices because their health plan negotiated prices with providers, leaving them with modest deductibles and coinsurance payments. Now many people are selecting consumer-directed health plans with much higher deductibles and somewhat lower monthly premiums. These plans require consumers to pay the first $1,000 to $10,000 in health care costs. As a result, patients are beginning to ask service providers for pricing information before they buy, and they are shopping for care to get the best price.

Here are several Web sites that offer consumers access and information on making the best buying decisions:

HealthGrades Inc. (www.healthgrades.com) is a health care ratings company that sells reports on the cost of fifty-five medical procedures. The costs are based on regional averages of payments made by health plans. Also available are physician reports that include the amount individual physicians are paid by Medicare for more than one-hundred types of procedures. Further, HealthGrades offers hospital ratings of twenty-eight procedures and diagnoses at more than 5,000 non-federal hospitals at no charge.

Humana Inc. has created a free Web site (www.familyhealthbudget.com) in partnership with the advocacy group Consumer Action. The site includes a family health budget planner and a variety of tools to help select the best health care plan. It also projects a family's annual health care spending.

WageWorks Inc. (www.wageworks.com) offers tax-advantaged spending accounts for health and dependent care. It also has a flexible spending account (FSA) calculator. Setting up a FSA allows employees to set aside a specified amount of money before taxes to pay for qualified medical expenses. The calculator assists consumers in estimating whether this type of account makes financial sense for them and how much cash they should add to their FSA.

eHealthInsurance (www.ehealthinsurance.com) is for individuals not covered by an employer health plan. This site includes a large selection of health plans for indviduals and shows a comparison of benefits and costs.

HealthDecisions.org offers benefits information on 1,300 health plans and thousands of health insurance agents and brokers by state.

Source: M. Singletary, "Before You Get Sick, Shop Around," *Washington Post*, Oct. 22, 2006, p. F1.

Consumer perceptions of products and services are also affected by *price cues*. Many sellers believe that prices should end in an odd number. Research has shown that consumers tend to process prices in a "left-to-right" manner rather than by rounding.[8] Price encoding in this fashion is important if there is a mental price break at the higher, rounded price. Another explanation for "9" endings is that they convey the notion of a discount or bargain.[9] The LASIK Vision Institute regularly runs newspaper ads with the headline "LASIK $499*." The asterisk explanation at the bottom of the ad details all of the rules related to this price, such as the following: Nidek laser only, price may increase based on type of treatment, price is per eye, and price is subject to change without notice. Prices that end with "0" and "5" are also commonly observed in the marketplace, as they are thought to be easier for consumers to process and retrieve from memory.[10]

Setting the Price

An organization must set a price when it develops a new product, introduces an existing product into a new distribution channel or geographical area, or enters bids on new contract work. For example, in 1989, Glaxo started marketing its drug Well-butrin (bupropion) to treat depression. By 1997 it had received FDA approval for bupropion as a treatment to help smoking cessation. To promote this new indication, Glaxo created a new name (Zyban), product appearance, and pricing structure.

In some markets, such as the auto industry, as many as eight *price points*, or price tiers, and levels can be found in the distribution channel. In this respect, health care is usually simpler, with manufacturer, wholesaler, and retailer levels constituting the usual pricing points.

To help an organization consider the many factors in setting its pricing policy, we describe a seven-step procedure: (1) selecting the pricing objective; (2) determining demand; (3) estimating costs; (4) analyzing competitors' costs, prices, and offers; (5) deciding whether to use price as a competitive strategy; (6) selecting a pricing method; and (7) selecting the final price.

Selecting the Pricing Objective. In deciding where it wants to position its market offering, a company can pursue any of five major objectives through its pricing: survival, maximum current profit, maximum market share, maximum market skim-ming, or product-quality leadership. A company's choice of objective is strategically important, because it usually cannot attain more than one objective simultaneously. For example, as mentioned previously, during the 1990s some managed care plans that pursued a maximum market strategy were surprised that maximum current profit did not follow.

Survival is a short-term objective that is appropriate for companies plagued with overcapacity, intense competition, or changing consumer wants. As long as prices cover variable costs and some fixed costs (discussed shortly), the company stays in business. Survival is obviously a short-run objective; in the long run, the firm must learn how to add value or face extinction.

To gain the *maximum current profit*, companies estimate the demand and costs associated with alternative prices, choosing the one that produces maximum current profit, cash flow, or rate of return on investment. In emphasizing *current* performance, the company may sacrifice *long-run* performance by underspending on brand building or ignoring competitors' long-run responses.

Organizations that choose the *maximum market share* objective believe that a higher sales volume will lead to lower unit costs and higher long-run profit. To obtain a high share, the organization will set a very low price. This tactic, called *marketing penetration pricing*, is appropriate when the market is highly price-sensitive and a low price stimulates market growth. Accumulated experience causes production and distribution costs to fall, and the lower price discourages competition. This practice should not be confused with illegal *predatory pricing*, whereby very large companies price below their production costs to drive small, more poorly financed firms out of business.

Companies unveiling a new technology favor setting high prices to maximize *market skimming;* that is, to gain as much revenue as possible in the short run. Pharmaceutical companies are frequent practitioners of market-skimming pricing, whereby prices start high and are slowly lowered over time when competitive offerings and generic substitutes become available. If the price is set too high, however, the product may fail to gain customers or may be excluded from formularies. Market skimming ideally makes sense when (1) a sufficient number of buyers have a high current demand, (2) the unit costs of producing a small volume are not so high that they cancel the advantage of charging what the traffic will bear, (3) the high initial price does not attract more competitors to the market, and (4) the high price communicates the image of a superior product.

Organizations that aim to be the *product quality leaders* in the market hope to produce "gold-standard quality" and charge premium prices.

Nonprofit and public organizations may adopt other pricing objectives. A hospital may try to set charges based on reference prices from a peer group, a cost-plus approach, or a price that will not stimulate public scrutiny. It may also price certain services at low or no cost to fulfill its charitable mission. A public health service agency may set a sliding scale with prices geared to client income levels.

Whatever the specific objective, companies that use price as a strategic tool will profit more than those that simply let prevalent market costs determine their pricing.

Determining Demand. Normally, demand and price are inversely related: the higher the price, the lower the demand. In the case of health care services and products, the quantity demanded does not always change with increased prices. We explain the reasons for this departure from classical economics in Chapter Four; you should recall that the role of third-party payers and the power of providers to induce demand are among the important reasons for this behavior. With the growth of high-deductible health plans and other increased out-of-pocket expenses, price *is* now beginning to have an increasing influence on consumer health care demand.

Price sensitivity. The first step in estimating demand is to understand what affects price sensitivity. Generally speaking, customers are most price-sensitive when products are very costly or bought frequently. The converse is also true: consumers are less price-sensitive to low-cost or infrequently purchased items. Further, they are also less price-sensitive when price is only a small part of the total charge to obtain, operate, and service the product over its lifetime. A seller can charge a higher price than competitors and still get the business if it can convince the customer that it offers the lowest *total cost of ownership* (TCO). Thus a pharmaceutical company can price its branded drug higher than its competitors' on the grounds that fewer pills are needed to treat a particular illness or its brand works much faster and therefore allows patients to return to their normal activity sooner.

Estimating demand. Organizations can use one of three methods to estimate customer demand. The first method is analyzing past data and their relationships to each other, such as prices, units sold, referrals, admissions, visits, and procedures. The second method is conducting field experiments to observe the effect of varying prices on the same products in different, but similar, markets. Even single-site organizations, such as individual hospitals and medical groups, may need to conduct such experiments. For example, an urgent care center could vary the prices of services offered and observe the effect on changes in volume. Organizations can also vary the prices of *similar* services and note any differences in volume. The third method is using prospective surveys to explore how likely consumers say they are to buy at different proposed prices.

The sensitivity of the volume change to alteration in price is called the *price elasticity of demand*. If demand change is minimal, with a small change in price, we say the demand is *inelastic*. Because of such factors as third-party insurance coverage, many health care products and services fit into this category. If demand changes with price, we say it is *elastic*. The greater the volume growth resulting from a price reduction, the larger is the positive price elasticity. (Conversely, if products sell more by *increasing* the price, we say elasticity is negative. Some luxury goods and services fit into this category.)

In addition to the price sensitivity factors just listed, demand is likely to be less elastic under the following conditions: (1) there are few or no substitutes or competitors, (2) buyers do not readily notice the higher price, (3) buyers are slow to change their buying habits, and (4) buyers think the higher prices are justified. An example of inelastic demand is the market for health care in a rural county with a single hospital; raising hospital prices may be economically feasible but politically difficult.

The elasticity may not be linear across a full range of prices. For example, consumers may not care about prices if they vary within a certain range; outside that range, behavior may change rapidly. The range of prices for which demand is inelastic is called the *price indifference band*, and firms obviously want to operate at the highest point in this range. The difficulty with employing this strategy in health care is that the price indifference band can be very difficult to estimate, because end-users share the effects of pricing changes with third-party payers. Specifically, third-party payers and patients may have different price elasticity behavior. For example, an insurance company may be very willing to pay the majority of the

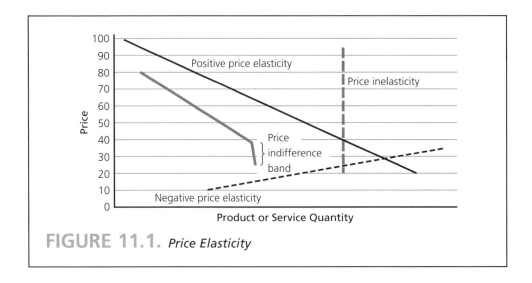

FIGURE 11.1. *Price Elasticity*

cost for a medication costing hundreds of dollars, but the patient may balk at filling a prescription with a $45 co-payment. As previously mentioned, with high-deductible health plans becoming more common, consumer sensitivity to price is increasing. These concepts are illustrated in Figure 11.1.

Finally, long-run price elasticity may differ from short-run elasticity. Consumers may initially continue to buy from a current supplier or provider after a price increase, but they may eventually switch after shopping for lower costs. In this case, demand is more elastic in the long run than in the short run. The reverse may also occur: consumers may drop a supplier after being notified of a price increase but return later when the competitor raises prices. This type of switching is common in the individual health insurance market when premium prices are raised annually. The distinction between short-run and long-run elasticity means that sellers will not know the total effect of a price change until time passes.

In measuring the price-demand relationship, the marketer must also control for various other factors that will influence results, such as competitive response by rivals, changes in prevalent economic conditions, changes in product characteristics, or changes in other marketing-mix factors besides price.

Estimating Costs. Demand sets a ceiling on the price the company can charge for its product or services, and costs set the floor: the organization needs to charge a price that covers its cost of producing, distributing, and selling the product, including a fair return for its effort and risk.

Types of cost and levels of production. A company's costs can be expressed in a number of ways. We can first differentiate between fixed and variable costs. *Fixed costs* are costs that do not vary with production or sales revenue, regardless of output and subject to capacity constraints. For example, to produce 100 units, the firm's fixed costs are constant. To produce units 101 to 200, the fixed costs may also be constant but at a higher level, reflecting additional investment in plant and equipment. *Variable costs* vary directly with the level of production. For example, in an emergency room, fixed costs are the heat, beds, computer system, and professional salaries. Variable costs are sutures, anesthetic, bandages, and medication. *Total costs* consist of the sum of the fixed and variable costs for any given level of volume. *Average cost* is equal to total costs divided by volume. Ideally, management will charge a price that exceeds average costs.

When no units are produced, the cost per unit is theoretically infinite. As more units are produced, the fixed costs are spread over more items and their contribution to each item becomes smaller and smaller. This decline is called an experience curve (or learning curve) and is the result of economies of scale or know-how or both. As production volume becomes very large, total cost approaches variable cost. This fact leads to two important management principles:

1. Whenever you have fixed costs, you cannot determine per unit costs without specifying a volume of output.

2. A firm cannot price below its variable cost and expect to stay in business for long.

See Figures 11.2 and 11.3 for graphic representations of these concepts.

Some firms do not realize the importance of these principles and price their products based on the *anticipated* costs that would result from large-volume production. Their idea is that low prices will drive higher sales, which in turn will enable the firm to lower costs by taking advantage of high-volume production. *Experience-curve pricing*, however, carries major risks: aggressive pricing may give the product a cheap image, competitors may lower *their* prices and cut into anticipated volume growth, and projected volumes may not be realized, with prices stuck at levels below what is financially sustainable.

Another, complementary way to view this issue is to consider the difference between direct and indirect costs. *Direct costs* can be traced to a service, organizational unit, or individual provider or manager. For example, in a consulting firm, salaries for associates assigned to work full-time for a partner are part of that partner's direct costs. In pharmaceutical manufacturing, the chemicals required to produce a discrete compound are the direct costs for that item. *Indirect costs* are all other types of costs and must be allocated to whatever or whoever produces revenue, such as services, products, organizational units, or individual providers or managers. For example, costs for a computer system must be allocated among the partners of a consulting firm. Administrative services (such as CEO salary) must be allocated among the different products of a pharmaceutical manufacturer. Figure 11.4 provides an example of how hospitals can allocate costs.

The allocation process can be straightforward, such as determining how many minutes of computer time each consulting partner's team uses. It can also be

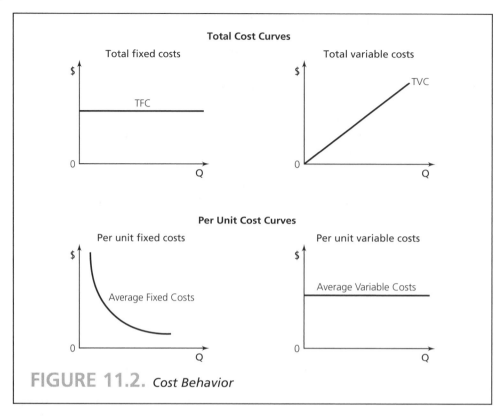

Total Cost Curves

Total fixed costs

Total variable costs

Per Unit Cost Curves

Per unit fixed costs

Per unit variable costs

FIGURE 11.2. *Cost Behavior*

Q = Number of units produced or volume of services provided.

complicated, such as distributing the cost of electricity. Some other examples of methods to allocate indirect costs to revenue centers include assignment by the percent of total company revenue the center generates, the portion of square feet a unit occupies, and the percentage of total full-time equivalents it employs. Because choosing the *method* of indirect cost allocation is a subjective process, it can be very contentious and can affect the marketing manager's ability to competitively price a product or service.

Health care marketers should also appreciate the special problems caused by the allocation method used by many hospitals in cost-based pricing. Since the start of the Medicare program in 1966, the federal government has required them to submit an annual cost report based on the expenses they incur in caring for this population. Because Medicare reimbursement was originally cost-based, hospitals used allocation methods that maximized their Medicare reimbursement; however, hospitals also used this report to price their services for private payers. Even though Medicare now pays hospitals on the basis of global payments (diagnosis related groups—DRGs), they

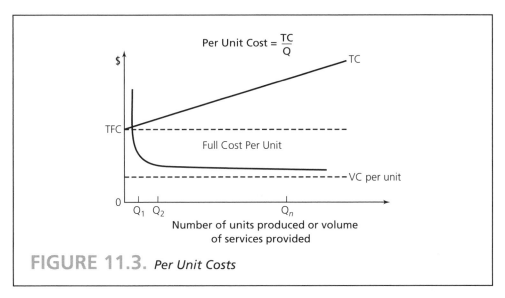

FIGURE 11.3. *Per Unit Costs*

Q = Number of units produced or volume of services provided.
TFC = Total fixed cost.
TC = Total cost.
VC = Variable cost.

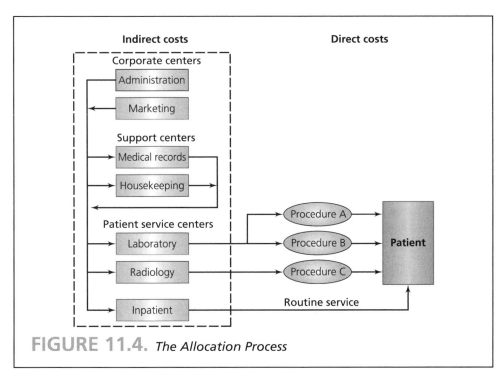

FIGURE 11.4. *The Allocation Process*

are still required to file this report, and many continue to use the same process to set prices for other payers. The problem with this pricing method is highlighted by the following example:

FOR EXAMPLE

Physicians employed by a hospital's psychiatric department experienced difficulty in competing on price with firms who specialized in delivering mental health benefits to managed care plans. The problem was that the hospital priced the department's services based on their Medicare cost report, which had little to do with the younger population the physicians were interested in treating. Similar problems result from hospital-based laboratories being unable to competitively price their services vis-à-vis national companies. The lesson is that marketing managers must understand the method of indirect cost allocation and its impact on product costs. Failure to argue for a more appropriate allocation of indirect costs can lead to product overpricing and market failure.

Activity-based cost accounting (ABC) is one method that attempts to make this assignment more fair and to more closely reflect the resources used in producing a revenue-generating product or service. Table 11.1 shows different methods that can be used to assign costs to various health care services in a hospital. (Explanations of the abbreviations are provided in the later section on government as a payer.)

An additional method in this category is *target costing*.[11] Market research is used to establish a new product's desired functions and its anticipated sales price. Deducting the desired profit margin from this price leaves the target cost that must be achieved. The objective is to deliver the product within the target cost range. If this goal is not possible, it may be necessary to stop development. Target costing is used by more sophisticated medical device manufacturers and rarely by health services providers.

An application of target costing is *cost-benefit analysis* and a special case, when applied to the pharmaceutical industry, is termed *pharmacoeconomic analysis*. Pharmacoeconomic analysis considers *total* disease costs, not just what is attributable to drug treatment. These costs include direct expenditures on such items as physician services, hospitalizations, diagnostic tests, and supplies. Unlike many other analyses, however, this method also includes collateral expenses, such as lost time from work and the economic cost of lost life (such as quality-adjusted life years, or QALYs). Pharmaceutical firms take these costs into consideration when pricing new therapeutic categories as well as competitively pricing new drugs against existing ones. Consider how cost-benefit analysis may be used in the following examples:

TABLE 11.1. Sample Activity Bases for Costing Techniques

Department	(Macro)	(Micro)
Operating room	Surgical case	Operating room minutes
Anesthesiology	Anesthesia case	Anesthesia case minutes
Postoperative rooms	Postoperative case	Post operating room minutes
Radiology	Exams	RVUs
Laboratory	Tests	RVUs
Physical therapy	Modalities	Treatment minutes
Isotopes	Treatments	RVUs
Blood bank	Transfusions	RVUs
Delivery room	Deliveries	Treatment minutes
Social service	Visits	Treatment hours or fractions of hours
Emergency room	Visits	Treatment minutes
Routine service	Patient days	Hours of care
Physician service	Charges	RBRVS
Ambulatory care	Visits; APCs	RVUs
Per procedure or per case	DRGs	Intensity of care or acuity levels

- An inexpensive drug used to treat high cholesterol requires frequent doctor visits and blood tests to prevent potential side effects.

- An inexpensive drug for treating high blood pressure often requires the addition of another medication to adequately treat this condition.

- An expensive diagnostic test has good predictive value for colon cancer and reduces the need for many colonoscopies without increasing the error rate for missed lesions.

- Merck sells a vaccine (Varivax) to prevent childhood chickenpox. The condition is usually not more than an annoyance for the patient, but causes many days of lost work for parents who must stay home with their children. The approval of the vaccine and its pricing were based on this socioeconomic cost rather than the cost or morbidity of the disease itself.

Analyzing Competitors' Costs, Prices, and Offers. Within the range of possible prices determined by market demand and company costs, the firm must take competitors' costs, prices, and possible price reactions into account. In conducting this analysis, the firm should especially consider the distinct features its product offers and whether they are valued by customers who are willing to pay extra. (The converse is also true; that is, the firm can charge less than a competitor if the other company's product includes features that do not add value.) Pharmaceutical companies often use this method when they introduce second-to-market products in a particular therapeutic category. Managed care plans also used this technique when they priced their plans just below those of traditional indemnity products. The practice of adjusting prices to keep them just under those of the competition is called *shadow pricing*.

Deciding Whether to Use Price as a Competitive Strategy. Given that sales of many goods and services *are* sensitive to price reductions, firms can cautiously use competitive pricing as a marketing strategy. For a full discussion of this issue, please see the internal rivalry section in Chapter Five.

Selecting a Pricing Method. The company can use these three Cs to price products: the *customers'* demand schedule, the *cost* function, and *competitors'* prices. To summarize three steps from the preceding discussion: (1) costs set a floor to the price, (2) competitors' prices and the price of substitutes provide an orienting point, and (3) customers' value assessment of unique features establishes the price ceiling. Companies select a pricing method that includes one or more of these three considerations.

We will examine four price-setting methods: markup pricing, target-return pricing, value pricing, and going-rate pricing. Although these techniques are often used by manufacturers of health care products, other health care sectors can also employ them.

Markup pricing. The most elementary pricing method is to add a standard *markup* to the product's cost, either a fixed amount or a percentage. However, any pricing method that ignores current demand, perceived value, and competition is not likely to lead to the optimal price for its producer. Further, the method works only if the marked-up price accurately predicts sales volume. (Recall that you must know sales volume to determine the per-unit allocation of fixed and indirect costs.) However, markup pricing continues to remain popular for at least three reasons. First, sellers can estimate production costs much more easily than demand. Second, when all firms in the industry use this pricing method, prices tend to be similar if their costs are similar. Price competition is therefore minimized. Third, many people believe that cost-plus pricing is fairer to both buyers and sellers. Sellers do not take advantage of buyers when the latter's demand increases and sellers earn a fair return on investment.

Target-return pricing. In target-return pricing, the firm determines the price that would yield its target rate of return on investment (ROI). (This method is also used by public utilities, which also need to make a fair return on investment.) In employing this method, the manufacturer must consider different prices and estimate their probable impacts on sales volume and profits.

Value pricing. An increasing number of companies base their price on the *customer's perceived value* of their product or service. We define *value* as either the lowest price for a desired product quality or the best product quality, given the price the customer is willing to pay. To communicate value and enhance its perception, firms use advertising and sales force methods along with other marketing-mix elements.

Perceived value is made up of such factors as the buyer's image of the product performance, the channel deliverables, warranty quality, customer support, and the company's reputation and trustworthiness. Each customer segment places a different priority on these different elements. Some will be *quality buyers* (our first value definition), others will be *price buyers* (our second value definition), and still others will be *loyal brand buyers*. Companies need different marketing strategies for each of these three groups. For quality buyers, companies must keep innovating, guided by active and frequent market research that tracks customer preference changes. For price buyers, companies need to offer basic products with reduced services. For loyal brand buyers, companies must invest in relationship building and customer intimacy.

These principles can be applied, for example, in the pharmaceutical industry. Because consumers regard pharmaceuticals in the same therapeutic class as equally efficacious, branded drugs that go "off patent" often fail to support their perceived value in comparison to generic equivalents. One approach to supporting brand-name pharmaceuticals is to draw on customer trust and familiarity with the company, the brand name, or both by producing "branded generic" or "branded over-the-counter" products. For instance, in the heartburn market, Tagamet and Zantac successfully used their brand identities when generic competitors appeared and this class of medication became available over the counter.

Going-rate pricing. In going-rate pricing, the organization bases its price largely on competitors' prices. When costs are difficult to measure or competitive response is uncertain, firms feel that the going price is a good solution because it is thought to reflect the industry's collective wisdom. This tactic is particularly used for "second-to-market" products for innovative technologies. For example, when Merck launched its offering (the now-withdrawn Vioxx) into the new category of Cox-2 inhibitors that treat arthritis, the pricing decision was framed by the first entrant, Celebrex. One cautionary note: price collusion is illegal, and the Federal Trade Commission and other governmental bodies closely scrutinize such deals as those between hospitals and physician practices as well as among product companies.

Selecting the Final Price. The methods described in the first six steps narrow the range from which an organization must select a price. In making its final decision, however, the firm must consider additional factors, including the impact of other marketing activities, overall organizational pricing policies, gain- and risk-sharing pricing, public perceptions, and the impact of price on other parties.

The influence of other marketing activities. The final price must take into account the brand's quality, positioning, and promotion relative to the competition. In a classic study, Farris and Reibstein examined the relationships among relative price, relative quality, and relative advertising for 227 consumer businesses, and found the following:

- Brands with average relative quality but high relative advertising budgets were able to charge premium prices. Consumers apparently were willing to pay higher prices for known products than for unknown products. This finding suggests a higher degree of trust with a familiar offering than with an unknown offering.

- Brands with high relative quality and high relative advertising obtained the highest prices. Conversely, brands with low quality and low advertising charged the lowest prices.

- The positive relationship between high prices and high advertising held most strongly in the later stages of the product life cycle for market leaders.[12]

These findings are especially important to the pharmaceutical industry, in which direct-to-consumer (DTC) advertising can strongly influence patient demand for a particular medication. For example, consider AstraZeneca's "Purple Pill" campaign for the premium-priced Nexium (used for heartburn, reflux, and peptic ulcer disease).

Organization pricing policies. A product pricing decision must involve internal as well as external environmental constraints. Many companies have internal policies that set price ranges or methods of relative pricing for their portfolio of products and services. For example, the maker of premium-quality wheelchairs would be reluctant to price one of its products significantly below others in its line; customers might wonder about its quality or, if they accept the quality, might then believe that the rest of the offerings are overpriced. Pricing policy is also important to allow salespeople a range in which they can negotiate with their customers.

Gain- and risk-sharing pricing. Buyers may resist accepting a seller's proposal because of a high perceived level of risk. In this case, the seller may offer to absorb part or all of the risk if the product does not deliver the full promised value. A pioneering example occurred in the 1990s when Baxter Healthcare, a medical products firm, proposed an information management system that would save a large hospital chain millions of dollars over eight years. When the chain hesitated, Baxter offered to guarantee the savings. If the savings turned out to be greater than promised, however, Baxter would also share some of the gain. This offer of mutual risk-sharing was accepted, and Baxter got the order. Pharmaceutical Benefit Management (PBM) companies may have similar arrangements with managed care companies with respect to pharmaceutical cost management.

Impact of price on other parties. Management must also consider the reactions of other stakeholders to the contemplated price.[13] For example, if distributors, dealers, and sales personnel believe they cannot make enough money with a given price, they may choose not to promote that particular product with potential clients. Companies must also ask these other pricing questions: How will competitors react? Will suppliers raise their prices when they see the company's price? Will the government intervene and prevent this price from being charged? How will public interest groups react to the high cost of a new product category, such as some biologicals?

Marketers also need to know the laws regulating pricing. Many federal and state statutes protect consumers against deceptive pricing practices. For example, it is illegal for a company to set artificially high "regular" prices and then announce a "sale" at prices close to previous everyday prices.

Adapting the Price

Companies usually do not set a single price, but rather develop a pricing structure that reflects variations in geographical demand and costs, market-segment requirements, purchase timing, order levels, delivery frequency, guarantees, service contracts, and other factors. As a result of discounts, allowances, and promotional support, a company rarely realizes the same profit from each unit of a product that it sells. Even service businesses may have different prices for different payers. For example, medical groups negotiate different fees with different insurance companies for the same services. We will now examine several price-adaptation strategies: geographical pricing, price discounts and allowances, promotional pricing, and differentiated pricing.

Geographical Pricing. In geographical pricing, the organization decides how much to charge different customers in different locations. Because services are usually consumed where they are delivered, this consideration applies primarily to products. A common example is the different prices for over-the-counter medications, which can vary by neighborhood. It can also apply to international pharmaceutical prices. Pharmaceutical companies traditionally sell the same drugs for higher prices in northern Europe than in Southern Europe, reflecting income differences. Unfortunately for these companies, this disparity has led to gray markets: Southern European wholesalers order extra quantities and sell them to wholesalers in Northern Europe, thus making an additional profit.

Price Discounts and Allowances. Most companies will adjust their list price and give discounts and allowances for early payment, volume purchases, and off-season buying.[14] Companies must proceed carefully, however, or they may find that their profits are much less than planned.[15] Sales management needs to monitor the proportion of customers who are receiving discounts, the average discount, and particular salespeople who are overrelying on discounting. Higher levels of management should conduct a *net price analysis* to arrive at the "real price" of their offering.

A word of caution on this practice comes from Kevin Clancy, chairman of Copernicus, a major marketing research and consulting firm. He found that only between 15 and 35 percent of buyers in most categories are price-sensitive. Because people with higher incomes and higher product involvement are more willing to pay for special features, enhanced customer service, added quality, more convenience, and the brand name, it can be a mistake for a strong, distinctive brand to plunge into price discounting to respond to low-price attacks.[16]

Discounting can be a useful tool if the company can gain value in return, such as when the customer agrees to sign a three-year contract, or is willing to order electronically (thus saving the company billing and collection expenses), or purchases in large quantities. If discounting without an offsetting benefit to the company becomes a routine tactic used to close business, the real price becomes highly subjective and affects the perception of product value and hence the company's reputation.

A further important consideration is required when pricing for government contracts, particularly for pharmaceuticals. To give lowest prices to programs such as Medicaid and the Veterans Health Administration, companies must track *net* prices to *all* customers; that is, factoring in volume discounts and rebates. Further, because Part B of Medicare pays providers based on *average* sales price, sellers must be able to calculate this amount for each product—again, net of volume discounts and rebates.

Promotional Pricing. Companies can use a number of pricing techniques to stimulate early purchase:

- *Loss-leader pricing:* Hospitals often cannot price their obstetrical services high enough to cover their expenses. Because women are the primary decision makers for the family's health care choices, investment in these services can help stimulate future hospital use when the need arises.

- *Special-event pricing:* Sellers will establish special prices to attract customers for special occasions, such as opening a new store, launching a new product line, or celebrating some other special event.

- *Seasonal discounts:* As is the case for many retail businesses, health care revenue cycles can be cyclical. To smooth demand, some firms offer special pricing during predictable downturns. For example, cosmetic dermatology services are often promoted in the spring and summer months.

- *Cash rebates:* Health care product companies offer cash rebates to encourage purchase of the manufacturer's products within a specified time period. Blood

glucose monitoring machines are one example of such a product. A more immediate type of rebate is a cash discount at the point of purchase; for example,
coupons that patients can use when they fill a physician's prescription at the
pharmacy.

- *Low-interest financing:*   Instead of cutting its price, the company can offer customers low-interest financing. This technique is particularly attractive for health
care information technology firms, because they price annual service contracts
based on a percentage of the system's sales price.

- *Longer payment terms:*   This tactic is used particularly by medical device and
pharmaceutical companies, which stretch loans over longer periods and thus
lower the monthly payments.

- *Warranties and service contracts:*   Companies can promote sales by adding a
free, low-cost, or extended warranty or service contract.

- *Psychological discounting:*   This strategy involves setting an artificially high
price and then offering the product at substantial savings. As mentioned earlier,
such tactics are investigated by the Federal Trade Commission and other organizations, such as Better Business Bureaus. However, discounts from normal
prices are a legitimate form of promotional pricing.

Promotional-pricing strategies should be used cautiously, because they are often a
zero-sum game. If they work, competitors copy them and they lose their effectiveness.
If they do not work, they waste money that could have been put into other marketing
tools, such as building up product quality and service or strengthening product image
through advertising.

Differentiated Pricing.   Companies often adjust their basic price to accommodate
differences in customers, products, and locations. *Price discrimination* occurs when
a company sells a product or service at two or more prices that do not reflect
a proportional difference in costs. In *first-degree price discrimination*, the seller
charges a separate price to each customer depending on the intensity of his or her
demand. In *second-degree price discrimination*, the seller charges less to buyers who
buy a larger volume. In *third-degree price discrimination*, the seller charges different
amounts to different classes of buyers, as in the following cases:

- *Customer-segment pricing:*   Different customer groups are charged different
prices for the same product or service. For instance, health plans often charge a
lower premium for students and a higher premium for senior citizens based on
their expected use of health care services. Another example is the pharmaceutical
companies that have agreed to price HIV-AIDS drugs at substantially lower
prices (sometimes zero) in poor African countries.

- *Product-form pricing:*   Different versions of the product are priced differently,
but not proportionately to their respective costs. A pharmaceutical company may
charge $75 for a thirty-day supply of a drug in a 5 mg dosage, whereas the 10 mg

dose will cost $110. (Some pharmaceutical companies *do* charge proportionately the same for different doses to avoid patients buying the larger sized pill and breaking it in half.)

■ *Image pricing:* Some organizations price the same product at two different levels based on different images held by different buyers. Consider the following example:

> In July [2000], Lilly got Food and Drug Administration approval to market Prozac under the new name Sarafem. The company is packaging the drug in pretty pink-and-lavender capsules, exclusively for women, most in their late twenties or early thirties. Says Laura Miller, a spokesperson for Lilly, "Women told us they wanted treatment that would differentiate PMDD [premenstrual dysphoric disorder] from depression."[17]

■ *Channel pricing:* Pricing for the same item can be different depending on the distribution channel. For instance, a ninety-day supply of medication is usually cheaper if purchased from a mail-order pharmacy than from the local drug store. Another example is "Doctors on Call." This firm contracts with local physicians to make house calls and charges prices that are considerably higher than traditionally charged when patients come to the physician's office.

■ *Location pricing:* The same product is priced differently at different locations even though the cost of offering at each location is the same. A tertiary care hospital that offers cosmetic surgery services in its urban facilities in Los Angeles may charge a higher price for the same procedures offered by its satellite facility in the resort town of Palm Springs. An international example is drug pricing differences in different countries, which can reflect regulatory or purchase price parity considerations.

■ *Time pricing:* Prices are varied by time of year or day of week. For example, if pharmacy traffic is slower midweek, it may offer discount prices on Wednesdays.

As mentioned earlier, although price discrimination is legal, predatory pricing—selling below cost with the intention of destroying competition—is unlawful.[18] Even if legal, some differentiated pricing may meet with a hostile reaction.

For price discrimination to work, certain conditions must exist. First, the market must be segmentable and the segments must show different intensities of demand. Second, members in the lower-price segment must not be able to resell the product to the higher-price segment. Again, this situation has been extremely problematic for the pharmaceutical industry; wholesalers in southern Europe sell their cheaper drugs to retail outlets in the north, where prices are higher. (This practice is legal in the European Union.) Third, competitors must not be able to undersell the firm in the higher-price segment. Fourth, the cost of segmenting and policing the market must not exceed the extra revenue derived from price discrimination. Fifth, the practice must not breed customer resentment and ill will. Finally, the particular form of price discrimination must not be illegal.[19]

Initiating and Responding to Price Changes

Organizations often face situations in which they need to change prices. We have discussed price cutting strategies; here we focus on price increases.

Initiating Price Increases. Other than the simple desire to increase profits, many organizations increase prices to *maintain* profits when they encounter cost inflation. To avoid customer antagonism, companies try to increase prices as few times as possible; however, in expectation of rising costs, they often raise their prices by *more* than they expect in the short run. This practice is called *anticipatory pricing*. A difficult task for marketers is deciding whether to raise a price sharply on a one-time basis or to raise it by small amounts over several periods. Generally, consumers prefer small price increases on a regular basis to sudden sharp increases.

Another factor causing price increases is *overdemand*. When a company cannot supply all of its customers, it can use one of the following techniques:

- *Delayed quotation pricing:* The company does not set a final price until the product is finished or delivered. This pricing is prevalent in industries with long production lead times. It is also used in economies that are experiencing rapid inflation.

- *Escalator clauses:* The company requires the customer to pay today's price and all or part of any inflation increase that takes place before delivery. An escalator clause bases price increases on some specified price index. Escalator clauses are found in contracts for major industrial projects like construction. It is also standard in property rent agreements.

- *Unbundling:* The company maintains its price but removes or prices separately one or more elements that were part of the former offer, such as free delivery or installation.

- *Reduction of discounts:* The company instructs its sales force not to offer its normal cash and quantity discounts.

- *Reduction of size:* The amount delivered to the customer is reduced, although the price remains the same. For example, the number of pills in a bottle of over-the-counter medication may be reduced while the package sells for the same price.

Reactions to Price Changes. Any price change can provoke a response from customers, competitors, distributors, suppliers, and even the government. Customers often question the motivation behind price changes[20] and can interpret them in different ways. In the case of a price reduction, they may think the item is about to be replaced by a new model, the item is faulty and is not selling well, the firm is in financial trouble, the price will come down even further, or the quality has been reduced. Conversely, a price increase, which would normally deter sales, may carry some positive meanings to customers, such as that the item is "hot" and represents an unusually good value.

Competitors are most likely to react to a price change when few firms offer the product, the product is homogeneous, and buyers are highly informed. In markets characterized by high product homogeneity, firms search for ways to augment value-added aspects of the product; if there truly are none, it will have to meet the price reduction. If one company raises its price in a homogeneous product market, other firms may not match it unless the increase will benefit the industry as a whole. Then the leader will have to roll back the increase.

In nonhomogeneous product markets, a firm has more latitude in its response. Companies can ask: Why did the competitor change the price? Was it to steal the market, to use excess capacity, to meet changing cost conditions, or to lead an industry-wide price change? Does the competitor plan to make the price change temporary or permanent? What will happen to our company's market share and profits if we do *not* respond? Are other companies going to respond? What are the competitor's and other firms' responses to each possible reaction likely to be?

Consider the following example of how premium pricing can succeed:

FOR EXAMPLE

In 1981, Glaxo (now GlaxoSmithKline) introduced its ulcer medication Zantac to attack Tagamet, the first ulcer treatment drug in its class. The conventional wisdom was that, as the "second one in," Glaxo should price Zantac 10 percent below Tagamet. CEO Paul Girolam knew that Zantac was superior to Tagamet in terms of fewer drug interactions and side effects and more convenient dosing. Glaxo introduced Zantac at a significant price premium over Tagamet and still gained the market-leader position.[21] By 1988 it was the world's best-selling prescription medication.

How can a firm anticipate a competitor's reactions? The company needs to research the competitor's current financial situation, recent sales, customer loyalty, and corporate objectives. For instance, if the competitor has a market-share objective, it is likely to match the price change.[22] On the other hand, if it has a profit-maximization objective, it may react by increasing the advertising budget or improving product quality.

Market leaders also frequently face aggressive price cutting by newer or smaller firms trying to build market share. The market leader can respond in several ways:

- *Maintain price and profit margin:* The leader can maintain its price and profit margin, believing that (1) it will lose too much profit if it reduced its price, (2) it will not lose much market share to the competitor, and (3) it could regain market share when necessary.

- *Maintain price and add value:* The leader can improve its product, services, or communications. The firm may find it cheaper to maintain price and spend money to improve perceived quality rather than cut price and operate at a lower margin. It can also draw on brand loyalty.

- *Reduce price:* The leader can lower its price to match the competitor's price. This strategy may be attractive if the firm needs to maintain a certain production volume to hold down its costs and also if it anticipates difficulty in regaining market share once it is lost.

- *Increase price and add brands:* The leader can raise its price and introduce new brands to bracket the attacking brand.

- *Launch a low-price line:* The leader can add lower-priced items to the line or create a separate, lower-priced brand.

The best response, of course, varies with the situation. The company has to consider the product's stage in the life cycle, its importance in the organization's portfolio, the competitor's intentions and resources, the market's price and quality sensitivity, the behavior of costs with volume, and the company's alternative opportunities. Because there may not be time for an extended analysis of alternatives when the attack occurs, the company should anticipate competitors' possible price changes and prepare contingent responses in advance.

GOVERNMENT PAYERS

When government becomes the payer, buyer power is introduced; that is, sellers who want to care for or provide products for patients covered by these plans must accept the amounts and payment methods the government sets. Because the Medicare program is a pervasive force, we will focus on that payer. The U.S. Congress sets the methods of payment and how rates will be increased (or decreased) over time, and the Centers for Medicare and Medicaid Services (CMS), a part of the Department of Health and Human Services, administers the pricing schemes. Prices are set based on what was done, what was given, and why; that is, by *procedure*, *product*, and *diagnosis*. To enable all parties to compare episodes of care, set prices, and expedite payment, a series of standardized codes has been developed by a variety of organizations. These codes are especially important because private payers also use them to set prices and make payments. The three most common coding systems are as follows:

- *Current Procedural Terminology 4th Edition* (CPT-4). This system (copyrighted by the American Medical Association) lists procedures, usually with a five-digit code. For example, a routine office visit is 99213, a chest X-ray (front and side views) is 71020, and total hip replacement is 27130. This coding scheme has been developed for U.S. use; other countries use their own methods.

- *Healthcare Common Procedural Coding System* (HCPCS). CMS issues and updates these codes annually. They include health care products (such as injectable pharmaceuticals, durable equipment and disposable medical supplies) as well as procedures and professional services (such as dentistry and temporary medical service codes). These codes are in the form of a letter followed by four digits. Examples include E0776 (IV pole), Q4005 (plaster for a long arm adult cast) and J0290 (injection of 500 mg ampicillin).

- *International Classification of Disease* (ICD). The World Health Organization develops this disease listing system, which countries may modify. The newest version is ICD-10, which came into use after 1994. The U.S. and a few other countries, however, still use a version called ICD-9CM (the "CM" stands for clinical modification). The U.S. conversion to ICD-10 is expected about 2012. Most ICD-9CM codes are three digits, followed by up to two more digits after a decimal point. For example, mildly elevated blood pressure (benign essential hypertension) is 401.1. (As an illustration of how different ICD-10 is, the same diagnosis would be designated I10).

These coding systems are used as the building blocks for other types of payment classifications. For example, physicians are paid for their services based on a Resource Based Relative Value Scale (RBRVS), a fee schedule that uses the CPT-4 coding system. Hospitals are paid on a diagnosis related group (DRG) scheme that relies on ICD-9CM codes. In addition to DRGs, the federal government sets many other fees according to a variety of prospective payment systems. The systems of payment that Medicare employs are briefly explained in Table 11.2. It is important for the health care marketers to understand these different reimbursement methods, because this will affect not only *their* companies' payments, but how their customers get paid for using these products and services. For example, Medicare will not pay a hospital extra for using a more expensive antibiotic to treat a pneumonia patient; with few exceptions, the DRG payment is a flat amount regardless of the number or costs of services or products delivered. For the hospital customer, therefore, the price needs to reflect some other aspect of value: either the product is superior to all others available (and is, thus, a standard of care) or it is clinically equivalent but saves the hospital money on some other dimension of care, such as a shorter stay or fewer tests.

Several additional considerations arise for pharmaceutical companies who price their products outside the United States. First, unlike the United States, most other countries consider drug prices when they decide whether to approve a drug for sale. (In the United States, *only* safety and efficacy are criteria.) This consideration is independent of the government's responsibility to pay for medications. The method these countries use to determine the price often depends on a comparison to prices for the same product (or therapeutic category) in other selected nations. The allowed price can be an average of those in the other countries or pegged to the lowest price in any of them. This process is often called *reference* (or *index*) *pricing*. In

TABLE 11.2. Medicare Payment Methods

Place of Service	Payment Method
Inpatient hospital	International Classification of Disease (ICD)-9 CM coding that determines a diagnosis related group (DRG). Global amount paid per hospital stay.
Outpatient hospital	Ambulatory Payment Category (APC)-Outpatient Prospective Payment System (OPPS) based on Current Procedural Terminology (CPT)-4 and Healthcare Common Procedural Coding System (HCPCS). Global amount paid per type of care, for example, emergency room visit or chemotherapy visit. May have more than one APC per encounter.
Ambulatory surgicenter (not hospital affiliated)	Nine payment categories. After 2008, new rates will be phased in linked to the APC methodology.
Skilled nursing facility	Resource Utilization Group (RUG-III)-Health Insurance Prospective Payment Systems (HIPPS). Pays on per diem basis.
Physician office*	CPT-4 or HCPCS codes that determine Resource Based Relative Value Scale (RBRVS) per service payment. For administration of medications, such as chemotherapy, reimbursement is based on Average Sales Price (ASP) plus 6 percent.
Pharmacies	Contracted rates with either a Medicare Managed Care Organization (under Part C) or Part D payer. Medicare beneficiaries who do not sign up for Part C or D pay out-of-pocket charges.
Hospice	Daily rates (per diems) based on level of service: routine home care, continuous attendance at home, inpatient respite care, and general inpatient care (for palliative treatment).
Home health care	Outcome and Assessment Information Set (OASIS)-Home Health Resource Groups (HHRG). Pays global amount for each sixty-day episode of care (adjusted downward for increments less than sixty days).

Notes: *CPT-4-based fees also apply to physician services in all other settings. This table expands the information in Table 3.1; we offer it again here for emphasis of these concepts.

this sense, the term has the same meaning as we described for consumer use. For example, in Canada, the Patented Medicines Prices Review Board determines if the prices the pharmaceutical companies want to charge are "excessive" by comparing the proposed price for medicines still on patent with the averages in France, Germany, Italy, Sweden, Switzerland, Great Britain, and the United States; it is then up to provincial health plans to negotiate with the drug companies.

Another example is when government sets overall cost targets and can demand variable pricing. In Australia, the government negotiates prices with pharmaceutical companies based on anticipated use. If the actual volume exceeds targets, the prices are lowered.

PRIVATE PAYERS

Before the company offers a new product, its actuaries estimate frequency of utilization for a variety of health care services for the target population. This service cost estimate is equivalent in the product sector to the "cost of goods sold." When the plan is on the market, managers will have actual cost data for this utilization—termed the *medical expense ratio*. This item should account for about 80 to 85 percent of the premiums that such firms charge. Managers must also estimate sales, general, and administrative (SG&A) expenses. These items usually make up about 10 to 15 percent of premiums. (The profit margin for these plans is usually 3 to 5 percent.)

As mentioned previously, the presence of health insurance adds complexity to health care pricing considerations. Because in this case *both* the insurance company and insured individuals or families are customers for health care services and products, the health care marketer must understand each party's payment responsibility and price accordingly. For example, we cited earlier the case in which an insurance company may be willing to pay for its portion of the cost of medications, yet patients do not fill or refill medications if they feel the cost is too high.[23] To understand how much the *consumer* is responsible for paying for health care, we define four terms:

- *Premium.* The amount the consumer pays to purchase an insurance product. A *certificate of insurance* specifies what it covers and how much of the expense that plan will pay. The rest is the consumer's responsibility.

- *Deductible.* The amount the consumer pays before the insurance starts to cover charges.

- *Coinsurance.* A *percent* of charges the patient pays; the remainder is the responsibility of the insurance company.

- *Co-payment.* The amount the consumer patient pays at *each* encounter, whether it is for receiving a service or buying a product (such as medication).

Two examples of how these terms are applied follow. When health insurance is responsible for *any* of the benefits, *all* of these terms should be used to determine the *total* consumer cost for a product or service. For example, Medicare has a Web site (www.medicare.gov) that will help its members select a private drug plan. After the user enters the member's medications, the search function combines premium, co-payment, and deductible expenses to rank the area plans according to total annual cost.

EXAMPLE OF THE APPLICATION OF OUT-OF-POCKET EXPENSES TO PAYMENT OF HEALTH CARE CHARGES

Your health plan covers "medically necessary" services and pharmaceuticals. The services are subject to an annual (calendar year) deductible of $200, 80/20 coinsurance (your insurance pays 80 percent and you pay 20 percent), $25 physician office visit co-payment (which does not count toward deductible, coinsurance, or out-of-pocket annual maximum payment), and a maximum out-of-pocket payment (after the deductible is met) of $1,000 per calendar year. (Pharmaceutical benefits are handled separately; these are addressed in the second example.) Hospital charges are covered in full.

You see a physician at the beginning of the year and are charged $150. It is an acceptable amount, according to a fee schedule upon which she and your insurance company have agreed. How much do you pay? First, you have a $25 office co-payment. Then, you determine whether you have satisfied your annual deductible. Because it is the beginning of a new year and your deductible is $200, you are responsible for the entire bill.

Unfortunately, your physician finds a problem that requires a return visit four weeks later. After that visit you have an allowable charge of $100. How much do you owe for that visit? Again, start with the $25 co-payment. Because you satisfied $150 of your $200 deductible during your last visit, you owe an additional $50. Now that you have reached your deductible limit, your coinsurance starts to apply. Of the remaining $50 of your bill, you pay 20 percent, or $10, and the insurance company pays the remaining $40.

Your doctor now tells you that you need surgery to correct the problem she found during the first visit. You have the surgery and review the physicians' charges (the only part of the bill for which you are responsible). Because the surgery was performed in the hospital, there is no office co-payment. The deductibles and coinsurance do, however, apply. The total of all physicians' charges (surgeon, anesthesiologist, pathologist, and radiologist) is $5,500. Because you have already satisfied your deductible, you are responsible for 20 percent of the $5,500 ($1,100). But you are only at risk for the first $1,000 of out-of-pocket expenses after your deductible is met. You already paid $10 for coinsurance at the last office visit. So you would pay $990. For the remainder, you pay only office co-payments, as you have met your annual out-of-pocket maximum.

Note: This example illustrates how out-of-pocket provisions *may* operate. Plans have diverse provisions. For example, the expenditures that apply to annual limits may be different, and co-payments are frequently not the same for all types of services.

EXAMPLE OF THE APPLICATION OF OUT-OF-POCKET EXPENSES TO PAYMENT FOR PHARMACEUTICALS

Your insurance plan covers pharmaceuticals that you can take by yourself (self-administered medications, like pills, and simple injections, like insulin). To hold down costs, the insurance company has contracted with an independent company (pharmaceutical benefit management company, or PBM) to administer these benefits. The PBM classifies the medications into three categories (or tiers) and assigns different co-payments to their purchase, depending on how much they cost the company relative to others in the same category. The first tier is all generic drugs, which carry a $10 co-payment for a thirty-day supply.[a] The second tier comprises brand-name drugs; for example, those for which the PBM has negotiated special considerations from the manufacturers in the form of rebates or lower prices. Tier 2 medications have a $25 co-payment for a thirty-day supply. Tier 3 consists of all other branded medications. The Tier 3 co-payment is $40 for a thirty-day supply. The listing of all these medications, their uses, and assigned tiers is called a *formulary*.[b]

Note: There are many different variations with respect to pharmaceutical coverage. For example, some plans have more than three tiers, depending on the extent of favorable manufacturer contracts, and others have eliminated co-payments and use coinsurance instead. Additionally, some plans may apply annual maximum out-of-pocket cost limits for drugs.

[a]Virtually all plans also provide patients with the opportunity to order ninety-day medication supplies by mail at less than the cost of three co-payments.

[b]In addition to U.S. companies, countries that provide pharmaceuticals to their citizens also use formularies and differential cost structures. The difference between the two is that in the United States the tiers are based on *medication cost;* other countries (Italy, for example) assign tiers by *effectiveness*.

In addition to the actuarial costs that we discussed earlier, insurance companies also take into account the patient's out-of-pocket costs (deductibles, co-payments, and coinsurance) when pricing their products. Because the majority of health care purchases are relatively low cost, even small increases in patients' up-front payments can cause large premium reductions. Insurance companies often compete on their ability to customize price points by varying the amounts and mix of out-of-pocket expenses.

Table 11.3 displays the common payment methods private insurance companies use in different settings. Health care marketers must understand these methods when pricing their products or services.

TABLE 11.3. Common Private Insurance Payment Methods

Place of Service	Payment Method
Inpatient hospital	Charges: Percentage discount on charges; per diem fees (most common) based on level of service, such as, intensive care, rehabilitation, maternity, or DRGs. Charges are issued according to standardized chargemaster coding.
Outpatient hospital	Charges: Percentage discount on charges; or global payments for episodes of care. Paid according to chargemaster and/or RBRVS code.
Ambulatory surgicenter (whether or not it is hospital affiliated)	Charges: Percentage discount on charges; or global payments for episodes of care. Paid according to chargemaster and/or RBRVS code.
Skilled nursing facility	Per diem fees.
Physician office*	CPT-4 or HCPCS codes that determine payments usually based on a percentage of RBRVS. For administration of medications, such as chemotherapy, reimbursement is based on a fee schedule based on ASP or Average Wholesale Price (AWP).
Pharmacies	Contracted rates with Pharmaceutical Benefit Management (PBMs) companies and/or Direct Manufacturer Contracts. Direct contracts usually include volume-based discounts.
Hospice	Per diem fees.
Home health care	Per visit fees.

Note: *CPT-4-based fees also apply to physician services in all other settings.

SUMMARY

There is much dissatisfaction with the prices of health care services. Consumers face rising co-payments and deductibles, employers are feeling the pinch of increasing premiums, hospitals and physicians feel they are not sufficiently reimbursed, and the government's bill for health care keeps rising. Most participants in the health care marketplace see little logic to how health care prices are determined and distributed to participants.

The task of setting prices in health care organizations differs depending on who is paying the bill: patients, government, private parties (insurers), or some combination of these stakeholders. The theory of setting appropriate prices for patients consists of seven steps: (1) selecting the pricing objective; (2) determining demand; (3) estimating costs; (4) analyzing competitors' costs, prices, and offers; (5) deciding whether to use price as a competitive strategy; (6) selecting a pricing method (such as markup pricing, target return pricing, value pricing, and going-rate pricing); and (7) selecting the final pricing.

However, the theory must be modified by the influence of other factors, such as the health care organization's brand strength, its pricing policies, government regulations, and the impact of price on other stakeholders.

Prices must undergo further adjustment to take into account geographical factors, price discounts and allowances, promotional pricing, and differentiated pricing.

The health care organization must also decide when to initiate a price increase or reduction as well as how to react to competitors' price initiatives.

The government reserves the right to set prices for payment under Medicare, Medicaid, and Veteran's Administration programs and has set up an elaborate system for price determination depending on the nature of the product or service and where it is provided.

Although private insurers set the medical conditions that they will cover and the prices they will pay, they often rely on government guidelines. Their goal is successfully competing against other private insurers to get contracts with employers and the government.

DISCUSSION QUESTIONS

1. You are the chief marketing officer of a market-leading, nonprofit health plan. The CFO and the head of risk assessment think that premium prices should be increased, but you want to first examine the elasticity of demand. How would you get such information? What findings would cause you to support a price increase, and what findings would cause you to drop the decision to raise prices?

2. Academic medical centers often compete with neighboring community hospitals for routine patient care services. What price-quality assumptions about health services do consumers make in deciding between two such hospitals? Are they

rational? Assuming that the monetary costs to use either facility are often equivalent, what are the nonmonetary costs facing consumers who use either hospital?

3. Pharmaceutical companies have received negative publicity for setting the prices of their medicines for life-threatening diseases as much as twenty or more times the cost of production. Luxury goods manufacturers also charge high prices; however, their products do not mean the difference between life and death, health and disability. What reasons could a pharmaceutical company use to justify their pricing?

CHAPTER

12

DESIGNING AND MANAGING HEALTH CARE MARKETING CHANNELS

LEARNING OBJECTIVES

In this chapter, we will address the following questions:

1. What is a marketing channel system and value network?
2. What functions and flow are performed by marketing channels?
3. How should effective health care delivery channels be designed?
4. What decisions do companies face in managing their channels?
5. How should channels be integrated and channel conflict managed?

OPENING EXAMPLE

Novant Health Decides to Build an Integrated Health Care Delivery Network   Novant Health was one of the many hospitals nationwide that implemented a breakthrough marketing channels strategy in the 1990s. This Winston-Salem, North Carolina–based health care system decided to create an integrated delivery network (IDN). Hospitals at the time believed that they could gain market share, increase operational efficiency, and ultimately reduce overall health care costs by participating in as many components of the health care system as possible.

A typical IDN brought together a range of health care organizations. For example, a horizontal channels integration strategy was used to merge with or create alliances with other hospitals. A vertical channels integration strategy was employed to invest in physician practices and health insurance plans. Hospitals nationwide purchased health clubs, laundries, laboratories, and even restaurants in the name of integrating their networks. As Novant and other health care systems discovered, however, reaching their IDN objectives was more of a challenge than they expected.

Novant was successful with its *horizontal* channels strategy. It merged Forsyth Medical Center in Winston-Salem with Presbyterian Healthcare in Charlotte, North Carolina—two flagship hospitals—along with their various health services affiliates. Additionally, Novant committed to building three additional hospitals in small communities in its secondary markets and to developing medical plazas in strategic market locations. Medical plazas are innovative channels that offer a mix of ambulatory services, based on a community's specific medical needs, that are designed for easy access to each other.

One part of the Novant *vertical* channels strategy in the early 1990s was the development of Partners Health Plans, an independent practice association (IPA) HMO. Novant learned, however, that operating a health plan was very different from managing a medical center. For example, although the health plan and hospital were managed independently, physicians and other providers often criticized the senior medical center management because of difficult provider contracting and reimbursement decisions by Partners.

Partners Health Plans was quite successful based on its financial performance, membership growth, and NCQA certification. Other factors, however, including pushback from competing hospitals, strained physician relationships, and the lack of scale needed to compete with national payers led Novant to a decision to sell Partners to BlueCross BlueShield of North Carolina.

Another component of the Novant vertical channels strategy was the integration of medical practices that included an estimated 800 physicians. Like many hospitals, Novant experienced financial and management challenges here as well; but unlike some other hospitals, it persevered and made changes based on its commitment to its physician integration strategy.

Understanding that its physician practices needed to be managed more like a multi-specialty group than a hospital clinic, Novant adapted and placed decision-making for these practices back in the hands of the physician groups. Network management leaders with strong practice management experience were also brought on board. Physician compensation was tied to patient activity instead of a straight salary. Novant also formed a joint venture with the physicians to address the increasing costs of medical malpractice insurance. This "risk retention group" provided more competitively priced malpractice insurance to the medical staff.

Over time, this approach to vertical channels integration improved financial results and allowed Novant to invest in additional clinical and management resources, such as new medical equipment and physician recruitment assistance.

Source: Interview with Bob Seehausen, SVP of business development and sales at Novant, Aug. 2007.

As the opening example illustrates, health care organizations today must build and manage a continuously evolving value network. This chapter will examine the strategic marketing and tactical issues related to health care service and product channels and their accompanying value networks.

OVERVIEW: MARKETING CHANNELS AND VALUE NETWORKS

Because health care service providers, as well as health care product firms, often do not sell their services and goods directly to end users, a set of intermediaries, or channel partners, perform a variety of functions needed to deliver them. These intermediaries function as marketing channels, service delivery networks, and distribution channels. *Marketing channels* are sets of interdependent organizations involved in the process of making a product or service available for use or consumption. In health care, they are the set of pathways a service benefit or product follows either before or after production. The endpoint in the pathway is the purchase and use by the final end user. The process of a family medicine physician referring a patient to a heart surgeon at an academic medical center for a coronary artery bypass graft is an example of a marketing channel that leads to service delivery. In another example, a Valium tablet purchased by a hospital from the manufacturer, Roche USA, is first sent from the pharmaceutical company's plant to a warehouse. A drug wholesaler, jobber, or hospital group purchasing organization, such as Premier, then delivers it to the hospital pharmacy. A doctor at the patient bedside orders the Valium, and a nurse brings the tablet to the patient on the unit who then takes it. Each member of the distribution process performs a valuable function.

The Importance of Channels

A *marketing channel system* is the particular set of organizational paths and relationships that a firm employs to reach potential buyers and induce them into actions leading to profitable sales. Marketing channel system structure and management decisions are critical because channel members can collectively earn margins that account for 30 to 50 percent of the ultimate selling price. Marketing channels also represent a substantial opportunity cost; not only must they *serve* markets, but they must also *make* markets.[1] A prime example is the role played by pharmaceutical benefit management (PBM) companies, which not only serve as wholesalers but also manage most of the managed care drug benefits in the United States.

The channels a company chooses affect all other marketing decisions. Pricing is influenced by the types and costs of distribution; costs are often higher for services and products that require many channel partners, because each member of the distribution chain needs to be compensated. The firm's sales force and advertising decisions depend on how much training and motivation dealers need. In addition, channel decisions involve relatively long-term commitments to its members as well as establishment of sets of policies and procedures to delineate mutual goals and responsibilities. When a hospital signs a network agreement with a physician group for endoscopic procedures, the hospital cannot buy them out the next day and replace them with a hospital-owned diagnostic center.

In managing its intermediaries, the organization must decide how much effort to devote to *push* versus *pull* marketing. A *push strategy* involves the organization using its sales force and resources to motivate intermediaries to carry, promote, and sell the product to end users. A push strategy is appropriate where there is low brand loyalty in a category, brand choice is made at the time of purchase, the product is an impulse item, and product benefits are well understood. Stryker uses a push strategy, supported by its sales force, that actually advises surgeons during operations on how to best use its orthopedic implants. A *pull strategy* involves the organization's use of advertising and promotion to motivate consumers to ask intermediaries for the product, thus motivating the intermediaries to order it. Pull strategy is appropriate when there is high brand loyalty and high involvement in the category, when people perceive differences between brands, and when customers choose the brand before they make a purchase. A direct-to-consumer (DTC) television ad for the drug Rozerem is a tactic supporting a pull strategy designed to have consumers go to their doctors and ask for this medication if they have trouble sleeping.

Top marketing organizations skillfully employ both push and pull strategies. United Healthcare, a managed care company, uses a push strategy when it motivates brokers and consultants to advise employers to include its plans in their employee health benefit choices. A pull strategy is used when the company advertises to consumers to both ask their employers for United Healthcare coverage and select it over the other health plans being offered.

Value Networks

The organization should first think of the target market and then design the supply chain backward from that point, a process called *demand chain planning*. An even broader view sees an organization at the center of a *value network* — a system of partnerships and alliances that it creates to source, augment, and deliver its offerings. A value network includes an organization's suppliers, its suppliers' suppliers, its immediate customers, and customers' end customers. A hospital value network, for example, includes relations running the gamut from physicians to equipment suppliers to government regulatory agencies. An organization needs to orchestrate these parties to enable it to deliver superior value to the target market.

Demand chain planning yields several insights. First, the organization can estimate whether more money is to be made upstream or downstream, which will guide decisions on backward or forward integration, respectively. Second, the firm becomes more aware of disturbances anywhere in the supply chain that might cause costs, prices, or supplies to change suddenly. Third, companies can go on-line with their channel partners to carry on faster and more accurate communications, transactions, and payments to reduce costs, speed up information transfer, and increase accuracy.

Marketers have traditionally focused on the side of the value network that looks toward the customer. In the future, they will increasingly participate in and influence their organizations' upstream activities and become network managers (see Field Note 12.1).

FIELD NOTE 12.1.

Tufts–New England Medical Center Builds a Value Network Tufts–New England Medical Center (Tufts–NEMC) merged with the LifeSpan Health System in 1997. After five years, this association was dissolved and Tufts–NEMC became independent again. The merger and return to independence left Tufts–NEMC in a bind. Over the five-year period it was merged with LifeSpan, hospital competitors in the Boston market had developed alliances with health plans and had also purchased a number of primary care physician practices. Tufts–NEMC was left with about forty scattered physicians in their own network, and it needed to develop a competitive value network with physicians quickly.

Tufts–NEMC leadership learned that Tufts University Medical School graduates were more likely to go into clinical practice than graduates of any other area medical school. This finding seemed to indicate that Tufts–NEMC could have a base of primary care physicians who naturally referred their patients to its medical specialists.

Secondary marketing research showed that the data needed to measure referral trends was not comprehensive and up-to-date. Primary marketing research with physicians reinforced the conclusion that (1) doctors refer patients to other *doctors* and not to hospitals, and (2) the primary care physicians who were Tufts grads did not know much about the Tufts–NEMC specialist physicians due to the recent management and medical staff changes.

Marketing research also found that a large number of hospitals in Boston used the same "high-quality care" positioning. Further, a Tufts–NEMC capability analysis revealed that the medical center's smaller scale operation could be used to its advantage. This more intimate environment naturally enabled Tufts–NEMC to provide its physicians with enhanced communications, easier access to patient and hospital information, and other tools such as convenient web-based continuing medical education programs.

Using this marketing intelligence and understanding of internal strength, Tufts–NEMC decided to position their nascent medical network as providing high-quality care in a more intimate and personal setting.

Tufts–NEMC also decided to boost physician referrals through the reorganization of the enterprise along clinical product lines. Services were organized into nine business units that were charged with identifying growth opportunities, care, and cost improvement initiatives and in some cases major restructuring. Today, the Tufts–NEMC physician value network has grown to include 220 primary care physicians and 550 specialists.

Source: Interview with Deb Joelson, SVP of market development and planning at Tufts–New England Medical Center, Sept. 2007.

THE ROLE OF MARKETING CHANNELS

Why would a service provider or a product manufacturer delegate some of the delivery or selling tasks to intermediaries when delegation means relinquishing some control over how and to whom the services and products are sold? Producers of services and products gain several advantages by using intermediaries:

■ *Many producers lack the financial resources to carry out direct marketing.* EMD Pharmaceuticals is always searching for appropriate "in-licensing" opportunities. The company's business development team actively solicits new compounds from smaller pharmaceutical developers that cannot afford to operate their own sales force. EMD salespeople add these new compounds to their list of products and split the revenue with the smaller drug developers.

■ *Producers who establish their own channels can often earn a greater return by increasing investment in their main business.* If a growing company earns a 20-percent rate of return on manufacturing and a 10-percent return on retailing, it does not make sense for it to do its own retailing.

■ *In some cases direct marketing simply is not feasible.* The Bayer Corporation would not find it practical to establish small retail drug and grocery stores throughout the world or to sell aspirin, vitamins, nasal spray, and other over-the-counter remedies by mail order. Bayer finds it easier to work through the extensive network of separate distribution organizations.

Intermediaries normally achieve superior efficiency in making goods widely available and accessible to target markets. Through their contacts, experience, specialization, and scale of operation, intermediaries usually offer the firm more than it can achieve on its own. According to Stern and his colleagues:

> *Intermediaries smooth the flow of goods and services. . . . This procedure is necessary in order to bridge the discrepancy between the assortment of goods and services generated by the producer and the assortment demanded by the consumer. The discrepancy results from the fact that manufacturers typically produce a large quantity of a limited variety of goods, whereas consumers usually desire only a limited quantity of a wide variety of goods.*[2]

To make health care more available and convenient, new channels are emerging, particularly in the establishment of services in retail and wholesale outlets. These new channels offer a combinations enhanced access, shorter waiting times, and lower prices (see Field Note 12.2 for examples).

FIELD NOTE 12.2.

Retail Health Care Delivery Systems   Take Care Health operates fifty-six health clinics in Chicago, Kansas City, Milwaukee, Pittsburgh, and St. Louis, and is a wholly-owned subsidiary of Walgreen Company. It plans to have more than 400 clinics inside Walgreens drugstores by the end of 2008. Take Care Health employs nurse practitioners to meet basic health care needs, without the need for an appointment. Take Care Health has an integrated electronic medical record system, physician record review, peer review, and compliance auditing to support quality care.

One of Take Care's primary competitors is MinuteClinic, which also treats common family illnesses such as strep throat and ear, eye, sinus, bladder, and bronchial infections. The fee for these services averages $59 per visit, and the patient's primary care physician receives a copy of the diagnostic and treatment record. MinuteClinic is a subsidiary of CVS Caremark Corporation, and it has installations in 250 CVS Pharmacies across the nation. MinuteClinic is the first and only retail health care provider to receive accreditation from the Joint Commission on Accreditation of Healthcare Organizations.

Another competitor, RediClinic, received funding from Revolution Health in 2005 to roll out its national network of clinics. Revolution Health was established by Steve Case who was a founder of AOL. RediClinic emphasizes the typical retail heath care services and also stresses preventive and screening services. Consumers can check their medical test results on-line through the RediClinic Web site. RediClinic is located in select H-B-E food stores, Wal-Mart stores, and Walgreens' stores in Texas, Virginia, Georgia, Arkansas, and Oklahoma.

Wal-Mart is also moving forward with its own plans for retail clinics. Wal-Mart will lease space in its stores to local or regional hospitals and other organizations that are independent of Wal-Mart. The move is a significant expansion of a pilot project begun

in September 2005. As of April 2007, seventy-six clinics were operating inside Wal-Marts in twelve states. In addition, Kroger and Publix supermarkets have begun testing walk-in clinics, as has the mass merchandiser Target.
Source: "Guidelines for In-Store Treatment," *Modern Healthcare*, Jan. 9, 2006, p. 32.

CHANNEL FUNCTIONS AND FLOWS

A marketing channel performs the work of moving services and goods from producers to consumers. It overcomes the time, place, and possession gaps that separate goods and services from those who need or want them. Members of the marketing channel perform a number of key functions, including the following:

- Gathering information about potential and current customers, competitors, and other actors and forces in the marketing environment.

- Developing and disseminating persuasive communications to stimulate purchasing.

- Reaching agreements on price and other terms so that transfer of ownership or possession can be affected.

- Placing orders with manufacturers.

- Acquiring the funds to finance inventories at different levels in the marketing channel.

- Assuming risks connected with carrying out channel work.

- Providing for the successive storage and movement of physical products.

- Providing for buyers' payment of their bills through banks and other financial institutions.

- Overseeing actual transfer of ownership from one organization or person to another.[3]

Some functions (like providing physical possession or title to goods) constitute a *forward flow* of activity from the organization to the customer; other functions (ordering and payment) constitute a *backward flow* from customers to the organization. Still others (information, negotiation, finance, and risk taking) occur in both directions. A simplified model of these three flows is presented in Field Note 12.3 for the marketing of a hospital orthopedic product line. Note that even for this straightforward example, the complexity of a health care service marketing channel is substantial.

FIELD NOTE 12.3.

Model of Three Channel Flows

1. *Physical Flow.*

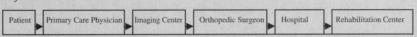

2. *Examples of Payment Flow (processes may occur sequentially or concurrently).* Insurance precertification, patient deductible and coinsurance, physician bills, imaging center bills, hospital bills, insurance reimbursement, physician write-off after reimbursement, hospital write-off after reimbursement, imaging center write-off after reimbursement, patient deductible and coinsurance for rehabilitation, rehabilitation bills, insurance reimbursement, rehabilitation write-offs after reimbursement.

3. *Examples of Information Flow (processes may occur sequentially or concurrently).* Patient to insurance precertification; insurance precertification to primary care physician and patient; primary care physician to imaging center; imaging center to primary care physician; primary care physician to orthopedic surgeon; orthopedic surgeon to hospital; orthopedic surgeon to rehabilitation center; orthopedic surgeon to primary care physician.

The question is often not *whether* various channel functions need to be performed, but rather *who* is to perform them. All channel functions have three things in common: they use up scarce resources, they can often be performed better through specialization, and they can be shifted among channel members. When the manufacturer shifts some functions to intermediaries, the producer's costs and prices are lower, but the intermediary must add a charge to cover *its* work. If the intermediaries are more efficient than the manufacturer, prices to consumers can be lower. If consumers perform some functions themselves, they should enjoy even lower prices. An obvious example of the latter is when patients come to the doctor's office for care versus the physician making a house call.

Marketing functions are more basic and stable than the institutions that perform them. Changes in channel institutions largely reflect the discovery of more efficient ways to combine or separate the economic functions that provide assortments of services and goods to target customers. For example, TelaDoc is a Dallas-based subscription service that connects consumers to its 175 participating physicians for medical advice by telephone. Instead of waiting to schedule an appointment, then paying up to $100, consumers can pay $35 per call along with an $18 setup fee and a $7 per month subscription fee. The service was launched in April 2005 and eventually had forty-one thousand registered customers who accounted for $1.7 million in revenue through February 2006. TelaDoc relies primarily on contracts with such membership organizations as the National Association of the Self-Employed and small health care insurers to draw its customers.

CHANNEL LEVELS

Because the producer and the final customer are part of every channel, we use the number of intermediary levels to designate the length of a channel.

A *zero-level channel* (also called a *direct-marketing channel*) consists of a producer selling directly to the final customer through door-to-door sales, mail order, telemarketing, TV selling, internet selling, and other methods. A *one-level channel* contains one selling intermediary, such as a retailer. A *two-level channel* contains two intermediaries, a *three-level channel* contains three intermediaries, and so on. From the producer's point of view, obtaining information about end users and exercising control becomes more difficult as the number of channel levels increases.

Channels normally describe a forward movement of services or products. One can also talk about *reverse-flow channels*, which bring products back for reuse (such as surgical instruments), refurbishing items for resale, or disposal of products and packaging.[4] For example, GE Healthcare will accept trade-ins and sell refurbished diagnostic equipment.

SERVICE SECTOR CHANNELS

Producers of health services and ideas also face the problem of making their output available and accessible to target populations. For example, cosmetic medicine companies such as Sleek MedSpa, Solana MedSpa, Sona MedSpa, and Radiance Medspa contract with physicians who oversee services and procedures that are often performed by a nurse or licensed technician. These treatments—which include injectable Botox and Restylane, peels and laser procedures, along with facials and therapeutic massage—are now moving into day spas in malls and other retail areas. Convenience (they are often open nights and weekends), ambience, and pampering are benefits that differentiate these medical spas from the typical physician's office. Although prices are often competitive with physicians' fees, in certain cities, like Los Angeles, there is strong price competition—a concept familiar to retailing but rare in medicine.

As the Internet and other technologies advance, health service organizations such as physician groups, hospitals, health insurance companies, and disease management firms operate through new channels. Blue Cross Blue Shield of North Carolina now enrolls more individual health insurance subscribers through their web portal than they enroll by telephone.

Another example of augmented service channels is Doctors Making Housecalls, based in central North Carolina. This medical group of six experienced, board-certified physicians provides care for patients aged 5 to 105 in their homes or offices. Their services are available from 7:00 AM to 7:00 PM and include urgent care for acute problems, routine care, and comprehensive care for chronic and complex conditions. In addition to physical examinations, they can draw blood and perform X-rays, EKGs, sonograms, Doppler studies, and Pap smears. Their goal is to improve access and quality of care by combining clinical excellence with uncommonly high levels of service and personalized attention, at an affordable price. Doctors Making Housecalls is "concierge medicine" with no annual fee; the group contracts with Medicare, files insurance claims with all commercial carriers, and accepts credit cards.

CHANNEL-DESIGN DECISIONS

Designing a marketing channel system involves analyzing customer needs, establishing channel objectives, identifying major channel alternatives, and evaluating major channel alternatives.

Analyzing Customers' Desired Service Output Levels

In designing the marketing channel, the marketer must understand the service output levels target customers desire. Channels produce five service outputs:

1. *Lot size:* The number of units the channel permits a typical customer to purchase on one occasion. In buying cars for its hospitals, HCA prefers a channel from which it can buy a large lot size; a household wants a channel that permits buying a lot size of one.

2. *Waiting and delivery time:* The average time customers of that channel wait for receipt of the goods or a service. Customers increasingly prefer faster and faster delivery channels. This feature is especially desirable in hospital emergency departments, where queuing is common and patients are often in pain.

3. *Spatial convenience:* The degree to which the marketing channel makes it easy for customers to purchase the product. As mentioned earlier, CVS is establishing MinuteClinics in its stores to make it easy for consumers to quickly receive minor medical care.

4. *Product variety:* The assortment breadth provided by the marketing channel. Normally, customers prefer a greater assortment because more choices increase the chance of finding what they need. Multi-specialty physician groups can treat individual patients for a variety of medical conditions without the patient having to leave the building; also, families can receive care at the same site and time.

5. *Service backup:* The add-on services (credit, delivery, installation, repairs) provided by the channel. The greater the service backup, the greater the work provided by the channel.[5]

Establishing Objectives and Constraints

Channel objectives should be measured in terms of targeted service output levels at the lowest possible cost.[6] Effective planning requires determining which market segments to serve, what level of service they expect, and the best channels for each.

Channel objectives vary with product characteristics. Perishable products require more direct marketing. Bulky products, such as building materials, require channels that minimize the shipping distance and the amount of handling. Nonstandardized products, such as custom-built machinery and specialized business forms, are sold directly by company sales representatives. Products requiring installation or maintenance services, such as heating and cooling systems, are usually sold and maintained by the company or by franchised dealers. High-unit-value products, such as MRIs and PET scanners, are often sold through a company sales force rather than intermediaries.

Channel design must take into account the strengths and weaknesses of different types of intermediaries. For example, contract sales reps who work with multiple pharmaceutical company clients are able to contact physicians at a low cost per customer, and the selling effort per customer is less intense than if company sales reps did the selling. Additionally, channel design is influenced by competitors' channels, economic conditions, and legal regulations and restrictions. U.S. law looks unfavorably on channel arrangements that may lessen competition or create a monopoly.

IDENTIFYING MAJOR CHANNEL ALTERNATIVES

There are many different options in selecting channels, and most organizations use a mix to cost-effectively reach different segments. A channel alternative is described by three elements: the types of intermediaries available, the number of intermediaries needed, and the terms and responsibilities of each channel member.

Types of Intermediaries

Some intermediaries—such as wholesalers and retailers—buy, take title to, and resell the merchandise; they are called *merchants*. Others—brokers, manufacturers' representatives, sales agents—who search for customers and may negotiate on the producer's behalf, but do not take title to the goods, are called *agents*. Still others—transportation companies, independent warehouses, banks, advertising agencies—who assist in the distribution process, but neither take title to goods nor negotiate purchases or sales, are called *facilitators*. These intermediaries help expand the channel possibilities.

An international example of channel expansion is IndUShealth, which provides American patients complex medical procedures in India at prices well below those offered at U.S. hospitals. The firm, founded in 2005 in Raleigh, North Carolina, coordinates overseas health care referrals for U.S. patients at three of India's top hospital systems: Wockhardt Hospitals, Ltd., in Mumbai and Indraprastha Apollo Hospitals and Escorts Heart Institute and Research Center located in New Delhi. The amount of savings varies by procedure, but InduShealth claims that the cost of the medical care it offers through its Indian partners is 70 to 80 percent lower than fees charged for the same care in the United States. The *Washington Post* reported that in 2004 a heart valve replacement surgery would cost up to $200,000 in the United States; the same procedure is about $10,000 at Escorts Heart Institute. Other examples of procedures available include hip resurfacing, knee replacement, coronary artery bypass grafts, and endoscopic disc removal.

Number of Intermediaries

In deciding how many intermediaries to use, companies can employ one of three strategies: exclusive, selective, and intensive distribution. *Exclusive distribution* means severely limiting the number of intermediaries. It is used when the producer wants to maintain control over the service level and outputs offered by the resellers. Often it involves *exclusive dealing* arrangements. By granting exclusive distribution, the producer hopes to obtain more dedicated and knowledgeable selling. It requires greater partnership between seller and reseller.

An example of a company that uses exclusive distribution is Quill Medical, which develops and commercializes innovative surgical products for wound closure and tissue management. These products, based on Quill's patented technology, enable surgical closures to "self-anchor" in tissue without the need for a suture. Products that employ these designs are expected to be useful across a range of surgical applications covering the fields of general, orthopedic, cosmetic, vascular, and endoscopic surgery. The company has an exclusive distribution alliance with Surgical Specialties Corporation, a leading provider of micro incision and wound closure technology. Under the alliance, Surgical Specialties sells Quill Medical's suture technology for aesthetic surgery under the trade name Contour ThreadLift, a minimally invasive product for lifting skin.

Selective distribution involves the use of more but fewer than all of the intermediaries who are willing to carry a particular product. It is used by established companies and by new companies seeking distributors. The company does not have to worry about too many outlets; it can gain adequate market coverage with more control and less cost than with an intensive distribution strategy.

An example of a firm that uses this approach is Expanscience Laboratories, an international pharmaceutical company based in France that specializes in dermo-cosmetics. Over the past fifty years, the company has relied on a selective distribution strategy for these products in selected pharmacies and, more recently, in a new category of distribution called *parapharmacies*. As the name suggests, a *parapharmacie* (the origin is French) is an offshoot of a pharmacy, but it focuses more on skin and hair care, along with vitamins, mineral supplements, and herbal teas. This selective distribution strategy is complemented by a selective sales strategy that targets certain prescribing physicians, midwives, and nurses.

Intensive distribution consists of the manufacturer placing the goods or services in as many outlets as possible. This plan is generally used for items such as over-the-counter medications like aspirin, first-aid products, vitamins, and other products that support the need for location convenience.

Rights and Responsibilities of Channel Members

The organization must determine the rights and responsibilities of participating channel members. To strengthen the linkages, each channel member must be treated respectfully and given the opportunity to be profitable or gain value.[7] The main elements in the "trade-relations mix" are price policies, conditions of sale, territorial rights, and specific services to be performed by each party.

Price policy calls for the organization to establish a price list and schedule of discounts and allowances that intermediaries see as equitable and sufficient. *Conditions of sale* refer to payment terms and guarantees. Most services- or goods-producing organizations grant cash discounts to distributors for early payments. Producers might also give distributors a guarantee against defective merchandise or price declines, which provides an incentive to buy larger quantities.

Distributors' territorial rights define not only *their* territories, but also the terms under which the organization will enfranchise other distributors. Distributors normally expect to receive full credit for all sales in their territory, whether or not *they* closed the specific deal.

Mutual services and responsibilities must be clearly communicated, especially in franchised and exclusive-agency channels. For example, American Ramp sells and rents ramps to consumers who use wheelchairs or who cannot climb stairs. This home health care organization enables consumers to be discharged earlier from hospitals and receive less expensive patient care in the home. They provide their franchisees with training, phone support, advertising, engineering support, and an accounting system. In return, franchisees are expected to pay a franchise fee, buy inventory, and purchase training, supplies, vehicles, and other equipment and services from approved suppliers.

EVALUATING THE MAJOR ALTERNATIVES

Once the organization has identified its major channel alternatives, it must evaluate each choice against appropriate economic, control, and adaptive criteria. From an economic perspective, each channel option will produce a different level of sales and costs. Figure 12.1 shows how six different sales channels perform in terms of the value added per sale and the cost per transaction. The next step is to estimate the costs of selling different volumes through each channel. Organizations that can move their customers to lower cost channels (such as moving from direct sales to web-based sales)—without losing sales, service quality, or customers—will gain a *channel advantage*.

The organization should also determine whether an in-house company sales force or a contracted sales agency will produce more sales. Using a sales agency poses a

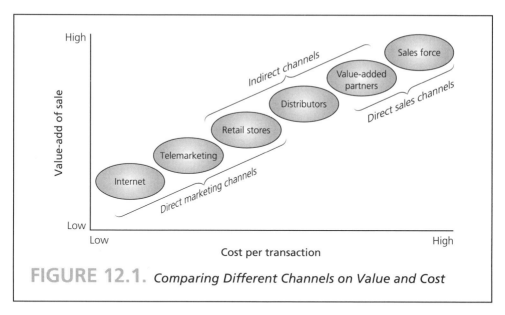

FIGURE 12.1. *Comparing Different Channels on Value and Cost*

Source: Kotler and Keller, *Marketing Management*, 12th ed. Upper Saddle River, N.J.: Prentice-Hall, 2006, p. 481.

control problem. A *sales agency* is an independent firm with a portfolio of different goods or services. As mentioned earlier, such an arrangement can lower the direct sales force cost; however, agents may concentrate more of their selling resources on the goods or services that are more easily sold or that generate greater profits to the agency. Therefore, agents also need appropriate incentives to master the more technical details of the company's product, handle its promotion materials effectively, and promote it equally with offerings from their other clients.

Although strong channel development requires that members make some degree of commitment to each other for a specified period of time, these commitments invariably lead to a decrease in the producer's ability to respond to a changing marketplace. The tradeoff is therefore between, on the one hand, stability and strength, and on the other, flexibility.

CHANNEL-MANAGEMENT DECISIONS

After an organization has chosen a channel alternative, individual intermediaries must be selected, trained, motivated, and evaluated. Marketers must also be ready to modify channel arrangements over time.

Selecting Channel Members

Organizations need to select their channel members carefully, because the channels represent the company to customers. Companies should evaluate channel members based on such characteristics as the number of years in business, growth and profit record, financial strength, cooperativeness, and service reputation. If the intermediaries are sales agents, producers should evaluate the number and character of other lines carried and the size and quality of the sales force. If the intermediaries want exclusive distribution rights, the producer should evaluate expertise, experience, locations, future growth potential, and the type of clientele they typically serve.

Training Channel Members

Organizations need to carefully plan and implement training programs for their intermediaries. For example, Misys Healthcare Systems, a market leader in health care IT, has a national program for its sales channel members called Misys Valued Partner or MVP. This program provides support to companies recognized as elite providers of Misys brand health care IT solutions that serve physician practices nationwide. To achieve MVP status, channel partners must complete a technical support training program and earn a specialized solution certification. As an authorized reseller of Misys Healthcare Systems solutions, the MVP offers its customers a fully integrated practice management solution including billing, scheduling, and electronic medical record services and products. When physicians purchase products from a Misys Healthcare Systems' MVP, they can be confident that the products and services are supported by the manufacturer. MVPs also have the assurance that Misys Healthcare Systems will not directly compete within their local markets.

Motivating Channel Members

Companies must regard their intermediaries in the same way they regard their end users; that is, identifying their needs and tailoring their channel positioning to provide them superior value. The organization should provide training, market research, and other capability-building programs to improve intermediaries' performance. The firm must constantly work to make the intermediaries their partners in a joint effort to satisfy customers.

In trying to forge long-term partnerships with distributors, however, sophisticated organizations must clearly communicate what they want in the areas of market coverage, inventory levels, marketing development, account solicitation, technical advice and services, and marketing information. In this respect, producers often see gaining intermediaries' cooperation as a huge challenge, and they vary in their ability to manage these distributors.[8] To garner cooperation, these producers may apply *channel power*, which is defined as the ability to alter channel members' behavior so that they take actions they would not otherwise have taken.[9] For example, producers can use channel power when they have a very desirable product over which distributors compete for the right to represent it to the market. When the product or service is not quite this desirable, more creative methods must be employed, such as customized compensation plans that can be aligned to elicit the desired behavior.

Evaluating Channel Members

Producers must periodically evaluate intermediaries' performance against such standards as sales-quota attainment, average inventory levels, customer delivery time, treatment of damaged and lost goods, and cooperation in promotional and training programs. A producer will occasionally discover that it is paying too much to particular intermediaries for what they are actually doing. One manufacturer that was compensating a distributor for holding inventories found that the inventories were actually held in a public warehouse at its expense. Producers should set up functional programs that pay specified amounts for the channel partner's performance of each agreed-upon service. Underperformers need to be counseled, retrained, remotivated, or terminated. See Field Note 12.4 for an example of how a company can work with its channel partners to improve quality and growth.

FIELD NOTE 12.4.

Evaluating Health Care Marketing Channel Intermediaries How important is it for marketers to evaluate and manage suppliers, wholesalers, retailers, and other intermediaries? They can start by determining how suppliers—and *their* suppliers—as well as distributors can influence the organization's performance. Respirics combines proprietary inhalation technology with powder drug formulation expertise to develop unique drug delivery solutions. Respirics needed to find the best manufacturing and distribution channel partners to make its asthma drug delivery product, MD Turbo, accessible to the target market and profitable for the company.

Respirics began searching for a design and manufacturing partner for MD Turbo by evaluating 165 applicants from all over the world. Six companies were culled from this research, and one was selected—Computime. This selection was based on price (the cost of producing MD Turbo in the United States was double the cost of producing the device in China) and Computime's "customer first" corporate culture.

Another important step is to translate companywide strategic goals and measurements into specific targets and measures for value-network members. The Computime marketing culture was put to the test when the initial manufactured lots had a failure rate of 7.5 percent. After Respirics explained that this rate was unacceptable, Computime's management enhanced the quality assurance process and tested 100 percent of the units produced. The result was a reduction to a 1 percent initial failure rate. Volume is now three hundred thousand units annually and is growing.

Another key criterion is how well an intermediary can support the company's drive for growth. Respirics also entered into a distribution arrangement with a biopharmaceutical company focused on the development and commercialization of late-stage respiratory disease products. The three objectives of this partnership were to have the distribution partner's sales force call on (1) national pharmacy companies and their retail outlets,

(2) high-prescribing physicians, such as allergists and pulmonologists, and (3) health insurance companies and other third-party payers (to secure reimbursement coverage for MD Turbo). Through its monitoring, Respirics learned that the partner unfortunately was not performing up to standards. It had been unable to build its sales force to the size needed to accomplish the objectives. Both parties are now working together to solve this problem.

Source: Interview with Gil Mott, CEO of Respirics, Sept. 2007.

MODIFYING CHANNEL ARRANGEMENTS

Channel arrangements must be periodically reviewed and modified when the distribution channel is not working as planned, consumer buying patterns change, the market expands, new competition arises, innovative distribution channels emerge, or the product moves into later stages in the product life cycle.

No marketing channel will remain effective over the whole product life cycle. Early buyers might be willing to pay for high value-added channels, but later buyers will switch to lower-cost channels. In competitive markets with low entry barriers, the optimal channel structure will inevitably change over time. The change could involve adding or dropping individual channel members, adding or dropping particular market channels, or developing a totally new way to sell goods.

Adding or dropping an individual channel member requires an incremental analysis to determine what the firm's profits would look like with and without this intermediary. Monetary costs of changes are not always immediately evident, and problems may initially present themselves with other channel members and customers. For example, eliminating a channel may erode sales if the market incorrectly infers that the product is in trouble or channel partners think they will be next in facing cutbacks. Channel members can also decide to end their alliance with producing organizations; for example, surgeons can decide to use the operating rooms of other hospitals if their repeated requests for new equipment and timely communications are not met by their current hospital. Further, producers may disrupt ultimate customer sales when channel members have personal and long-standing relationships with end users. This situation is particularly prevalent in the hospital supply sector in Japan.

The most difficult decision involves revising the overall channel strategy.[10] Distribution channels can become outmoded over time as a gap arises between the existing distribution system and the ideal system that would satisfy target customers' (and producers') needs and desires. In the 1990s, Medic Computer Systems, a prominent physician information systems company, realized a significant percentage of its total sales revenue as an IBM value-added reseller (VAR), reselling midrange computer hardware. This revenue has declined markedly, because physicians can now purchase high-performance desktop PCs by phone, in a large commercial outlet or over the Web.

CHANNEL DYNAMICS

As new wholesaling and retailing institutions emerge, new channel systems evolve. We now look at the recent growth of vertical, horizontal, and multi-channel marketing systems and see how these systems cooperate, conflict, and compete.

Vertical Marketing Systems

One of the most significant recent channel developments is the rise of vertical marketing systems.[11] A *conventional marketing channel* comprises an independent producer, wholesaler(s), and retailer(s). Each is a separate business seeking to maximize its own profits, even if this goal reduces profit for the system as a whole. No channel member has complete or substantial control over other members.

A *vertical marketing system* (VMS), by contrast, comprises the producer, wholesaler(s), and retailer(s) acting as a unified system. One channel member, the *channel captain*, owns the others, franchises them, or has so much power that they all cooperate. The channel captain can be the producer, the wholesaler, or the retailer. VMSs arose as a result of strong channel members' attempts to control channel behavior and eliminate the conflict that results when independent members pursue their own objectives. VMSs achieve economies through size, bargaining power, and elimination of duplicated services. They have become the dominant mode of distribution in the U.S. consumer marketplace, serving between 70 and 80 percent of the total market. The three types of VMS are corporate, administered, and contractual.

A *corporate VMS* combines successive stages of production and distribution under single ownership. For example, many academic medical centers obtain over 50 percent of their hospital admissions from physicians who belong to the faculty practice plan.

An *administered VMS* coordinates successive stages of production and distribution through the size and power of one of the members. Manufacturers of a dominant brand are able to secure strong trade cooperation and support from resellers. Integrated delivery networks (IDNs) are another example. These health care service entities are often led by a hospital that has either purchased or created alliances with physician practices. Other entities—including ambulatory surgery centers, rehabilitation clinics, urgent care centers and, more rarely, an insurance company or a medical school—can also be IDN partners. The stated objective of many IDNs is to make health care more cost-effective through controlling as many providers and payers as possible. In reality, measuring and realizing these cost savings has been a challenge in many cases.

A *contractual VMS* consists of independent firms at different levels of production and distribution integrating their programs on a contractual basis to obtain more economies or sales impact than they could achieve alone. Johnston and Lawrence call them "value-adding partnerships" (VAPs).[12] Contractual VMSs are of three types:

■ *Wholesaler-sponsored voluntary chains* organize groups of independent retailers to help them compete with large chain organizations by standardizing selling practices and achieving buying economies. North Carolina Mutual Wholesale Drug Company, also known as Mutual Drug, is an independent wholesaler and distributor in North Carolina, South Carolina, and Virginia. Formed as a cooperative, Mutual Drug is owned and managed by pharmacists. Group buying, merchandising, government relations, and consumer advertising are some of the benefits of belonging to this wholesaler group.

- *Retailer cooperatives* arise when the stores take the initiative and organize a new business entity to carry on wholesaling and possibly some production. Members concentrate their purchases through the retailer co-op and plan their advertising jointly. Members share in profits in proportion to their purchases. The Independent Natural Food Retailers Association (INFRA) is a cooperative owned and governed by visionary retailers in the health foods industry. INFRA brings together retailers from all regions of the country to share resources, build market share, and strengthen their position in the industry. Retailers share operational solutions, provide a conduit and structure for strong industry partnerships, and leverage combined purchasing power.

- *Franchise organizations* are created when a channel member called a *franchisor* links several successive stages in the production-distribution process. The traditional system is the *producer-sponsored retailer franchise*. The dealers are independent businesspeople who agree to meet specified conditions of sales and services. AccuDiagnostics is a full-service third-party administrator providing drug, alcohol, steroid, and DNA testing as well as consultation to businesses, schools, government agencies, and private citizens. Individuals purchase a franchise to perform these services and are given training and limited marketing support. These arrangements also include *manufacturer-sponsored wholesaler franchises*, whereby a producer licenses wholesalers to buy its product components for resale to retailers in local markets. The *service-firm-sponsored retailer franchise* organizes a whole system to bring its service efficiently to consumers.

Horizontal Marketing Systems

Another channel development is the *horizontal marketing system*, in which two or more unrelated organizations combine resources or programs to exploit an emerging marketing opportunity in a business that is somewhat familiar for at least one of the partners. Each organization alone either (1) lacks the capital, delivery capability, know-how, production, or marketing resources to venture by itself or (2) is risk-averse. For example, as previously mentioned, pharmacy chains Walgreens and CVS Caremark contracted with provider organizations to furnish convenient in-store care. Subsequently, they purchased these organizations.

Multi-Channel Marketing Systems

In the past, many organizations sold to a single market through a single channel. Today, with the proliferation of customer segments and channel possibilities, more organizations have adopted multi-channel marketing. *Multi-channel marketing* occurs when a single firm uses two or more marketing channels to reach one or more customer segments. As an example, hospitals have traditionally relied on physicians for patient referrals for diagnostic tests, outpatient procedures, inpatient admissions, and for other services. Hospitals now use multi-channel marketing strategies that also encourage patients to ask physicians for referrals, patient self-referrals, and referrals by third-party payers. As mentioned earlier, health insurance companies traditionally often signed up members through brokers, but direct-to-consumer advertising now encourages on-line or phone enrollment.

By adding more channels, organizations can gain three important benefits: increased market coverage, lower channel cost (such as selling by phone or on-line rather than through personal visits to small customers), and more customized selling—such as adding a technical sales force to sell more complex equipment.

Conflict, Cooperation, and Competition

Despite the advantages of multi-channel marketing, even well-designed and managed channels can experience some conflict. *Channel conflict* is generated when one channel member's actions prevent the channel from achieving its goal. *Channel cooperation* occurs when members are brought together to advance the goals of the channel, even when member goals may be incompatible.[13] For example, recall the opening example in Chapter Five regarding Humana. That company was, at one time, both a hospital and an HMO firm. Hospitals traditionally make their money filling beds, whereas HMOs make money by keeping those beds empty. The task of management was to coordinate those competing channels for overall company benefit. An example of *channel competition* is when two channel partners attempt to sell a product to the same prospect at the same time. Sometimes this competition is the result of poor communication. Misys, a physician information system company, had a value-added reseller agreement with IBM. Misys installed its software on IBM computers and resold the systems to hospitals. Channel competition occurred when IBM and Misys salespeople encountered each other as competitors for a particular hospital account.

Types of Conflict and Competition. *Vertical channel conflict* occurs with clashes between different levels within the same channel. A hospital in the Southeast came into conflict with its gastroenterologists in trying to enforce new policies on service, pricing, and scheduling endoscopic procedures. The physicians reacted to the hospital's lack of interest in negotiating by building their own independent endoscopy center.

Horizontal channel conflict involves differences among members at the same level within the channel. In the 1980s, the national hospital chain HCA decided to brand all of its owned facilities with the HCA logo. Because not all of the hospitals offered the same level of care or participated in the voluntary, corporate quality-improvement programs, channel conflict arose when the higher-performing units were tied by the new brand identity to lower-performing ones.

Multi-channel conflict exists when the organization has established two or more channels that sell to the same market. Multi-channel conflict is likely to be especially intense when the members of one channel can offer a lower price (based on larger volume) or work with a lower margin. Insurance brokers who represent Blue Cross Blue Shield have certain latitude in configuring and pricing insurance products for their corporate customers. These prices are not always in line with those offered by Blue Cross Blue Shield direct salespeople, thus creating a conflict between the channels.

Causes of Channel Conflict. One major cause of conflict is *goal incompatibility*. The manufacturer may want to achieve rapid market penetration through a low-price policy. Dealers, in contrast, may prefer to work with high margins and pursue short-run profitability. Sometimes conflict arises from *unclear roles and rights*. HP may sell personal computers to pharmaceutical companies through its own sales force, but its licensed dealers may also be trying to sell to these same companies. Territory boundaries and credit for sales also often produce conflict.

Further, conflict can stem from *differences in perception*. For example, when the producer is optimistic about the short-term economic outlook, it would like dealers to carry higher inventory, but dealers may be more pessimistic about the sales forecast and want to keep inventory small. Conflict might also arise because of the intermediaries' *dependence* on the manufacturer. The fortunes of exclusive dealers are profoundly affected by the manufacturer's product and pricing decisions.

Managing Channel Conflict. Some channel conflict can be constructive and lead to more dynamic adaptation to a changing environment. Above a certain threshold, however, conflict can have negative results. The challenge is not to eliminate conflict but to constructively manage it. Several mechanisms exist for effective channel conflict management.[14] One is the adoption of superordinate goals. Channel members come to an agreement on the fundamental goal they are jointly seeking, whether it is survival, market share, high quality, or customer satisfaction. This consensus process usually occurs when the channel faces an outside threat, such as a more efficient competing channel, an adverse piece of legislation, or a shift in consumer desires.

A useful method to achieve this goal is to exchange persons between two or more channel levels. For example, at Biomet, the orthopedic specialty company, executives might agree to work for a short time in some distributorships, and some distributor owners might work in Biomet's distributor policy department. The objective is to have the participants grow to better understand, appreciate, and trust the other's point of view.

Co-optation is an effort by one organization to win the support of the leaders of another organization by including them in such groups as advisory councils and boards of directors. As long as the initiating organization treats the leaders seriously and listens to their opinions, co-optation can reduce conflict; but the initiating organization may have to compromise on its policies and plans to win their support.

Whether conflict is chronic or acute, the parties may have to resort to diplomacy, mediation, or arbitration. *Diplomacy* takes place when each side sends a person or group to meet with his or her counterpart to resolve the conflict. *Mediation* means resorting to a neutral third party who is skilled in conciliating the two parties' interests. *Arbitration* occurs when the two parties agree to present their arguments to one or more arbitrators and accept the arbitration decision. If those methods fail, the result can be prolonged, expensive *litigation*.

LEGAL AND ETHICAL ISSUES IN CHANNEL RELATIONS

For the most part, companies are legally free to develop whatever channel arrangements suit them. In fact, the law seeks to prevent companies from using exclusionary tactics that might keep competitors from using a channel.

Many producers like to develop exclusive channels for their products. A strategy in which the seller allows only certain outlets to carry its products is called *exclusive distribution*. When the seller requires that these dealers not handle competitors' products, it is called *exclusive dealing*. Both parties benefit from exclusive arrangements: the seller obtains more loyal and dependable outlets, and the dealers obtain a steady source of supply of special products and stronger seller support. Exclusive arrangements are legal as long as both parties enter into the agreement voluntarily and they do not substantially lessen competition or tend to create a monopoly.

Exclusive dealing often includes exclusive territorial agreements. The producer may agree not to sell to other dealers in a given area, or the buyer may agree to sell only in its own territory. The first practice increases dealer enthusiasm and commitment and is perfectly lawful—a seller has no legal obligation to sell through more outlets than it wishes. The second practice, wherein the producer tries to keep a dealer from selling outside its territory, has become a contentious legal issue.

The producer of a strong brand sometimes sells it to dealers only if they will take some or all of the rest of the line. This practice is called *full-line forcing*. Such *tying agreements* are not necessarily illegal, but they do violate U.S. law if they tend to lessen competition substantially.

Producers are free to select their dealers, but their right to terminate dealers is somewhat restricted. In general, sellers can drop dealers "for cause," but they cannot drop dealers if, for example, the dealers refuse to cooperate in a doubtful legal arrangement, such as exclusive dealing or tying agreements.

SUMMARY

Delivering efficient health care services involves the cooperation of a complex set of channel members. Between producers and final users stand one or more marketing channels consisting of a host of marketing intermediaries that perform a variety of functions, the most important being information provision, promotion, negotiation, ordering, financing, risk taking, physical possession, payment, and assuming title.

Marketing channels can consist of any number of intermediaries, depending on the function that needs to be performed. Deciding which type or types of channel to use calls for analyzing customer needs, establishing channel objectives, and identifying and evaluating the major alternatives, including the types and numbers of intermediaries involved in the channel.

Any party setting up a channel must be prepared to train, motivate, and evaluate the other channel members and alter channel arrangements when required. The goal is to build a long-term partnership that will be profitable for all channel members. What's important is that channel members have a clear sense of their responsibilities and benefits. Ill-defined terms of engagement can exacerbate the normal frictions that prevail among channel members, particularly among physicians, hospitals, employers, and health insurers.

All marketing channels have the potential for conflict and competition resulting from such sources as goal conflict and poorly defined roles and rights. Organizations can manage conflict by striving for superordinate goals that reward all the channel participants.

DISCUSSION QUESTIONS

1. Critics of rising health care costs often criticize the large number of channel intermediaries, claiming they cause higher prices for goods and services. Do intermediaries increase or reduce the cost of health care products and services? Would consumers be better off or worse off if there were fewer intermediaries in the health care market?

2. The number of retail store-based basic primary care clinics is increasing. This health care distribution innovation is simple, and there are low barriers of entry into this market. Why was this distribution strategy not implemented sooner? What other types of new health care distribution strategies could be successful?

3. You are the marketing vice president for an excellent hospital in India that is targeting U.S. and European patients. You understand that it is imperative to have a distribution plan that takes into account cultural factors. List the factors that will affect your plan and how you will adapt your plan to each factor.

4. Your small orthopedic implant company has traditionally distributed its products through wholesalers and distributors, but your vice president of marketing has recommended adding a direct web-based distribution channel. As the CEO, you are concerned that this change will result in channel conflict. What are the benefits and drawbacks of this strategy? How do you think clients, wholesalers and distributors, and competitors will react if this strategy is implemented?

CHAPTER

13

DESIGNING AND MANAGING INTEGRATED MARKETING COMMUNICATIONS

LEARNING OBJECTIVES

In this chapter, we will address the following questions:

1. What is the role of marketing communications?
2. What are the major elements making up the marketing communications process?
3. What are the eight major steps in developing effective communications?
4. What are the alternative methods of setting the communications budget?
5. What are the major communication tools making up the communications mix?
6. How can the organization develop an effective integrated marketing communications program?

OPENING EXAMPLE

Social Marketing Communications Strategy Used to Save Lives in Myanmar

The Joint United Nations Program on HIV/AIDS (UNAIDS) estimated that at least 530,000 individuals were infected with HIV in Myanmar (Burma) in 2000. The virus had spread from sex workers, intravenous drug users, and other high-risk groups to the general population. Population Services International (PSI) decided to address this growing problem through culturally sensitive marketing messages.

PSI is a nonprofit social marketing organization that partners with the private sector in more than sixty developing countries to promote products and services for low-income and vulnerable populations. The focus of these initiatives is on malaria, reproductive health, child survival, and HIV. One of PSI's major points of differentiation from other health care foundations is that its products and services are sold at subsidized prices rather than given away. This approach is attractive to commercial partners who are able to sell their products at a profit. It also motivates participants to comply with program procedures because it places a tangible value on PSI products and services.

Promoting condoms was initially very difficult because the military regime that runs Myanmar considered condom possession evidence of prostitution; and they felt that promoting condoms would encourage promiscuity. To overcome this hurdle, PSI launched an HIV/AIDS prevention branding campaign in 2003 that was geared to the local, conservative culture by developing a unique condom brand name and image. PSI chose the Burmese names "Aphaw" ("trusted companion") for the brand and chose a "Pothinnyo" ("chameleon") wearing a traditional man's sun hat as the brand image. Chameleons are very common in Myanmar, and young boys who see them often watch for the reptile to move its head, while chanting: "Pothinnyo, nod your head if you want a girl." PSI coined the slogan: "Pothinnyo, nod your head if you want an Aphaw." Humor was used to diffuse this somewhat stigmatized product. The PSI branding was successful; in three years, 82 percent of urban Burmese became aware of the Aphaw pothinnyo, and nearly all linked it to HIV/AIDS prevention.

PSI has relied on targeted marketing that continues to result in changes to the high-risk behaviors of those most in danger of HIV/AIDS. Since the initial launch of its condom social marketing program in 1996, PSI has distributed 25 million condoms; disseminated more than thirty-five different types of information, education, and communications materials; and reached millions of people across Myanmar with the information they need to protect themselves from HIV/AIDS. Sales of PSI's Aphaw condom have grown every year since 1997, while public and commercial sector condom distribution have also increased. The total condom market has increased in Myanmar from 4.4 million units in 1997 to 16.4 million units in 2000. PSI supplies about 75 percent of all the condoms used in Myanmar with heavy subsidies. The subsidies allow the condoms to be sold at less than one-third of their production cost and make them more affordable to the cash-strapped population.

PSI has continued to build partnerships with local industry associations and business groups to promote condom distribution efforts. Extensive religious networks have also been tapped to develop communications materials and to train community members, especially youth. PSI has broadened is promotion strategy to collaborate with famous cultural troupes to produce traveling theatrical performances using traditional opera, dance, theater, and comedy to educate small communities at risk of HIV/AIDS. Moreover, PSI has developed *Happy Travelers*—the first soap opera ever produced in Myanmar. This ten-part series follows the dramatic story of a group of families affected by HIV/AIDS and airs on national television.

This success is vindication of PSI's decision to set up shop in Myanmar more than a decade ago, in spite of criticism from pro-democracy groups that its presence could help prop up the repressive military regime.

Sources: PSI Web site [http://www.psi.org] and A. Kazmin, "Business Life: A Chameleon Enlists in War on AIDS," *Financial Times*, Feb. 20, 2006.

Modern marketing calls for more than developing a good product, pricing it attractively, and making it accessible. Companies must also communicate with present and potential stakeholders and the general public. For most companies, the question is not whether to communicate but rather what to say, how to say it, to whom, and how often. But communications gets harder and harder as more and more companies clamor to grab consumers' increasingly divided attention. To effectively reach target markets and build brand equity, holistic marketers are creatively employing multiple forms of communications.

Marketing communications can have a huge payoff to companies. This chapter describes how communications work, what marketing communications can do for a company, and how holistic marketers combine and integrate marketing communications. While this chapter looks at the different forms of mass (nonpersonal) communications (advertising, sales promotion, events and experiences, and public relations and publicity), Chapter Fourteen examines the different forms of personal communications (personal selling and direct marketing).

OVERVIEW: THE ROLE OF MARKETING COMMUNICATIONS

Marketing communications are the tools firms use to relate the benefits, positioning, and characters of their brands to consumers. Marketing communications, therefore,

- Represent the "voice" of the brand
- Are the primary vehicles used to establish a dialogue and build relationships with consumers

- Tell or show consumers how and why a product is used, by what kind of person, and where and when

- Inform consumers about who makes the product and what the company and brand represent

- Can give consumers an incentive or reward for trial or usage

- Allow companies to link their brands to other people, places, events, brands, experiences, feelings, and things

In these ways, marketing communications can contribute to brand equity by establishing the brand in memory and crafting a brand image. As Figure 13.1 shows, communications contribute to brand equity by creating brand awareness, crafting a brand image, eliciting brand responses, and facilitating a stronger consumer-brand connection.

MARKETING COMMUNICATIONS AND BRAND EQUITY

Although advertising is often a central element of a marketing communications program, it is usually not the only one, or even the most important one, in terms of

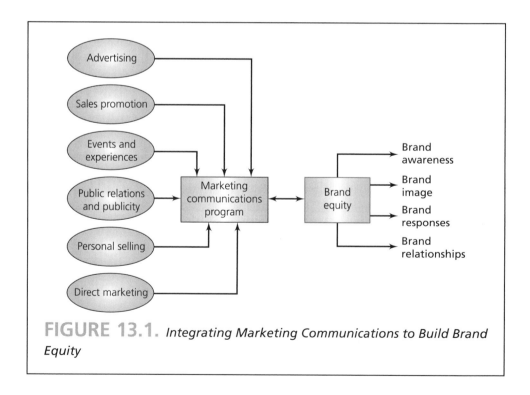

FIGURE 13.1. *Integrating Marketing Communications to Build Brand Equity*

building brand equity. The *marketing communications mix* consists of six major modes of communication:

- *Advertising:* Any paid form of nonpersonal presentation and promotion of ideas, goods, or services by an identified sponsor

- *Sales promotion:* A variety of short-term incentives to encourage trial or purchase of a product or service

- *Events and experiences:* Company-sponsored activities and programs designed to create daily or special brand-related interactions

- *Public relations and publicity:* A variety of programs designed to promote or protect a company's image or its individual products

- *Personal selling:* Face-to-face interaction with one or more prospective purchasers for the purpose of making presentations, answering questions, and procuring orders

- *Direct marketing:* Use of mail, telephone, fax, e-mail, or Internet to communicate directly with or solicit response or dialogue from specific customers and prospects[1]

Organizational communication goes beyond those specific platforms. The product's styling and price, the shape and color of the package, the manner and dress of individuals delivering the service, the physical surroundings and decor, the company's stationery—all communicate something to buyers. Every *brand contact* delivers an impression that can strengthen or weaken a customer's view of the organization.

Marketing communications activities contribute to brand equity in many ways: by creating awareness of the brand, linking the right associations to the brand image in consumers' memory, eliciting positive brand judgments or feelings, and, ideally, facilitating a stronger consumer-brand connection.

One implication of the concept of brand equity is that the manner in which brand associations are formed does not matter—only their resulting strength, favorability, and uniqueness. For example, Children's Hospital Boston runs a television ad that shows parents telling poignant stories about how the institution is saving children's lives. From this communication, potential customers can relate to the concepts of "medical research," "brilliant doctors," and "heroic decisions," thus developing a strong and favorable brand association with the hospital. Children's Hospital Boston also sponsors pediatric health tips on-line on *Yahoo Health*, creating an additional impression of a knowledgeable, caring partner for parents.

All marketing communications activities must be integrated to deliver a consistent message and achieve the strategic positioning. Brand awareness is a function of the number of brand-related exposures and experiences that have been accumulated by the consumer.[2] Thus, *anything* that causes the consumer to notice and pay attention to the brand can increase brand awareness, at least in terms of brand recognition. The starting point in planning marketing communications is an audit of all the potential interactions that customers in the target market may have with the brand and the company. For example, someone interested in purchasing cosmetic surgery might talk to others, see television ads, read articles, look for information on the Internet, and observe friends who have had similar procedures. Marketers need to assess which experiences and impressions will have the most influence at each stage of the buying process. This understanding will help them allocate communications dollars more efficiently and design and implement the right communication programs.

Armed with consumer insights, marketing communications can then be judged according to their ability to build brand equity and drive brand sales. For example, how well does a proposed hospital ad campaign contribute to awareness or creating, maintaining, or strengthening brand associations? Does a hospital sponsorship of a 10K road race to raise research money for cancer cause consumers to have more favorable brand judgments and feelings about a hospital? To what extent does an exercise health promotion campaign by the American Heart Association encourage consumers to exercise more?

From the perspective of building brand equity, marketers should evaluate *all* the different possible communication options that are available according to effectiveness criteria (how well does it work?) as well as efficiency considerations (how well does it work given the cost?). This broad view of brand building activities is especially relevant when considering marketing communications strategies to improve brand awareness.

COMMUNICATIONS PROCESS MODELS

Macro and micro models provide useful structures to help marketers understand the fundamental elements of effective communication.

Macro Model of the Communications Process

Figure 13.2 shows a macro communications model with nine elements. Two of the elements represent the major parties in a communication—the sender and the receiver. Two other elements represent the major communications tools—the message and the media used to send the message. Four of the elements represent major communications functions—message *encoding, decoding, response*, and *feedback*. The ninth element in the system is *noise*, or random and competing messages that can interfere with the intended communication.[3]

The model emphasizes the key factors in effective communication. Senders must know what audiences they want to reach and what responses they want to get. They must encode their messages so that the target audience can decode them. They must transmit the message through media that reach the target audience, and they must develop feedback channels to monitor the responses. The more the sender's field of experience overlaps with that of the receiver, the more effective the message is likely to be.

Note that selective attention, distortion, and retention processes may be operating during communication.

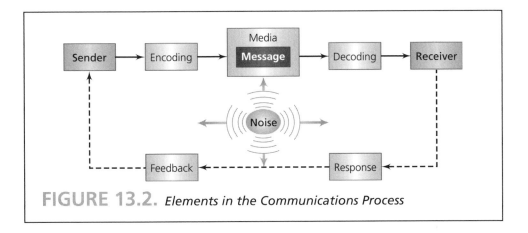

FIGURE 13.2. *Elements in the Communications Process*

- *Selective attention:* People filter messages to avoid sensory overload. If you are typical, you are bombarded by about 1,600 commercial messages a day, of which you consciously notice about 80, and about 12 provoke either a positive or negative reaction. Selective attention explains why advertisers sometimes go to great lengths to grab audience attention through emotions using fear, music, or sex appeal or using bold headlines promising something, such as "How to Eliminate Your Wrinkles."

- *Selective distortion:* Receivers of messages will hear and process what fits into their belief systems. As a result, receivers often add things to the message that are not there and do not notice some things that are there. The communicator's task is to strive for simplicity, clarity, interest, and the right amount of repetition to get the main points across.

- *Selective retention:* People will retain in long-term memory only a small fraction of the messages that reach them. If the receiver's initial attitude toward the object is positive, and he or she rehearses support arguments, the message is likely to be accepted and have high recall. If the initial attitude is negative, and the person rehearses counter arguments, the message is likely to be rejected but to stay in long-term memory.

Micro Model of Consumer Responses

Micro models of marketing communications concentrate on consumers' specific responses to communications. Figure 13.3 summarizes four classic *response hierarchy models*.

All these models assume that in evaluating a marketing communications message, the buyer passes through cognitive, affective, and behavioral stages, in that order. This "learn-feel-do" sequence is appropriate when the audience has high involvement with a product category perceived to have high differentiation, as in

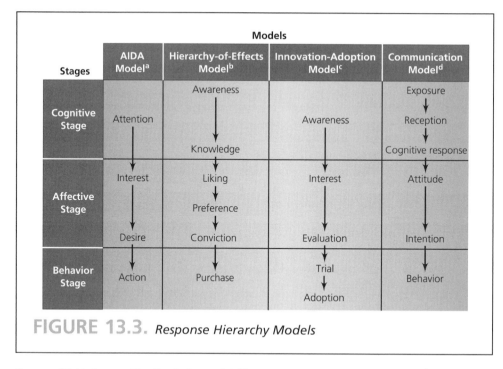

FIGURE 13.3. *Response Hierarchy Models*

Sources: [a]E. K. Strong, *The Psychology of Selling*, New York: McGraw-Hill, 1925; [b]R. J. Lavidge and G. A. Steiner, "A Model of Predictive Measurements of Advertising Effectiveness," *Journal of Marketing*, Oct. 1961, p. 61; [c]E. M. Rogers, *Diffusion of Innovation*, New York: Free Press, 1962; [d]various sources.

purchasing cosmetic surgery or an assisted living property. An alternative sequence, "do-feel-learn," is relevant when the audience has high involvement but perceives little or no differentiation within the product category, as in purchasing hospital emergency services or cholesterol-lowering medication. A third sequence, "learn-do-feel," is relevant when the audience has low involvement and perceives little differentiation within the product category, as in purchasing travel vaccine or health insurance. By choosing the right sequence, the marketer can do a better job of planning communications.[4]

DEVELOPING EFFECTIVE COMMUNICATIONS

Effective communications require eight steps:

1. Identify the target audience

2. Determine the objectives

3. Design the communications

4. Select the communications channels

5. Establish the budget

6. Choose the media mix

7. Measure results

8. Manage the integrated marketing communications process

Identify the Target Audience

The process must start with a clear target audience in mind. The target audience includes the potential buyers of the organization's products, current users, deciders or influencers, individuals, groups, particular publics, or the general public. The target audience is a critical influence on the communicator's decisions about what to say, how to say it, when to say it, where to say it, and to whom to say it.

A major part of audience analysis is assessing the current image of the company, its products, and its competitors. *Image* is the set of beliefs, ideas, and impressions a person holds regarding an object. People's attitudes and actions toward an object are highly conditioned by that object's image.

The first step is to measure the target audience's knowledge of the object, using the *familiarity scale:*

| Never | Heard of | Know a | Know a Fair | Know Very |
| Heard of | Only | Little Bit | Amount | Well |

If most respondents circle only the first two categories, the challenge is to build greater awareness.

Respondents who are familiar with the product can then be asked how they feel toward it, using the *favorability scale:*

| Very | Somewhat | Somewhat | Very | |
| Unfavorable | Unfavorable | Indifferent | Favorable | Favorable |

If most respondents check the first two categories, then the organization must overcome a negative image problem.

The two scales can be combined to develop insight into the nature of the communications challenge. Suppose area residents are asked about their familiarity with and attitudes toward four local hospitals: A, B, C, and D. Hospital A has the most positive image: most people know it and like it. Hospital B is less familiar to most people, but those who know it like it. Hospital C is viewed negatively by those who know it, but—fortunately for the hospital—not too many people know it. Hospital D is seen as a poor hospital, and everyone knows it.

Each hospital faces a different communications task. Hospital A must work at maintaining its good reputation and high awareness. Hospital B must gain the attention of more people. Hospital C must find out why people dislike it and must take steps to improve its quality while keeping a low profile. Hospital D should lower its profile, improve its quality, and then seek public attention.

FOR EXAMPLE

Conducting an Image Analysis

Every brand manager should research the specific content of the product's image. The most popular tool for this research is the *semantic differential*, a five-step process detailed in the following list.[5]

1. *Developing a set of relevant dimensions.* The researcher asks people to identify the dimensions they would use in thinking about the object: "What things do you think of when you consider a hospital?" If someone suggests "quality of medical care," this dimension is turned into a five- or seven-point bipolar adjective scale, with "inferior medical care" at one end and "superior medical care" at the other. A set of additional dimensions for a hospital is shown.

2. *Reducing the set of relevant dimensions.* The number of dimensions should be reduced to avoid respondent fatigue.

3. *Administering the instrument to a sample of respondents.* The respondents are asked to rate one object at a time. The bipolar adjectives should be randomly arranged so that the unfavorable adjectives are not all listed on one side.

4. *Averaging the results.* Figure 13.4 shows the results of averaging the respondents' pictures of hospitals A, B, and C (hospital D is omitted). Each hospital's image is represented by a vertical "line of means" that summarizes average perception of that hospital. Hospital A is seen as a large, modern, friendly, and superior hospital. Hospital C, in contrast, is seen as small, dated, impersonal, and inferior.

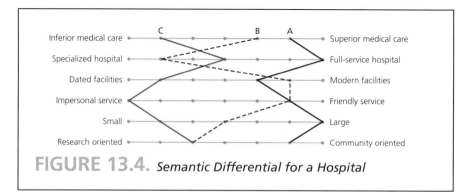

FIGURE 13.4. *Semantic Differential for a Hospital*

Note: A, B, and C refer to the hospitals in the example.
Source: Kotler, *Marketing Management*, 11th ed. Upper Saddle River, N.J.: Prentice-Hall, 2003, p. 567.

5. *Checking on the image variance.* Because each image profile is a line of means, it does not reveal image variability. Did everyone see Hospital B this way, or was there considerable variation? In the first case, we would say that the image is highly specific; in the second case, highly diffused. Some organizations prefer a diffused image so that different groups will see the organization in different ways.

Images are "sticky," and they tend to persist long after the organization has changed. Image persistence is explained by the fact that once people have a certain image, they perceive what is consistent with it. It will take highly disconfirming information to raise doubts and open their minds, especially when people do not have continuous or new firsthand experiences with the changed item, as is often the case for health care services and products that are used sporadically.

Determine the Communications Objectives

Rossiter and Percy identify four possible communications objectives, as follows:[6]

- *Category need:* Consumers recognize a product or service category in which they have a need. Communicating a new class of health care product, such as when Viagra became available, always begins with a statement that establishes the category need.

- *Brand awareness:* Consumers identify, recognize, or recall the name of a brand within the category. Recognition is easier to achieve than recall; but recall is important outside the store, whereas brand recognition is important inside the store. Brand awareness provides a foundation for brand equity.

- *Brand attitude:* Consumers evaluate whether a particular brand might meet a currently relevant need. Relevant brand needs may be *negatively originated* (problem removal, problem avoidance, incomplete satisfaction, normal depletion) or *positively oriented* (sensory gratification, intellectual stimulation, or social approval).

- *Brand purchase intention:* Consumers give self-instructions to purchase the brand or to take purchase-related action.

The most effective communications often achieve multiple objectives.

Design the Communications

Defining the communications to achieve the desired response will require solving three problems: what to say (*message strategy*), how to say it (*creative strategy*), and who should say it (*message source*).

Message Strategy. In determining message strategy, management searches for appeals, themes, or ideas that will tie into the brand positioning and help to establish points-of-parity or points-of-difference. Some of these points may be related directly to product or service performance, such as the quality, economy, or value of the brand. Others may relate to more extrinsic considerations, such as the perception of the brand as contemporary, popular, or traditional. It is widely believed that industrial buyers are most responsive to performance messages. They are knowledgeable about the product, trained to recognize value, and accountable to others for their choices. Consumers, when they buy certain big-ticket items, also tend to gather information and estimate benefits.

Creative Strategy. Communication effectiveness depends on how a message is being expressed as well as the content of the message itself. An ineffective communication may reflect the fact that the wrong message was used or that the right message was just being expressed poorly. *Creative strategies* are the approaches that marketers employ to express their messages; they are how marketers translate their messages into a specific communication. Creative strategies can be broadly classified as involving either "informational" or "transformational" appeals.[7]

An *informational appeal* rationally elaborates on product or service attributes or benefits. Examples of informational creative strategies in advertising are: *problem-solution ads* (Excedrin stops headache pain quickly), *product demonstration ads* (Effergrip Denture Adhesive Cream can withstand the pressure of biting into an apple), *product comparison ads* (Crestor, the cholesterol-lowering drug, prices all dosages the same, compared with Lipitor, which has higher prices for higher doses), and *testimonials* from an unknown or celebrity endorser (Cheryl Ladd, formerly of the TV show *Charlie's Angels*, subtly promoting hormone replacement therapy drugs made by Wyeth Pharmaceuticals). Informational appeals assume the consumer rationally processes the communication so that logic and reason rule. Exhibit 13.1 summarizes a hospital print ad campaign focused on informing consumers about the proficiency of its physicians. Figures 13.5 and 13.6 present newspaper advertising and direct-mail invitations that were part of the campaign.

The research of Hovland, Lumsdaine, and Sheffield has shed much light on informational appeals and their relation to conclusion drawing, one-sided versus two-sided arguments, and order of presentation.[8] Some early experiments supported stating conclusions for the audience rather than allowing the viewer to reach his or her own. Subsequent research, however, indicates that the best ads ask questions and allow readers and viewers to form their own conclusions.[9] Conclusion drawing can cause negative reactions if the communicator is seen as untrustworthy or the issue is seen as too simple or too highly personal. Drawing too explicit a conclusion can also limit appeal or acceptance. Some stimulus ambiguity can lead to a broader market definition and more spontaneous purchases.

Although one-sided presentations that praise a product might seem more effective than two-sided arguments that also mention shortcomings, two-sided messages may be more appropriate when some negative association must be overcome. In this spirit, Listerine ran the message "Listerine tastes bad twice a day."[10] Two-sided messages are more effective with more educated audiences and those who are

EXHIBIT 13.1. Consumer Print Campaign Promoting Hospital Physician Staff

HOSPITAL

Prince William Hospital

LOCATION

Manassas, Virginia

SITUATION

Affluent newcomers used to big-city health care options are seeking a better quality of life in Prince William County, contributing to record-breaking population growth. Prince William Health System is carrying out a plan to expand its services and facilities to gain market share in this highly competitive health care environment.

CHALLENGE

Convince these health care-savvy newcomers that they don't need to drive past Prince William Hospital and head toward Washington, D.C., for medical care.

SOLUTION

Knowing that physicians act as a gateway for patients to use hospital services, the Franklin Street advertising agency developed a marketing plan to promote qualified physicians who would have a halo effect on the entire hospital. The creative strategy involved developing newspaper ad and direct mail templates that featured a different specialty each quarter. Newspaper ads focused on innovative procedures the physicians were using and invited consumers to seminars. A direct-mail piece, which was targeted toward affluent communities, covered a broader health topic and included invitations to privately held seminars.

RESULTS

After the media ran, first-time visits to Prince William Hospital's Web site increased 28 percent and returning visits increased 16 percent. The physician seminars experienced record-breaking attendance. Calls to the Physician Finder service, which was promoted heavily through the campaign, rose 24 percent.

Source: Franklin Street Marketing, 2007.

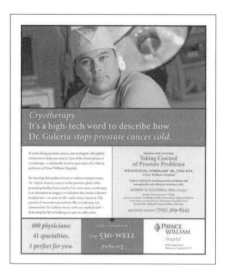 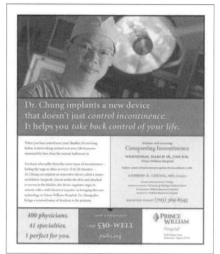

FIGURE 13.5. *Newspaper Advertisements*

initially opposed to the product.[11] The reader should note that in some cases, such as direct-to-consumer advertising of prescription pharmaceuticals, two-sided advertising is a legal requirement. Further, such disclosure may mitigate potential legal problems in case of adverse reactions.

The *order* in which arguments are presented is also important.[12] In the case of a one-sided message, presenting the strongest argument first has the advantage of arousing attention and interest. This method is important in newspapers and other media whose audience often does not attend to the whole message. With a captive audience, however, a climactic presentation might be more effective. In the case of a two-sided message, if the audience is initially opposed, the communicator might start with the other side's argument and conclude with his or her strongest argument.[13]

A *transformational appeal* elaborates on a non-product-related benefit or image. It might depict what kind of person uses a brand (Claritin allergy tablets ads show different types of people before and after taking the drug to help them with allergies) or what kind of experience results from the delivery of a service brand (as when Methodist Hospital in Houston advertised to compassionate, mission-driven people to recruit them to work as nurses with their "Leading Medicine" multimedia campaign). Transformational appeals often attempt to stir up negative or positive emotions that will motivate purchase. Many communicators use negative appeals such as fear, guilt, and shame to get people to do things (brush their teeth, have an annual health checkup) or stop doing things (smoking, abusing alcohol, or overeating). Fear appeals work best when they are not too strong. Research indicates that

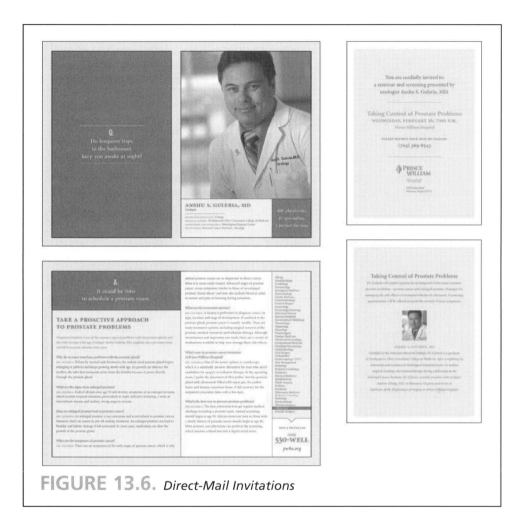

FIGURE 13.6. *Direct-Mail Invitations*

neither extremely strong nor extremely weak fear appeals are as effective as moderate ones. Furthermore, fear appeals work better when source credibility is high and when the communication promises to relieve, in a believable and efficient way, the fear it arouses.[14] Messages are most persuasive when they are moderately discrepant with what the audience believes. Messages that state only what the audience already believes at best only reinforce beliefs; if the messages are too discrepant, they will be counter-argued and disbelieved.

Communicators also use positive emotional appeals such as humor, love, pride, and joy. Motivational or "borrowed interest" devices—such as the presence of cute babies, frisky puppies, popular music, or provocative sex appeals—are often employed to attract consumer attention and raise their involvement with an ad.

Such techniques are thought to be necessary in the tough new media environment characterized by low-involvement consumer processing and much competing ad and programming clutter. One challenge in arriving at the best creative strategy is figuring out how to "break through the clutter" to attract the attention of consumers—but still be able to deliver the intended message.

Message Source. Many communications do not use a source beyond the company itself. Others use known or unknown people. Messages delivered by attractive or popular sources can potentially achieve higher attention and recall, which is why advertisers often use celebrities as spokespeople. Celebrities are likely to be effective when they personify a key product attribute. The three factors underlying source credibility are expertise, trustworthiness, and likability.[15] *Expertise* is the specialized knowledge the communicator possesses to back the claim. *Trustworthiness* is related to how objective and honest the source is perceived to be. Friends are trusted more than strangers or salespeople, and people who are not paid to endorse a product are viewed as more trustworthy than people who are paid.[16] *Likability* describes the source's attractiveness. Qualities like candor, humor, and naturalness make a source more likable.

The most highly credible source would be a person who scores high on all three dimensions. Pharmaceutical companies want doctors to testify about product benefits because doctors have high credibility. Antidrug crusaders will use ex-drug addicts because they have higher credibility for students than teachers do. Television news anchor Katie Couric does public service announcements for colon cancer screening; part of her effectiveness is based on the potentially curable, undiagnosed colon cancer that caused her husband's death in his forties.

If a person has a positive attitude toward a source and a message, or a negative attitude toward both, a state of *congruity* is said to exist. What happens if the person holds one attitude toward the source and the opposite toward the message? Suppose a consumer hears a likable celebrity praising a brand that she dislikes? Osgood and Tannenbaum posit that *attitude change will take place in the direction of increasing the amount of congruity between the two evaluations*.[17] The consumer will end up respecting the celebrity somewhat less or respecting the brand somewhat more. If she encounters the same celebrity praising other disliked brands, she will eventually develop a negative view of the celebrity and maintain her negative attitudes toward the brands. The *principle of congruity* implies that communicators can use their good image to reduce some negative feelings toward a brand but might, in the process, lose some of the audience's esteem.

Companies that sell their products to different cultures or in different countries must be prepared to vary their messages. First, they must decide whether the product is appropriate for a country. Second, they must make sure the targeted market segment is both legal and customary. Third, they must decide if the style of the ad is acceptable. Fourth, they must decide whether ads should be created at headquarters or locally.

Ads featuring actual physicians, or even actors wearing white coats who could be mistaken for physicians, were not allowed by the Federal Trade Commission for many years. The rules have changed; now portraying doctors in ads is in style, as evidenced by a multi-media ad campaign for a New York health plan. (See Field Note 13.1.)

FIELD NOTE 13.1.

Physicians Play Starring Roles in Repositioning a Health Plan   Does a health plan known for its affordable monthly premiums also have lower quality doctors? This marketing problem faced management at Group Health, Inc. (G.H.I.), in New York City. The reality was that although G.H.I. premiums were relatively cheap compared to other plans in the area, G.H.I. actually had a number of world-class physicians in its network. Management decided to use advertising to correct this misperception of G.H.I.

The plan felt that consumer attitudes toward plan physicians was a key determinant for those selecting health insurance. Management needed to shift the G.H.I. positioning in the minds of its target market from "affordability" to "access to world-class doctors." With the help of its advertising agency, the plan decided to feature three of its doctors in advertisements that would emphasize that its physicians were outstanding. Three G.H.I. specialists were selected in orthopedics, cardiology, and allergy. All three had been named to the list of New York's "Best Doctors" by *New York* magazine. Television spots were created with each of the three physicians encountering typical New York residents near familiar local landmarks. The overarching concept was to communicate that the G.H.I. network had excellent local doctors who would be available to the average New Yorker if they ever needed them.

For example, one spot shows a middle-aged man, Eddie, eating at a diner. The announcer says, "This is Eddie. Thirty-six years, and never took a sick day." As Eddie leaves the diner, he forgets to take his cap. Dr. Lynn Perry-Böttinger, the featured G.H.I. cardiologist at New York Presbyterian Hospital, returns the cap to Eddie. Another ad shows a man named Dave running through Central Park. The announcer explains, "This is Dave. He made a resolution this year, and so far, he's keeping it." Dave runs past G.H.I. surgeon Dr. Joseph Zuckerman, who is professor and chairman of orthopedic surgery at New York University Hospital for Joint Diseases.

The commercials were shown to consumers in focus groups before they were aired. This qualitative research indicated that the ads would do what they were supposed to do—change the perception of G.H.I. from a lower-cost, lower-quality health plan to a lower-cost, higher-quality health plan. Following the qualitative research, radio, print, web-based, and outdoor media were added to the campaign. Media spending for the campaign was estimated to be between $3 million and $5 million.

Source: S. Elliott, "Doctor, Doctor, Give Me the News," *New York Times*, May 1, 2006.

Select the Communication Channels

Selecting efficient channels to carry the message becomes more difficult as channels of communication become more fragmented and cluttered.

Personal Communication Channels. *Personal communication channels* involve two or more persons communicating directly with each other face-to-face, person-to-audience, over the telephone, or through e-mail. Instant messaging and independent sites to collect consumer reviews are other means of growing importance in recent years. Personal communication channels derive their effectiveness through individualized presentation and feedback. We will discuss this subject in detail in Chapter Fourteen.

Nonpersonal Communication Channels. *Nonpersonal channels* are communications directed to more than one person; they include media, sales promotions, events and experiences, and public relations.

- *Media* consist of print media (newspapers and magazines), broadcast media (radio and television), network media (telephone, cable, satellite, wireless), electronic media (audiotape, videotape, CD-ROM, Web site), and display media (billboards, signs, posters). Most nonpersonal messages come through paid media.

- *Sales promotions* consist of consumer promotions (such as samples, coupons, and premiums), trade promotions (such as advertising and display allowances), and business and sales-force promotions (contests for sales reps).

- *Events and experiences* include sports, arts, entertainment, and "cause" events, as well as less formal activities that create novel brand interactions with consumers.

- *Public relations* include communications directed internally to employees of the company or externally to consumers, other firms, the government, and media.

Much of the recent growth of nonpersonal channels has been with events and experiences (discussed later in this chapter). A company can build its brand image through creating or sponsoring various events. Event marketers have favored sports events and are now using other venues such as art museums, zoos, and ice shows to entertain clients and employees. HCA, the leading for-profit hospital chain, sponsors symphony concerts, stage performances, and art exhibits. Blue Cross Blue Shield of North Carolina is an active sponsor of the former Stanley Cup Champion Carolina Hurricanes ice hockey team; and Pfizer Canada is one of the Principal Founders of Centre iSci, Montreal's new interactive science and entertainment complex.

Events can create attention, although whether they have a lasting effect on brand awareness, knowledge, or preference will vary considerably, depending on the quality of the product, the event itself, its execution, and how often these may recur.

Integration of Communication Channels. Although personal communication is often more effective than nonpersonal mass communication, mass media could be the major means of *stimulating* personal communication. Mass communications affect personal attitudes and behavior through a two-step, flow-of-communication process. Ideas often flow from radio, television, and print to opinion leaders and from these to the less media-involved population groups. This two-step flow has several implications. First, the influence of mass media is dominated by thought leaders—people whose opinions the public seeks or who carry their opinions to others. Second, this process demonstrates that people interact primarily within their own social groups and acquire ideas from their group's opinion leaders. Third, two-step communication suggests that mass communicators should direct messages specifically to thought leaders and let them carry the message to others.[18] Communications by and between a particular group, using customer-generated media, can be found with pediatric cancer patients. (See Field Note 13.2.)

FIELD NOTE 13.2.

Customer-Generated Media: Using Web Communication to Heal   Customer-generated media (CGM) are used by customers to influence other customers. A greater diversity of people can be influential in reaching others with their opinions than through the two-step flow of communication models. For example, young patients with cancer and other serious illnesses often feel alone and have trouble emotionally coping with their disease. *USA Today* reports that the Internet is now permitting patients to interact with one another and share their stories.

Some patients have begun creating blogs or posting messages to discussion boards; others are recording their personal experiences in podcasts that can be downloaded to iPods and other portable audio players. Personal Web pages, *Facebook* and *MySpace* "walls," and other social networking technologies are part of the life fabric of the newest generation of cancer patients. Sites of particular interest to them, including teenswithcancer.org and planetcancer.org, are geared toward young adults. Teens use the web-based venues to discuss their resentment of medications or to speak freely about concerns without worrying about "fitting in." Some hospitals, including Memorial Sloan-Kettering Cancer Center in New York City, are promoting use of the sites by providing internet access at the bedside and even allowing young patients to use cell phones to send text messages from within the hospital. Supporters say the technology allows young patients to stay connected with their friends and schools, as well as to interact with and gain support from other cancer patients. Even with the most advanced technology, a teenage girl with bone cancer said she is reluctant to really bond with other young patients because they all have cancer and "something could happen to them."
Source: L. Szabo, "Kids with Cancer Bond On-line," *USA Today*, Apr. 10, 2006.

Establish the Total Marketing Communications Budget

One of the most difficult marketing decisions is determining how much to spend on promotion. John Wanamaker, the department-store magnate, once said, "I know that half of my advertising is wasted, but I don't know which half." Industries and companies vary considerably in how much they spend on promotion. Expenditures might amount to 30 to 50 percent of sales in the cosmetics industry and 5 to 10 percent in the industrial-equipment industry. Even within the same industry segment, there can be a large variation. There are four common methods for deciding on a budget: affordable, percentage-of-sales, competitive-parity, and objective-and-task.

Affordable Method. Many companies set the promotion budget at what they think the company can afford. The affordable method completely ignores the role of promotion as an investment and the immediate impact of promotion on sales volume. It leads to an uncertain annual budget, which makes long-range planning difficult.

Percentage-of-Sales Method. Many companies set promotion expenditures at a specified percentage of sales (either current or anticipated) or of the sales price. Schonfeld & Associates publishes an annual market research report that forecasts advertising spending as a percentage of net sales by industry and by company. According to the 2007 report, the health care industry was expected to spend 3.4 percent of net sales on advertising, but with a great deal of variation among sectors. More specifically, the pharmaceutical industry was projected to increase spending 10.5 percent in 2007 and exceed $24 billion. The biotech and electro-medical apparatus sectors showed a growth in advertising spending of over 10 percent.[19]

Supporters believe that this method links promotion expenditures to the movement of corporate sales over the business cycle, focuses attention on the interrelationship of promotion and selling price and unit profit, and encourages stability when competing firms spend approximately the same percentage of their sales on promotion. Conversely, the percentage-of-sales method views sales as the determiner of promotion rather than as the result. It leads to a budget set by the availability of funds rather than by market opportunities, discourages experimentation with countercyclical promotion or aggressive spending, and interferes with long-range planning. Finally, it does not encourage building the promotion budget by determining what each product and territory deserves. There is no logical basis for choosing the specific percentage method; companies engage in this practice for historical reasons or to follow what competitors are doing.

Competitive-Parity Method. Some companies set their promotion budget to achieve share-of-voice parity with competitors. Proponents of this method argue that competitors' expenditures represent the collective wisdom of the industry and that maintaining competitive parity prevents promotion wars. Neither argument is valid. Company reputations, resources, opportunities, and objectives differ so much that comparing promotion budgets is not an appropriate guide. Furthermore, there is no evidence that budgets based on competitive parity discourage promotional wars.

Objective-and-Task Method. The objective-and-task method calls on marketers to develop promotion budgets by defining specific objectives, determining the tasks that must be performed to achieve these objectives, and estimating the costs of performing these tasks. The sum of these costs is the proposed promotion budget.

For example, suppose UCLA Medical Center wants to introduce a new sports medicine service for the casual athlete. The objective-and-task method employs six steps to establish a promotion budget.

1. *Establish the market-share goal.* The organization estimates the total number of potential users of this service and sets a target of attracting, say, 8 percent of the market.

2. *Determine the percentage of the market that should be reached by advertising.* Marketers identify a media mix and media weights needed to reach a specific percentage of the total target market. UCLA hopes to reach 80 percent of the prospects with the advertising message.

3. *Determine the percentage of aware prospects who should be persuaded to try the brand.* UCLA would be pleased if 25 percent of aware prospects tried the sports medicine service, based on estimates that 40 percent of all those who tried the service would become loyal users. This target is the market goal.

4. *Determine the number of advertising impressions per 1-percent trial rate.* UCLA estimates that forty advertising impressions, or exposures to a message, for every 1 percent of the target population would bring about a 25-percent trial rate.

5. *Determine the number of gross rating points that must be purchased.* A gross rating point is one exposure to 1 percent of the target population. Because UCLA wants to achieve forty exposures to 80 percent of the population, it will want to buy 3,200 gross rating points.

6. *Determine the necessary advertising budget on the basis of the average cost of buying a gross rating point.* To expose 1 percent of the target population to one impression costs an average of $3,277. Therefore, 3,200 gross rating points would cost $10,486,400 (= $3,277 × 3,200) in the introductory year. The sports medicine service would therefore need to generate at least $10.5 million in profit to reach breakeven expenses from this promotion investment alone. If this level of profit is not expected, then a different or lower-cost promotion investment should be considered.

The objective-and-task method has the advantage of requiring management to spell out its assumptions about the relationships among dollars spent, exposure levels, trial rates, and regular usage. A major question is how much weight marketing communications should receive in relation to alternatives such as product improvement, lower prices, or better service. In theory, the total communications budget should be established so that the marginal profit from the last communication dollar just equals the marginal profit from the last dollar in the best noncommunication use. Implementing this principle, however, is not easy.

Choose the Media Mix

Companies must allocate the marketing communications budget over the six major modes of communication—advertising, sales promotion, public relations and publicity, events and experiences, personal selling (sales force), and direct marketing. The following sections discuss the first four of these modes in depth; then personal selling and direct marketing are overviewed, with a detailed discussion to follow in Chapter Fourteen. We then complete our discussion of the eight steps of developing effective communications, with a consideration of steps 7 and 8.

Within the same industry, companies can differ considerably in their media and channel choices. For example, Tufts-New England Medical Center in Boston concentrates its promotional funds on media relations, whereas Massachusetts General spends heavily on advertising. Between or within similar organizations the product itself can drive communication mix strategies. Consider pharmaceutical companies that invest heavily in direct-to-consumer television spots for certain products while relying on medical journal ads for others. Further, product stage can determine the appropriate mix. For example, during initial launch of a product, a medical device company may want to focus on personal contact with potential high-use physicians while buying mass media ads to raise consumer awareness of the device's benefit. Once the product is more established, more general communications can be used to maintain brand awareness. Organizations are always searching for ways to gain efficiency by replacing one promotional tool with others. For example, many pharmaceutical companies are replacing some field sales activity with ads and direct mail. The substitutability among promotional tools explains why marketing functions must be coordinated and constantly evaluated.

ADVERTISING

Advertising is any paid form of nonpersonal presentation and promotion of ideas, goods, or services by an identified sponsor. Ads can be a cost-effective way to disseminate messages, whether to build brand preference for Pfizer pharmaceuticals or to educate people to lower their cholesterol. Most organizations use an outside agency to help create advertising campaigns and to select and purchase media. Advertising agencies are redefining themselves as *communication companies* and assisting clients in improving their overall communication effectiveness.

When the U.S. Supreme Court ruled in 1975 that professional associations were subject to antitrust laws, organizations—such as the American Medical Association—changed their restrictions on advertising by members. This ruling was followed by other U.S. Supreme Court decisions in 1980 and 1982 that further clarified that restricting advertising was illegal, and physicians and hospitals have been freely advertising ever since. We note, however, that it is legal for these organizations to publish their ethical codes outlining what is professionally acceptable; for example, accurately listing credentials and prohibiting false or exaggerated claims.

Advertising can be used to establish a long-term image for a product (Sucrets sore throat lozenges) or trigger quick sales (a LASIK Vision Institute sale ad for "the first 1,000 eyes"). Advertising can also efficiently reach geographically dispersed buyers. Certain forms of advertising (TV advertising) can require a large budget; other forms (newspaper advertising) are less costly. Research indicates that the presence of advertising alone might have an effect on sales: consumers might believe that a heavily advertised brand must offer "good value."[20] Health care services advertising, however, may provoke a different response. Consumers may think that a doctor who advertises needs more patients—"If he were a good doctor he would not need to solicit patients." Although the many forms and uses of advertising make generalizations difficult,[21] the following qualities can be noted:

- *Pervasiveness:* Advertising permits the seller to repeat a message many times. It also allows the buyer to receive and compare the messages of various competitors. Large-scale advertising says something positive about the seller's size, power, and success.

- *Amplified expressiveness:* Advertising provides opportunities for dramatizing the organization and its products through the artful use of print, sound, and color.

- *Impersonality:* The audience does not feel obligated to pay attention or respond to advertising. Advertising is a monologue in front of—not a dialogue with—the audience.

Developing and Managing an Advertising Program

In developing an advertising program, marketing managers must always start by identifying the target market and buyer motives. Then they can make the five major decisions, known as "the five M's of communication":

Mission: What are the advertising objectives?

Money: How much can be spent?

Message: What message should be sent?

Media: What media should be used?

Measurement: How should the results be evaluated?

These decisions are summarized in Figure 13.7 and described in the following sections.

Setting the Advertising Objectives

The advertising goals and objectives must flow from prior decisions on the target market, brand positioning, and the marketing program. An effective *advertising objective* is a specific communication task and achievement level to be accomplished with a specific audience in a specific period. Advertising objectives can be classified

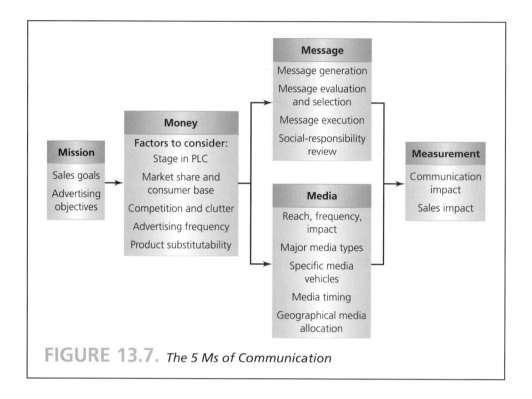

FIGURE 13.7. *The 5 Ms of Communication*

according to their aim: to inform, persuade, remind, or reinforce. They aim at different stages in the *response hierarchy model* presented earlier in this chapter in Figure 13.3.

Informative advertising aims to create brand awareness and knowledge of new products or new features of existing products. The National Ovarian Cancer Coalition uses television public service announcements to increase awareness of ovarian cancer and correct common misconceptions about this disease (see Field Note 13.3). *Persuasive advertising* aims to create liking, preference, conviction about, and purchase of a product or service. Some persuasive advertising uses comparative advertising, which makes an explicit comparison of the attributes of two or more brands. Braun compares its Oral B electric toothbrushes to two competitors in its television ads. *Reminder advertising* aims to stimulate repeat purchase of products and services. Four-color Humana health insurance ads in magazines are intended to remind employees to select Humana when they are in an open enrollment period at work. *Reinforcement advertising* aims to convince current purchasers that they have made the right choice. M. D. Anderson Medical Center ads often depict satisfied patients enjoying simple pleasures and crediting M. D. Anderson for treating their cancers and saving their lives.

FIELD NOTE 13.3.

National Ovarian Cancer Coalition "Breaks the Silence" According to the American Cancer Society, each year more than twenty thousand women are diagnosed with ovarian cancer and more than fifteen thousand will die from the disease, making it the deadliest of all reproductive cancers. Because its symptoms are subtle and frequently mimic other common medical problems, more than 70 percent of cases go unnoticed until the cancer has spread to other regions of the abdomen, when it's most difficult to treat; the chance of living for five years after a later diagnosis is between 20 and 25 percent. If caught earlier, the five-year survival rate for ovarian cancer is 85 to 90 percent.

The National Ovarian Cancer Coalition (NOCC) conducted an online survey in March and April 2006, and just over one thousand women aged forty and older chose to respond to the survey. Only 15 percent of women who responded were familiar with the symptoms of ovarian cancer; 82 percent had never talked to their doctor about the symptoms and risk factors of ovarian cancer; and 67 percent incorrectly believed that a yearly Pap test is effective in the diagnosis of ovarian cancer. Additionally, a media publication audit found that an estimated 14,500 articles on ovarian cancer were published, compared with 96,300 articles devoted to breast cancer.

In response to this low awareness of ovarian cancer and its impact on diagnosis timing and survival rates, NOCC and San Francisco-based public relations firm WeissComm Partners decided to help jumpstart a public dialogue in 2006. Their strategies were as follows:

- Create a compelling umbrella campaign to generate consistent dialogue over an extended period of time at the national and local levels.

- Identify appropriate third-party partners to resonate with younger women through targeted communications channels.

- Leverage NOCC's grassroots infrastructure of nearly eighty local divisions to generate dialogue at the community level throughout the country.

NOCC used a comprehensive range of public relations tactics to support its strategies, which included the following:

- *Updating the NOCC corporate identity to resonate with a younger target audience.* NOCC asked John Magnan, an artist with a personal connection to ovarian cancer, to create a wooden sculpture that honors and personifies the personal triumphs of women battling the disease. This sculpture was the creative inspiration for a new NOCC logo.

- *Identifying a corporate partner to reach women of all ages through creative channels and a captive environment.* NOCC formalized a copromotion partnership with

PureOlogy Serious Colour Care, a company that has made ovarian cancer education part of its mission and one of the few to offer an entire carcinogen-free hair care product line. Together, NOCC and PureOlogy created educational "salon literature" including brochures, posters and product tags that were distributed through ten thousand hair salons across the country in September and October 2006. The company also donated a percentage of proceeds from the sales of certain products to NOCC during these same months. Additionally, PureOlogy actively promoted its relationship with NOCC and dedication to raising awareness of ovarian cancer though its ongoing media outreach to health and beauty reporters.

- *Enlisting a hip celebrity personality with a sincere connection to ovarian cancer to extend the reach of the message*. WeissComm identified and secured Eva LaRue, cast member of CBS's hit show *CSI: Miami* and former *All My Children* star, as the national face and voice for NOCC's first television public service announcement (PSA) that was released in conjunction with Ovarian Cancer Awareness Month in September. As NOCC's national spokeswoman, Eva LaRue—who lost her grandmother and great-grandmother to ovarian cancer—extended the reach of her PSA messages through ongoing national media outreach.

- *Conducting a Satellite Media Tour (SMT) with a physician and an ovarian cancer survivor to reach local morning show and syndicated national radio show audiences throughout the country*.

- *Extended reach through NOCC's eighty divisions by providing them with hands-on training and turnkey toolkits for launching "Break the Silence" initiatives in their communities through local media outreach*.

The post-program results of this effort will not be measured for some time, but the implementation measures included the following:

- Forty-four million media impressions through combined television, radio, PSA, and print placements. Media vehicles included UPI Newswire, *Healthy Living, Saturday Evening Post*, and Medstar Health System syndicated television coverage.

- A 38-percent increase in the number of ovarian cancer stories between June and September 2006 (4,459) compared to same time period in 2005 (3,238).

The advertising objective should emerge from a thorough analysis of the current marketing situation. If the product class is mature, the company is the market leader, and brand usage is low, the proper objective should be to stimulate more usage. If the product class is new and the company is not the market leader, but the brand is superior to that of the leader, then the proper objective is to convince the market of the brand's value and differentiation and to generate trial.

Deciding on the Advertising Budget

Earlier we discussed the methods for determining the promotion budget. Here we present five environmental issues the marketing manager must consider when setting the advertising budget:[22]

- *Product life cycle stage.* New products typically receive large advertising budgets to build awareness and to gain consumer trial. Established brands usually are supported with lower advertising budgets as a ratio to sales.[23]

- *Market share and consumer base.* To maintain their competitive position, high-market-share brands usually require less advertising expenditure as a percentage of sales. The converse is also true: building share requires larger expenditures. On a cost-per-impression basis, it is less expensive to reach consumers of a widely used brand than to reach consumers of low-share brands.

- *Competition and clutter.* In a market with a large number of competitors and high advertising spending, a brand must advertise more heavily to be heard. Even simple clutter from advertisements not directly competitive to the brand creates a need for heavier advertising.

- *Advertising frequency.* The number of repetitions needed to put across the brand's message to consumers has an important impact on the advertising budget and varies with such factors as understanding brand use, familiarity with brand identity, and simplicity or complexity of the message. For example, newer oral contraceptives reduce the number of menstrual periods to few to none per year. Although women are familiar with product characteristics, the brand names and features when first introduced were new and required frequent message exposure.

- *Product substitutability.* Brands in less well-differentiated or commodity-like product classes (such as over-the-counter pain relievers and cotton swabs) require heavy advertising to establish a differential image. Advertising is also important for a brand that can offer unique benefits or features.

Developing the Advertising Campaign

In designing and evaluating an ad campaign, it is important to distinguish the message strategy or positioning (what will be conveyed about the brand) from its creative strategy (how it expresses the brand claims). Advertisers follow three steps to develop a message strategy: message generation and evaluation, creative development and execution, and social responsibility review.

Message Generation and Evaluation. An effective ad normally focuses on one or two core selling propositions. As part of refining the brand positioning, the advertiser should conduct market research to determine which appeal works best with its target audience. The research should be summarized in a creative brief, typically covering one or two pages, covering an elaboration of the positioning statement and including the following elements: key message, target audience, communication objectives (to do, to know, to believe), benefits to promise, supports for the promise, and selected media. All the team members working on the campaign need to agree on the creative brief before moving forward.

Creative Development and Execution.   The ad message's impact depends not only on *what* is said, but also, and often more importantly, on *how* it is said. Message execution can be decisive when brand positioning for competitors is similar. Next, the advertiser can prepare a copy strategy statement describing the objective, content, support, and tone of the desired ad. Advertisers must also consider the specific advantages and disadvantages of each medium as they develop the creative strategy. Television reaches a broad spectrum of consumers, but it can be expensive; print ads can provide detailed product information, yet print media are fairly passive; radio reaches 96 percent of all Americans aged twelve and older, and it is relatively inexpensive, but the lack of visual images and the passive nature of consumer processing are disadvantages.

Social Responsibility Review.   Advertisers and their agencies must be sure advertising does not overstep social and legal norms. Under U.S. law, companies must not do any of the following: engage in false or deceptive advertising; make false claims, such as stating that a product cures something when it does not; create ads that have the capacity to deceive, even though no one may actually be deceived; practice bait-and-switch advertising that attracts buyers under false pretenses; or claim product superiority without valid supporting evidence. To be socially responsible, advertisers must be careful not to offend the general public as well as any ethnic, racial minority, or special-interest groups. Stakeholder opinions about the social value of advertising may differ. For example, although pharmaceutical companies and some disease advocacy groups claim direct-to-consumer (DTC) drug advertisements are effective educational programs, payers and many physicians have criticized these campaigns as encouraging consumers to seek drugs that they may not really need. Field Note 13.4 provides an example of a DTC campaign; the reader can make up his or her own mind about its purported educational value.

FIELD NOTE 13.4.

DTC Advertising and the Case of Roche's Tamiflu   The drug company Roche started its advertising campaign for the prescription antiviral drug Tamiflu at Thanksgiving. The flu affects forty million people every year and the tablet is designed to be taken at the first sign of symptoms to lessen its severity and duration. But was Roche guilty of "creating" demand for a relatively expensive drug that has been shown to have only modest clinical effectiveness?

The ad campaign began at Thanksgiving because it coincided with the potential beginning of the flu season. It included light-hearted advertisements in print publications, trailers in movie theaters, television spots, Web site banner ads, and signs inside airports to attract the attention of families who were traveling to holiday destinations. The ads featured the penguins from the Warner Bros. animated movie *Happy Feet* that opened nationwide the previous week.

The unbranded advertising did *not* mention Tamiflu by name, but it focused on increasing awareness of disease-fighting options. Roche believes that consumers do not realize that there are treatment and prevention options.

The Centers for Disease Control has noted that "the single best way to prevent the flu" is through a vaccine that is given prior to flu exposure. The Food and Drug Administration, which approved Tamiflu in 1999, permits its use to "reduce the chance" of getting the flu during an outbreak or shorten its impact for those who are infected. The Roche-sponsored flufacts.com Web site suggests patients ask doctors for the antiviral just in case they may have a future need for it.

Roche has been criticized by members of the medical profession who contend that Tamiflu has only modest benefits. These doctors also worry that if consumers take antivirals indiscriminately, the virus will build up a resistance to them that could undermine their effectiveness in the case of a widespread flu outbreak.

In the fall of 2005, there was an international avian flu outbreak, and Tamiflu prescriptions in the United States rose seven-fold. Consumers appeared to be purchasing Tamiflu as a preventive measure to store in their medicine cabinets in case the avian flu made it to their city. The recommended dosage for Tamiflu is two tablets per day. The price for ten tablets on an Internet pharmacy site is about $100, and the generic version of Tamiflu is now available for $45.

Source: D. Henderson, "Heads Shaking at Flu Drug Ads," *Boston Globe*, Nov. 1, 2006.

Drug advertising, especially television advertising, can educate patients about new drugs, inform them about silent health conditions, and trigger conversations between doctors and patients. The investment in DTC ads by pharmaceutical companies also has a positive return on investment by increasing the number of prescriptions that doctors write. Every dollar spent on drug advertising creates an extra $4.20 in drug sales, according to a 2005 Kaiser Family Foundation study. Doctors also tend to write eight times more prescriptions in a single year for heavily advertised drugs, according to the Government Accountability Office (GAO).

The opposite view of DTC advertising comes from studies like the one by Weissman and colleagues.[24] Their research found no widespread adverse health effects resulting from drug ads aimed at consumers, but they stated that society still needs to weigh in on the consequences of this advertising. A national telephone survey about health care experiences associated with direct-to-consumer advertising of prescription drugs found that among the 35 percent of the sample who had a physician visit during which DTC was discussed, 25 percent received a new diagnosis and 43 percent were considered high priority according to authoritative sources. More than half also reported actions taken by their physician other than prescribing the advertised drug. Despite concerns about DTC's negative consequences, the researchers found no differences in health effects between patients who took advertised drugs and those who took other prescription drugs. Still, concerns remain. Since the Food and Drug Administration allowed pharmaceutical companies to begin drug advertising on television in 1997, Schering-Plough has aggressively pitched its allergy drug Claritin, spending as much as $185 million in one year. AstraZeneca spent $257 million in a year promoting its acid reduction treatment Nexium. The GAO estimated total DTC spending to be $4.5 billion dollars for 2006. Because of aggressive advertising of such drugs as the painkiller Vioxx (which generated huge profits but was later found to subject thousands of Americans to heart attack risks), consumer drug advertising is facing scrutiny from Congress, consumers, and physicians.

The physician backlash included six resolutions to curb drug ads, which were proposed during the American Medical Association's annual meeting in 2005. In response, the Pharmaceutical Research and Manufacturers of America (PhRMA), the drug industry's lobbying arm, unveiled voluntary guiding principles for advertising in July 2005. PhRMA's document includes a request that companies discuss new drugs with doctors before launching advertising that targets consumers. To adapt to these guidelines and outside pressures, drug companies are reconsidering how they market drugs and explain their risks. For example, Bristol Myers Squibb agreed to withhold any DTC advertising until twelve months after a new drug is launched; Pfizer and Johnson & Johnson settled on a six-month wait. Also, some companies have rolled out new campaigns that sell their brand, rather than an individual product. For instance, Merck is spending roughly $20 million to tell consumers about the role its research played in ending childhood diseases including measles, mumps, and rubella. Forty percent of Merck's new ads also inform patients of programs offering discounted drugs, and patient assistance requests have climbed.

Deciding on Media

The advertiser's next task is to choose the appropriate media to carry the message. The steps here are (1) deciding on desired reach, frequency, and impact; (2) choosing among major media types; (3) selecting specific media vehicles; and (4) deciding on media timing.

Deciding on Reach, Frequency, and Impact. *Media selection* means finding the most cost-effective media to deliver the desired number and type of exposures to the target audience. The advertiser is seeking a specified advertising objective and response from the target audience—for example, a target level of product trial. The rate of product trial will depend on, among other things, the level of brand awareness. The effect on audience awareness depends on the exposures' reach, frequency, and impact:

- *Reach:* The number of different persons or households exposed to a particular media schedule at least once during a specified time period.

- *Frequency:* The number of times within the specified time period that an average person or household is exposed to the message.

- *Impact:* The qualitative value of an exposure through a given medium (thus, a hospital information system ad in *Modern Healthcare* would have a higher impact than in the *Weekly Standard* magazine).

Although audience awareness will be greater with higher reach, frequency, and impact, the media planner must determine the most cost-effective combination. Reach is most important when launching new products, flanker brands, extensions of well-known brands, or infrequently purchased brands or in going after an undefined target market. Frequency is most important when there are strong competitors, a complex story to tell, high consumer resistance, or a frequent-purchase cycle.[25]

Many advertisers believe a target audience needs a large number of exposures for the advertising to work. The job of repetition is partly to put the message into permanent memory. The higher the forgetting rate associated with a brand, product category, or message, the higher the warranted level of repetition. Others doubt the value of high frequency. They believe that after people see the same ad a few times, they either act on it, get irritated by it, or stop noticing it. In other words, ads wear out and viewers tune out.

Choosing Among Major Media Types. The media planner must know the capabilities of the major advertising media types to deliver reach, frequency, and impact. The major advertising media along with their advantages and limitations are profiled in Table 13.1.

Media planners make their choice among media categories by considering the following variables:

- *The target-audience's media habits.* For example, radio, television, and the Web are effective media for reaching teenagers; newspapers and certain magazines are more effective for reaching seniors.

- *Product characteristics.* Media types have different potentials for product demonstration, visualization, explanation, believability, and color.

- *Message characteristics.* A message announcing a major event tomorrow will require radio, TV, or newspaper. A message containing a great deal of technical data might require specialized magazines or mailings.

- *Cost.* Television is typically very expensive, whereas radio advertising is relatively inexpensive. What counts is the cost per thousand exposures to a relevant audience.

Alternative Advertising Options. For a long time, television was the dominant medium. In recent years, however, researchers have noticed reduced effectiveness

TABLE 13.1. **Advertising Media: Their Costs, Advantages, and Limitations**

Medium	Advantages	Limitations
Newspapers	Flexibility; timeliness; good local market coverage; broad acceptance; high believability	Short life; poor reproduction quality; small "pass-along" audience
Television	Combines sight, sound, and motion; appealing to the senses; high attention; high reach	High absolute cost; high clutter; fleeting exposure; less audience selectivity
Direct mail	Audience selectivity; flexibility; no ad competition within the same medium; personalization	Relatively high cost; "junk mail" image
Radio	Mass use; high geographic and demographic selectivity; low cost	Audio presentation only; lower attention than television; nonstandardized rate structure; fleeting exposure
Magazines	High geographic and demographic selectivity; credibility and prestige; high-quality reproduction; long life; good pass-along readership	Long ad purchase lead time; some waste circulation; no guarantee of position without premium price
Outdoor	Flexibility; high repeat exposure; low cost; low competition	Limited audience selectivity; creative limitations
Yellow Pages	Excellent local coverage; high believability; wide reach; low cost	High competition; long ad purchase lead time; creative limitations

(Table 13.1 continued)

Medium	Advantages	Limitations
Newsletters	Very high selectivity; full control; interactive opportunities; relative low costs	Costs could run away
Brochures	Flexibility; full control; can dramatize messages	Overproduction could lead to runaway costs
Telephone	Many users; opportunity to give a personal touch	Relative high cost unless volunteers are used
Internet	High selectivity; interactive possibilities; relatively low cost	Relatively new medium with a low number of users in some countries or regions

due to increased commercial clutter, increased zipping and zapping of commercials aided by TiVo and Replay TV, and smaller audiences per channel owing to the growth in cable and satellite TV and VCRs. Furthermore, television advertising costs have risen faster than other media costs. Marketers are increasingly looking to go beyond traditional media to find more cost-effective alternatives.[26]

Place advertising, also called out-of-home advertising, is a broadly defined category that captures many different advertising forms outside traditional media. Marketers are using creative and unexpected ad placements that they hope will grab consumers' attention. The rationale for this practice is that it might be better to reach people in diverse settings, such as where they work, play, and, of course, shop. Some of the options available include billboards, public spaces (such as sports arenas, parking meters, buses, and subway stations), product placement, and point-of-purchase locations. Advertisers now can buy space not only in stadiums and arenas, but on garbage cans, bicycle racks, parking meters, airport luggage carousels, elevators, gasoline pumps, airline snacks, shopping carts, and supermarket produce, such as tiny labels on apples, bananas, and eggs. The main advantage of nontraditional media is that a very targeted and captive audience can often be reached in a cost-effective manner. Because out-of-home ads must be quickly processed, however, the message must be simple and direct. Strategically, out-of-home advertising is often more effective at enhancing brand awareness or reinforcing brand image than creating new brand associations.

These new marketing strategies and tactics must ultimately be judged for how they enhance brand equity, as unique ad placements designed to break through clutter may also be perceived as invasive and obtrusive. Consumer backlash has occurred when people see ads in traditionally ad-free spaces, such as in schools, on police cruisers, and in doctors' waiting rooms. A successful example of this advertising tactic is Chicago-based Northwestern Memorial Hospital's use of bus wraps. These signs, covering the outside of city buses, bore different Northwestern Memorial ad slogans and phone numbers. The ads generated consumer call volumes that met the hospital's objectives.

The media planner searches for the most cost-effective vehicles within each chosen media type, relying on measurement services that provide estimates of audience size, composition, and media cost. Audience size can be measured according to

- Circulation—the number of physical units carrying the advertising
- Audience—the number of people exposed to the vehicle (with pass-on readership, a print vehicle's audience is larger than circulation figures suggest)
- Effective audience—the number of people with target audience characteristics exposed to the vehicle
- Effective ad-exposed audience—the number of people with target audience characteristics who actually saw the ad

Knowing the audience size, media planners calculate the cost per thousand persons reached by a vehicle. If a full-page, four-color ad in *Newsweek* costs $200,000 and *Newsweek*'s estimated readership is 3.1 million people, the cost of exposing the ad to 1,000 persons is approximately $65. The same ad in *Business Week* may cost $70,000 but reach only 970,000 persons—at a cost-per-thousand of $72. The media planner ranks each magazine by cost-per-thousand and favors magazines with the lowest cost-per-thousand for reaching target consumers. The magazines themselves often put together a "reader profile" for their advertisers, summarizing the characteristics of the magazine's readers with respect to age, income, residence, marital status, and leisure activities.

Deciding on Media Timing. In choosing media, the advertiser faces both macro and micro scheduling challenges. The macro challenge involves scheduling the advertising in relation to seasons and the business cycle. For example, if 70 percent of a product's sales occur between June and September, the firm can vary its advertising expenditures to follow the seasonal pattern, to oppose the seasonal pattern, or to be constant throughout the year. Although hospitals very often go into an ad-spending hiatus in the June through August summer months, consumers continue to make health care buying decisions and form images of hospitals during this period. By contrast, health insurance plans anticipate employer open enrollment periods starting in November and advertise around this schedule.

The micro challenge calls for allocating advertising expenditures within a short episode to obtain maximum impact. Over a given period, advertising messages can be concentrated ("burst" advertising), dispersed continuously, or dispersed intermittently. The advertiser must decide whether to schedule advertising messages with a level, rising, falling, or alternating frequency.

In launching a new product, the advertiser has to choose among ad continuity, concentration, flighting, and pulsing. *Continuity* is achieved by scheduling exposures evenly throughout a given period. Generally, advertisers use continuous advertising in an expanding market with frequently purchased items, and in tightly defined buyer categories. *Concentration* calls for spending all the advertising dollars in a single period; it is more appropriate for products with one selling season or holiday. *Flighting* calls for advertising for some period, followed by a hiatus with no advertising, followed by a second period of advertising activity. It is used when funding is limited or the purchase cycle is relatively infrequent, and with seasonally purchased items. Health care purchases that fall into the seasonal category include elective surgeries and eyeglasses; spending on these items tend to occur at the end of the year to use up money in flexible spending accounts or to take advantage of lower out-of-pocket costs because annual deductibles have been met. *Pulsing* is continuous advertising at low intensity levels, reinforced periodically by waves of heavier activity. Those who favor pulsing believe that the audience will learn the message more thoroughly by this method and money can be saved.

A firm must decide how to allocate its advertising budget over space as well as over time. The company makes *national buys* when it places ads on national TV networks or in nationally circulated magazines. It makes *spot buys* when it buys TV time in just a few markets or in regional editions of magazines. These markets are called *areas of dominant influence* (ADIs) or *designated marketing areas* (DMAs). The company makes local buys when it advertises in local newspapers, radio, or outdoor sites.

Evaluating Advertising Effectiveness

Good planning and control of advertising depends on measures of advertising effectiveness. Advertisers should measure not only the communication effect of an ad— that is, its potential effect on awareness, knowledge, or preference—but also how it affects utilization and revenue. Hospitals have particular difficulty in measuring advertising effectiveness because individual patients purchase their services relatively infrequently. Additionally, most hospitals do not have the information systems to identify particular patients who may be motivated by the advertising to actually use their services.

Communication-effect research seeks to determine whether an ad is communicating effectively. Also called *copy testing*, it can be done before an ad is placed with the media (pretesting) and after it is placed (posttesting). There are three major methods of advertising pretesting. The *consumer feedback method* asks consumers for their reactions to a proposed ad. *Portfolio tests* ask consumers to view or listen to a portfolio of advertisements, taking as much time as they need. Consumers are then asked to recall all the ads and their content, aided or unaided by the interviewer. Recall level indicates an ad's ability to stand out and to have its message understood and remembered. Vanderbilt University Medical Center conducted consumer focus groups with the main purpose of determining if consumers found value in a hospital that had sophisticated health information systems. The Medical Center's advertising agency also prepared twenty different positioning statements related to information systems, and the group members were asked to rank them in order of preference. The results of the research were used in the development of a consumer advertising campaign based on health information systems.

Laboratory tests use equipment to measure physiological reactions to an ad, including heartbeat, blood pressure, pupil dilation, galvanic skin response, and perspiration measurement. Alternatively, consumers may be asked to turn a knob to indicate their moment-to-moment liking or interest while viewing sequenced material.[27]

These tests measure attention-getting power but reveal nothing about impact on beliefs, attitudes, intentions, or message retention.

Sales-effect research is complex because sales are influenced by many factors beyond advertising, such as the product's features, price, and availability, as well as competitors' actions. The sales impact is easiest to measure in direct-marketing situations and hardest to measure in brand or corporate image-building advertising.

Companies are generally interested in finding out whether they are over-spending or under-spending on advertising. A company's *share of advertising expenditures* produces a *share of voice* (percentage of company advertising of that product compared to all advertising of that product) that earns a *share of consumers' minds and hearts* and, ultimately, a *share of market*.

Researchers try to measure the sales impact through analyzing either historical or experimental data. The *historical approach* involves correlating past sales to past advertising expenditures using advanced statistical techniques.[28]

Other researchers use an *experimental design* to measure advertising's sales impact. A growing number of researchers are striving to measure the sales effect of advertising expenditures instead of settling for communication-effect measures.

SALES PROMOTION

Sales promotion, a key ingredient in marketing campaigns, consists of a diverse collection of incentive tools, mostly short term, designed to stimulate quicker or greater purchase of particular products or services by consumers or the trade.[29]

Whereas advertising offers a *reason* to buy, sales promotion offers an *incentive* to buy. Sales promotion includes tools for *consumer promotion* (samples, coupons, cash refund offers, prices off, premiums, prizes, patronage rewards, free trials, warranties, tie-in promotions, cross-promotions, point-of-purchase displays, and demonstrations), *trade promotion* (prices off, advertising and display allowances, and free goods), and *business* and *sales-force promotion* (trade shows and conventions, contests for sales reps, and specialty advertising).

Purpose of Sales Promotion

Sales-promotion tools vary in their specific objectives. A free sample stimulates consumer trial, whereas a free management-advisory service aims at cementing a long-term relationship with a retailer.

Sellers use incentive-type promotions to attract new triers, to reward loyal customers, and to increase the repurchase rates of occasional users. Sales promotions often attract brand switchers, who are primarily looking for low price, good value, or premiums. Sales promotions generally are unlikely to turn them into loyal users, although they may be induced to make some subsequent purchases.[30]

Sales promotions used in markets of high brand similarity can produce a high sales response in the short run but little permanent gain in market share. In markets of high brand dissimilarity, sales promotions may be able to alter market shares permanently.

Major Decisions in Sales Promotion

In using sales promotion, a company must establish its objectives, select the tools, develop the program, pretest the program, implement and control it, and evaluate the results.

Establishing Objectives. Sales-promotion objectives are derived from broader promotion objectives, which are derived from more basic marketing objectives developed for the product. For consumers, objectives include encouraging purchase of larger-sized units, building trial among nonusers, and attracting switchers away from competitors' brands. Ideally, promotions with consumers would have short-run sales impact as well as long-run brand equity effects. For wholesalers, objectives include persuading retailers to carry new items and higher levels of inventory, incentivizing off-season buying, encouraging stocking of related items, offsetting competitive promotions, building brand loyalty, and gaining entry into new retail outlets. For the sales force, objectives include encouraging support of a new product or model, encouraging more prospecting, and stimulating off-season sales.[31]

Selecting Consumer-Promotion Tools. The promotion planner should take into account the type of market, sales-promotion objectives, competitive conditions, and each tool's cost-effectiveness. We can distinguish between sales-promotion tools that are "consumer-franchise building," which reinforce the consumer's brand preference, and those that are not. The former impart a selling message along with the deal, as in the case of free samples, frequency awards, coupons when they include a selling message, and premiums when they are related to the product. Sales-promotion tools that typically are not consumer-franchise building include price-off packs, consumer premiums not related to a product, contests and sweepstakes, consumer refund offers, and trade allowances. Consumer franchise building promotions offer the best of both worlds—building brand equity while moving product.

Selecting Trade-Promotion Tools. Manufacturers use a number of trade-promotion tools. Surprisingly, a higher proportion of the promotion pie is devoted to trade-promotion tools (46.9 percent) than to consumer promotion (27.9 percent). Manufacturers award money to the trade (1) to persuade the retailer or wholesaler to carry the brand; (2) to persuade the retailer or wholesaler to carry more units than the normal amount; (3) to induce retailers to promote the brand by featuring, display, and price reductions; and (4) to stimulate retailers and their sales clerks to push the product.

Developing the Program. In planning sales-promotion programs, marketers are increasingly blending several media into a total campaign concept. In deciding to use a particular incentive, marketers have several factors to consider. First, they must determine the *size* of the incentive. A certain minimum is necessary to attract customer attention if the promotion is to succeed. Second, the marketing manager must establish *conditions* for participation. Incentives might be offered to everyone or to select groups. Third, the marketer has to decide on the *duration* of promotion. According to one researcher, the optimal frequency is about three weeks per quarter, and optimal duration is the length of the average purchase cycle.[32] Fourth, the marketer must choose a *distribution vehicle*. A discount coupon can be distributed in the package, in stores, by mail, or in advertising.

Fifth, the marketing manager must establish the *timing* of promotion. Finally, the marketer must determine the *total sales-promotion budget*. The cost of a particular promotion consists of the administrative cost (printing, mailing, and promoting the deal) and the incentive cost (cost of premium or cents-off, including redemption costs), multiplied by the expected number of units that will be sold on the deal. In the case of a coupon deal, the cost would take into account the fact that only a fraction of the consumers will redeem the coupons.

Pretesting, Implementing, Controlling, and Evaluating the Program

Although most sales-promotion programs are designed on the basis of the marketer's experience, pretests can be conducted to determine if the tools are appropriate, the incentive size optimal, and the presentation method efficient. Consumers can be asked to rate or rank different possible deals, or trial tests can be run in limited geographic areas.

To evaluate the program, manufacturers can use three methods: sales data, consumer surveys, and experiments. The first method involves using scanner sales data. Marketers can analyze the types of people who took advantage of the promotion, what they bought before the promotion, and how they behaved later toward the brand and other brands. Did the promotion attract new triers and also stimulate more purchasing by existing customers?

In general, sales promotions work best when they attract competitors' customers to try a superior product and these customers switch. If the company's product is not superior, the brand's share is likely to return to its prepromotion level. If more information is needed, *consumer surveys* can be conducted to learn how many recall the promotion, what they thought of it, how many took advantage of it, and how the promotion affected subsequent brand-choice behavior.[33] Sales promotions can also be evaluated through *experiments* that vary such attributes as incentive value, duration, and distribution media. For example, coupons can be sent to half of the households in a consumer panel. Scanner data can be used to track whether the coupons led more people to buy the product immediately and in the future.

Beyond the cost of specific promotions, management must recognize additional costs. First, promotions might decrease long-run brand loyalty by making more consumers deal-prone rather than advertising-prone. Second, promotions can be more expensive than they appear. Some are inevitably distributed to the wrong consumers. Third, there are the costs of special production runs, extra sales-force effort, and handling requirements. Finally, certain promotions irritate retailers, who may demand extra trade allowances or refuse to cooperate.[34]

Sales promotion tactics are used for over-the-counter health care products sold at drug stores, grocery stores, and mass merchandisers. They are also used by pharmaceutical companies to promote physician trials of new medications or enhance use of existing drugs. For example, a drug rep will supply a physician with coupons to give to patients when prescribing certain medications. These coupons provide four types of patient benefits: free medication (such as thirty free pills or waiver of co-payment when the prescription is filled), discount on the cost of purchase, an offer for a value-added service (such as phone counseling on diet for diabetic patients), or discounts on related products that are tie-ins with other companies (for example, test strips for diabetic patients so they can check their blood sugars).

PUBLIC RELATIONS AND PUBLICITY

Public relations has been the traditional promotional tool of choice for health care service marketers. Before hospitals had "marketing" departments, they had public relations departments primarily to act as a go-between with the media and the community. Academic medical centers relied on their news and public affairs departments to send releases to the media that proclaimed advances in medical research. The appeal of public relations and publicity is based on three distinctive qualities: (1) high credibility (news stories and features are more authentic and credible to readers than ads), (2) ability to catch buyers off guard (reaching prospects who prefer to avoid salespeople and advertisements), and (3) dramatization (the potential for dramatizing a company or product with a story).

Not only must the organization relate beneficially to customers, suppliers, and dealers, but it must also relate to a large number of interested publics. A *public* is any group that has an actual or potential interest in or impact on an organization's ability to achieve its objectives. *Public relations* (PR) involves a variety of programs designed to promote or protect a company's image or its individual products.

The wise company takes concrete steps to manage successful relations with its key publics. Most companies have a public relations department that monitors the attitudes of the organization's stakeholders and distributes information and communications to build goodwill. The best PR departments spend time counseling top management to adopt positive programs and to eliminate questionable practices so that negative publicity does not arise in the first place. They perform the following five functions:

- *Press relations:* Presenting news and information about the organization in the most positive light

- *Product publicity:* Sponsoring efforts to publicize specific products

- *Corporate communication:* Promoting understanding of the organization through internal and external communications

- *Lobbying:* Dealing with legislators and government officials to promote or defeat legislation and regulation

- *Counseling:* Advising management about public issues and company positions and image during both good times and crises

Marketing Public Relations

Many companies are turning to *marketing public relations* (MPR) to directly support corporate or product promotion and image making. MPR, like financial PR and community PR, serves a special constituency—namely, the marketing department.[35]

The old name for MPR was *publicity*, which was seen as the task of securing editorial space—as opposed to paid space—in print and broadcast media to promote or "hype" a product, service, idea, place, person, or organization. MPR goes beyond simple publicity and plays an important role in the following tasks:

- *Assisting in the launch of new products.* At the successful introduction of a new heart center at a hospital in the Midwest, employees gathered outside to form a "live" human heart, and aerial photos and video were shot.

- *Assisting in repositioning a mature product.* Pfizer Consumer Healthcare (subsequently purchased by Johnson & Johnson) prepared a news campaign around Listerine PocketMist, a "portable shower" for the mouth in the latest repositioning for this antiseptic mouth wash. (Listerine was invented in the nineteenth century as a powerful surgical antiseptic. It was later sold, in a distilled form, as a floor cleaner and a cure for gonorrhea. Listerine became successful only in the 1920s when it was positioned as a solution for "chronic halitosis," the faux medical term that the Listerine advertising group created in 1921 to describe bad breath. By naming and thus creating a medical condition for which consumers now felt they needed a cure, Listerine created a market for their mouthwash.)

- *Building interest in a product category.* Companies and trade associations have used MPR to rebuild interest in categories where attention has declined. For example, the Immunization Action Council creates and distributes educational materials for health professionals and the public that enhance the delivery of safe and effective immunization services.

- *Influencing specific target groups.* Established in 1978 in response to the health care crisis in the Puerto Rican community, the Hispanic Health Council (HHC) is a community-based, nonprofit organization located in Hartford, Connecticut. HC's unique organizational model integrates public advocacy, high-level community-based research, and research-based service to provide outstanding care to the poor and underserved.

- *Defending products that have encountered public problems.* PR professionals must be adept at managing crises. The HealthSouth rehabilitation company had extremely bad press in the 1990s due to alleged management fraud. It launched a PR campaign focused on good corporate governance and high standards of business conduct and ethics that helped it become relisted on the New York Stock Exchange in 2006.

- *Building the corporate image in a way that reflects favorably on its products.* Art Collins, chairman and CEO of medical device maker Medtronic, gives non-marketing speeches and presentations to help create an innovative image for his company.

As the power of mass advertising weakens, marketing managers are turning more to MPR to build awareness and brand knowledge in a cost-effective manner that reaches local communities and specific groups. The company does not pay for the space or time obtained in the media, only for a staff to develop and circulate the stories and manage certain events. If the organization develops an interesting story, it could be picked up by the media and result in millions of dollars in equivalent advertising. Some experts say that consumers are five times more likely to be influenced by editorial copy than by advertising.

Major Decisions in Marketing Public Relations

In considering when and how to use MPR, management must establish the marketing objectives, choose the PR messages and vehicles, implement the plan carefully, and evaluate the results:

- *Establishing the marketing objectives:* MPR can *build awareness* by placing stories in the media to bring attention to a product, service, person, organization, or idea; *add credibility* by communicating the message in an editorial context; boost sales-force and dealer enthusiasm; and *hold down promotion cost*, because MPR costs less than media advertising. MPR is increasingly borrowing the techniques and technology of direct-response marketing to reach target audience members one-on-one.

■ *Choosing messages and vehicles:* The MPR manager must identify or develop interesting stories to tell about the product. Suppose a relatively unknown hospital wants more visibility. The MPR practitioner will search for possible stories. Do any physicians with admitting privileges have unusual backgrounds, or are any working on unusual medical research grants? Are any new and unusual patient services being offered? If there are no interesting stories, the MPR practitioner should propose newsworthy events the hospital could sponsor. Here the challenge is to *create* news. PR ideas include hosting major patient care meetings, inviting expert or celebrity speakers, and developing news conferences. Each event is an opportunity to develop a multitude of stories directed at different audiences.

■ *Implementing and evaluating the plan:* MPR's contribution to the bottom line is difficult to measure because it is used along with other promotional tools. The easiest measure of MPR effectiveness is the number of *exposures* carried by the media. Publicists supply the client with a clippings book showing all the media that have carried news about the product and a summary statement. This measure is not very satisfying because it contains no indication of how many people actually read, heard, or recalled the message and what they thought afterward; nor does it contain information on the net audience reached, because publications overlap in readership. Because publicity's goal is reach, not frequency, it would be more useful to know the number of unduplicated exposures. Once the marketer has taken these steps, the tools listed in Field Note 13.5 can be employed to implement them.

FIELD NOTE 13.5.

Major Tools in Marketing Public Relations

■ *Publications:* Companies rely extensively on published materials to reach and influence their target markets. These include annual reports, brochures, articles, company newsletters and magazines, and audiovisual materials.

■ *Events:* Companies can draw attention to new products or other company activities by arranging special events that will reach the target publics, such as news conferences, seminars, outings, trade shows, exhibits, contests and competitions, and anniversaries.

■ *Sponsorships:* Companies can promote their brands and corporate name by sponsoring sports and cultural events and highly regarded causes.

■ *News:* One of the major tasks of PR professionals is to find or create favorable news about the company, its products, and its people, and to get the media to accept press releases and attend press conferences.

- *Speeches:* Increasingly, company executives must field questions from the media or give talks at trade associations or sales meetings; these appearances can build the company's image.

- *Public-service activities:* Companies can build goodwill by contributing money and time to good causes.

- *Identity media:* Companies need a visual identity that the public immediately recognizes. The visual identity is carried by company logos, stationery, brochures, signs, business forms, business cards, buildings, uniforms, and dress codes.[36]

The best measure of success of an MPR campaign is the resulting change in product awareness, comprehension, or attitude after allowing for the effect of other promotional tools. These improvements can be measured by using statistically valid and reliable pre-MPR and post-MPR surveys. Sales-and-profit impact is of course the most satisfactory measure. For example, new patients who make appointments with a physician practice can be asked how they learned about the practice and its services. The MPR campaign will have a positive return-on-investment if enough new or incremental patients mention that they came to the practice based on exposure to the MPR campaign.

Many health services organizations do not actually measure campaign outcomes. A 2004 survey of hospital planners and marketers conducted by The Advisory Board Company compiled their main objections to calculating ROI on marketing tactics. The results are shown in Table 13.2.[37]

Health care service organizations *can*, however, benefit from borrowing the marketing decision frameworks, performance measures, and campaign effectiveness metrics that are more common among health care consumer product companies. For example, health care consumer product companies typically measure market share using consumer purchase data compiled by A. C. Nielsen. They also measure advertising recall, brand awareness and preference, and product purchase to measure advertising effectiveness and ROI.

EVENTS AND EXPERIENCES

A thoughtfully chosen event or experience that is relevant to the product or service can get the consumer personally involved. Events and experiences are "live" and are naturally very engaging physically and emotionally. They are also less obtrusive and are a "soft sell." Most hospitals host community health fairs to conduct basic blood pressure, cholesterol, and other simple screenings and to distribute healthy lifestyle information.

TABLE 13.2. **Main Obstacles to Calculating ROI on Marketing Tactics**

Cannot isolate effect of different campaigns from other factors	77.4%
Complex consumer decisions make ROI difficult	51.4%
Cannot show short-term effects of long-term campaigns	48.6%
Poor data quality and access to the data	47.3%
Metrics do not reflect long-term effects of campaigns	45.9%
Metrics do not reflect campaign performance	34.2%
Cannot connect campaigns with hospital goals	13.0%

Source: "2004 Survey of Planners and Marketers: Summary Results from the Marketing and Planning Leadership Council's On-line Poll." Washington, D.C.: The Advisory Board Company, Fall 2004, p. 7.

According to the IEG Sponsorship Report, $14.9 billion is projected to be spent on sponsorships in North America during 2007, with 66 percent of this going to sports; another 11 percent to entertainment tours and attractions; 5 percent to festivals, fairs, and annual events; 5 percent to the arts; and 10 percent to cause marketing. The health care and hospital industry is expected to spend 13 percent of the total spent in 2007.[38]

Through its involvement with events, the sponsoring health care provider, by becoming part of a special and more personally relevant moment in consumer lives, can broaden and deepen its relationship with its target market.

It should also be recognized that consumers can have daily experiences with brands that may impact their brand attitudes and beliefs. *Atmospheres* are "packaged environments" that create or reinforce the buyer's leanings toward product purchase. Plastic surgeons' offices are decorated with Oriental rugs and mahogany furniture to communicate luxury, stability, and success.[39]

Events Objectives

Marketers report a number of reasons why they sponsor events:

- *Identifying with a particular target market or life style.* Marketers can link their brands to events popular with either a select or a broad group of consumers. Customers can be targeted geographically, demographically, psychographically, or behaviorally. Events can be chosen based on attendees' attitudes toward and usage of certain products or brands.

- *Increasing awareness of company or product name.* Sponsorship often offers sustained exposure to a brand—a necessary condition to build brand recognition. By skillfully choosing sponsorship events or activities, marketers can enhance identification with a product and thus brand recall.

- *Creating or reinforcing consumer perceptions of key brand image associations.* Events themselves have associations that help to create or reinforce brand associations.

- *Enhancing corporate image dimensions.* Sponsorship is seen as much more of a soft sell and a means to improve perceptions that the company is likable, prestigious, and the like. The marketer often hopes that consumers will credit the company for its sponsorship and favor it in later product choices.

- *Creating experiences and evoking feelings.* Events can also be included as part of an experiential marketing program. The feelings engendered by an exciting or rewarding event may also indirectly link to the brand. Marketers can also use the Web to provide further event support and additional experiences.

- *Express commitment to the community or on social issues.* Often called *cause-related marketing*, these sponsorships frequently involve corporate tie-ins with nonprofit organizations and charities. Avon has strengthened its ties to its female target market through its Avon Breast Cancer Crusade fundraising efforts and events.

- *Entertain key clients or reward key employees.* Many events feature lavish hospitality tents and other special services or activities that are available only for sponsors and their guests. Involving clients with the event in these ways and others can engender goodwill and establish valuable business contacts. From an employee perspective, events can build participation and morale or be used as an incentive.

- *Permit merchandising or promotional opportunities.* Many marketers tie in contests or sweepstakes, in-store merchandising, direct response, or other marketing activities with their event. Kaiser Permanente—the Oakland, California–based health plan—has used a long-term events strategy to deliver its healthy living marketing messages.

FOR EXAMPLE

Health care giant Kaiser Permanente spent an estimated high-six-figure sum on new sponsorships in support of its "Thrive" ad campaign in 2006. One of the nonprofit organization's sponsorship agreements was with USA Diving, giving it the official health care sponsorship of the U.S. National Diving Championships. Kaiser also signed deals with local properties in its nine-state operating territory. These sponsorships include sponsorship of the Los Angeles and Napa Valley triathlons and "presenting" status for the inaugural Disneyland Half Marathon Weekend and the NFL Cleveland Browns Foundation Golf Outing.
Source: IEG Sponsor Report, Feb. 13, 2006.

Despite these potential advantages, there are a number of possible disadvantages to sponsorship. The success of an event can be unpredictable and out of the control of the sponsor. Although many consumers will credit sponsors for providing necessary financial assistance to make an event possible, some consumers may still resent the commercialization of events through sponsorship.

Major Decisions with Events

Developing successful sponsored events involves (1) choosing the appropriate events, (2) designing the optimal sponsorship program for the event, and (3) measuring the effects of events.[40]

Choosing Event Opportunities. Because of the huge cost involved and the number of event opportunities, many marketers are becoming much more strategic about the events with which they will get involved and the manner in which they will do so. There are a number of potential guidelines for choosing events. The marketing objectives and communication strategy that have been defined for the brand must be met by the event. The audience delivered by the event must match the target market of the brand. The event must have sufficient awareness, possess the desired image, and be capable of creating the desired effects with that target market. Consumers must make favorable attributions to the sponsor for its event involvement.

An ideal event might be one that

- Has an audience that closely matches the ideal target market
- Generates much favorable attention
- Is unique but not encumbered with many sponsors
- Lends itself to ancillary marketing activities
- Reflects or even enhances the brand or corporate image of the sponsor

Designing Event Sponsorship Programs. Many marketers believe that it is the marketing program accompanying an event sponsorship that ultimately determines its success. A sponsor can strategically identify itself at an event in a number of ways, including banners, signs, and programs. For more significant and broader impact, however, sponsors typically supplement such activities with samples, prizes, advertising, retail promotions, publicity, and so on. Marketers often note that at least two to three times the amount of the sponsorship expenditure should be spent on related marketing activities. *Event creation* is a particularly important skill in publicizing fundraising drives for nonprofit organizations. Fundraisers have developed a large repertoire of special events, including anniversary celebrations, art exhibits, auctions, benefit evenings, bingo games, book sales, cake sales, contests, dances, dinners, fairs, fashion shows, parties in unusual places, phoneathons, rummage sales, tours, and walkathons. No sooner is one type of event created, such as a walkathon, than competitors spawn new versions, such as readathons, bikeathons, and jogathons.[41]

CIGNA has consistently supported the March of Dimes through its annual walkathon. This long-term commitment builds a solid bond that benefits CIGNA's image and also builds a sense of community among CIGNA employees who do the actual walking during the event.

As a company that works to improve the health of its members, CIGNA's goals are well aligned with those of the March of Dimes. By reducing premature births through supporting March of Dimes information, education, and research initiatives, CIGNA can help families and communities affected by premature birth and reduce its costs of care for this high-risk group.

FOR EXAMPLE

In 2007, for the thirteenth consecutive year, a team of CIGNA employees walked shoulder to shoulder with the March of Dimes in its fight against premature birth. CIGNA was once again a national corporate sponsor of the March of Dimes 2007 WalkAmerica campaign.

CIGNA employees from across the country held special events, collected pledges, and walked miles to raise money for education and research to reduce prematurity and help babies get the healthiest start possible. CIGNA aimed to add to the $19 million it had raised thus far for the March of Dimes.

Source: J. Hartling, "CIGNA Again Joins March of Dimes as National Corporate Sponsor," *PR Newswire*, Apr. 18, 2007.

Measuring Sponsorship Activities

As with public relations, measurement of events is difficult. There are two basic approaches to measuring the effects of sponsorship activities: the *supply-side* method focuses on potential exposure to the brand by assessing the extent of media coverage; the *demand-side* method focuses on reported exposure from consumers. We examine each in turn.

Supply-Side Measures of Sponsorship Effects. Supply-side methods attempt to approximate the amount of time or space devoted in media coverage of an event. For example, the number of seconds that the brand is clearly visible on a television screen or column inches of press clippings covering an event that mention the brand can be estimated. This measure of potential impressions delivered by an event sponsorship is then translated into an equivalent value in advertising dollars according to the fees associated in actually advertising in the particular media vehicle. Some industry consultants have estimated that thirty seconds of TV logo exposure can be worth as much as 25 percent of the cost of a thirty-second TV ad spot.

Although supply-side exposure methods provide quantifiable measures, their validity can be questioned. The difficulty lies in the fact that equating media coverage with advertising exposure ignores the content of the respective communications that consumers receive. The advertiser uses media space and time to communicate a strategically designed message. Media coverage and telecasts only expose the brand and won't necessarily embellish its meaning in any direct way. Although some public relations professionals maintain that positive editorial coverage can be worth five to ten times the advertising equivalency value, it is rare that sponsorship affords the brand such favorable treatment.[42]

Demand-Side Measures of Sponsorship Effects. An alternative measurement approach is the "demand side" method that attempts to identify the effects that sponsorship has on consumers' brand knowledge. Thus, tracking or custom surveys can explore the ability of the event sponsorship to impact awareness, attitudes, or even sales. Event spectators can be identified and surveyed after the event to measure sponsor recall of the event as well as attitudes and intentions toward the sponsor as a result.

In the next chapter, we will discuss both personal selling and direct marketing in depth; a brief overview of these important communication tools follows.

Personal selling is the most effective tool at later stages of the buying process, particularly in building up buyer preference, conviction, and action. Qualities of personal selling are (1) personal interaction (an experiential interaction between two or more people); (2) cultivation of relationships, ranging from a matter-of-fact selling relationship to a deep personal friendship; and (3) response (the buyer feels under some obligation for having listened to the sales talk). Personal selling is very important to health care organizations such as pharmaceutical firms, medical device firms, and health plans; hospitals and physician groups also benefit from personal selling in slightly different forms.

The many forms of *direct marketing* —direct mail, telemarketing, internet marketing—share three distinctive characteristics; all are (1) customized (the message can be prepared to appeal to the particular individual), (2) current (the message can be prepared or modified rapidly), and (3) interactive (the message can evolve based on the recipient's response to it).

FACTORS IN SETTING THE MARKETING COMMUNICATIONS MIX

Organizations must consider several factors in developing their communication mix: type of product market, consumer readiness to make a purchase, and stage in the product life cycle. The organization's market position is also important. Also, consumer and business markets tend to require different promotional allocations. Although advertising is used less than sales calls in business markets, it still plays a significant role in introducing the organization and its products, explaining product features, generating sales leads, legitimizing the firm and its products, and reassuring customers about purchases. Personal selling can also be effective in consumer markets, by helping to persuade dealers to buy more stock and display more of the product, build dealer enthusiasm, sign up more dealers, and grow sales at existing accounts.

Promotional tools vary in cost-effectiveness at different stages of buyer readiness. Advertising and publicity are most important in the awareness-building stage. Customer comprehension is primarily affected by advertising and personal selling. Closing the sale is influenced mostly by personal selling and sales promotion. Reordering is also affected mostly by personal selling and sales promotion, and somewhat by reminder advertising.

Promotional tools also vary in cost-effectiveness at different stages of the product life cycle. Advertising and publicity have the highest cost-effectiveness in the introduction stage, followed by personal selling to gain distribution coverage and sales promotion to induce trial. In the growth stage, demand gains its own momentum through word of mouth, and the intensity of use of all tools can be reduced. In the maturity stage, sales promotion, advertising, and personal selling all grow more important in that order. The decline stage calls for strong sales promotions, reduced advertising and publicity, and salespeople who give the product only minimal attention.

MEASURING THE COMMUNICATIONS RESULTS

Senior managers want to know the *outcomes* and *revenues* resulting from their communications investments. More often, however, their communications directors supply only *outputs* and *expenses:* press clipping counts, numbers of ads placed, and media costs. The communications directors may also use intermediate outputs such as reach and frequency, recall and recognition scores, persuasion changes, and cost-per-thousand calculations. Ultimately, behavior change measures capture the real payoff from communications.

After implementing the plan, the communications director must measure its impact on the target audience. Members of the target audience are asked whether they recognize or recall the message, how many times they saw it, what points they recall, how they felt about the message, and their previous and current attitudes toward the product and company. The communicator should also collect behavioral measures of audience response, such as how many people bought the product, liked it, and talked to others about it. Hospital executives should demand to know how many new admissions resulted from their multimillion-dollar advertising campaign. This measure is often difficult to obtain without thoughtful investment in management information system infrastructure, but without this information the return on promotional investments cannot be accurately appreciated.

Consider the following examples: Suppose that 80 percent of the consumers in the total market are aware of brand A, 60 percent have tried it, and only 20 percent who have tried it are satisfied. These findings indicate that the communications program is effective in creating awareness, but the product fails to meet consumer expectations. By contrast, assume you found that only 40 percent of the consumers in the total market are aware of brand B, and only 30 percent have tried it, but 80 percent of those who have tried it are satisfied. In this case, the communications program needs to be strengthened to take advantage of the brand's power.

MANAGING THE INTEGRATED MARKETING COMMUNICATIONS PROCESS

According to Northwestern University's Medill Journalism School, *integrated marketing communications* (IMC) is the management of all organizational communications that builds positive relationships with potential customers and stakeholders, including employees, legislators, the media, the financial community, and other segments of the public. A similar definition by the American Association of Advertising Agencies also recognizes the added value of a comprehensive plan. Such a plan evaluates the strategic roles of a variety of communications disciplines—for example, general advertising, direct response, sales promotion, and public relations—and combines them to provide clarity, consistency, and maximum impact through the seamless integration of discrete messages.

Unfortunately, many organizations still rely on one or two communication tools to achieve their communications aims. This practice persists in spite of the fragmenting of mass markets into a multitude of mini-markets, each requiring its own approach; the proliferation of new types of media; and the growing sophistication of consumers. The wide range of communication tools, messages, and audiences makes it imperative that companies move toward IMC. Companies must adopt a 360-degree view of consumers to fully understand all the different ways in which communications can impact consumer behavior in their daily lives.

ORDINATING MEDIA

coordination can occur across and within media types. Personal and nonpersonal communication channels should be combined to achieve maximum impact.

Instead of using a single tool in a one-shot effort, a more powerful approach is the multiple-vehicle, multiple-stage campaign, such as the following sequence:

News campaign about a new health care service→Paid ad with a response mechanism→Direct mail→Outbound telemarketing→Face-to-face sales call→ Ongoing communication.

Multiple media deployed within a tightly defined time frame can increase message reach and impact. Research has also shown that promotions can be more effective when combined with advertising.[43] The awareness and attitudes created by advertising campaigns can improve the success of more direct sales pitches. Many companies are coordinating their on-line and off-line communication activities. For example, listing web addresses in ads (especially print) and on packages allows people to more fully explore a company's products, find distribution locations, and access more product or service information. Yale-New Haven Medical Center uses small newspaper banner ads with its phone number and web address to drive traffic to its Web site. The purpose is to forge direct customer relationships, strengthen customer loyalty, and follow up with targeted direct-mail promotional efforts based on consumer interest in particular diseases and medical issues.

IMPLEMENTING INTEGRATED MARKETING COMMUNICATIONS

Integrated marketing communications can produce stronger message consistency and greater sales impact. It forces management to think about every way in which the customer comes in contact with the company, how the company communicates its positioning, the relative importance of each vehicle, and timing issues. It gives the marketing manager the responsibility to unify the company's brand images and messages as they come through thousands of company activities. IMC should improve the company's ability to reach the right customers with the right messages at the right time and in the right place.[44] IMC also provides a way of directing the whole marketing process instead of focusing on its individual parts.

Professor Kevin Keller of Dartmouth College provides the following criteria for judging how integrated an IMC program is:[45]

■ *Coverage* relates to the proportion of the audience that is reached by each communication option employed, as well as how much overlap exists among communication options. In other words, to what extent do different communication options reach the designated target market and the same or different consumers making up that market?

■ *Contribution* relates to the inherent ability of a marketing communications effort to create the desired response from consumers in the absence of exposure to any other contact option. How much does a communication affect how consumers process the message, and how well does it build awareness, enhance the image, elicit responses, and induce sales?

- *Commonality* relates to the extent to which *common* associations are reinforced across communication options; that is, the extent to which meaning is consistent in all of the information conveyed by different communication options. The consistency and cohesiveness of the brand image is important because it determines how easily existing associations and responses can be recalled and how easily additional associations and responses can become linked to the brand in memory. For example, DTC television advertising of branded drugs is not legal in Canada. Because most Canadians have access to American channels, however, pharmaceutical companies can run commercials with the same look without naming the product, to reinforce their message.

- *Complementarity* relates to the extent to which *different* associations and linkages are emphasized across communication options. Communication options are often more effective when used in tandem. Different brand associations may be most effectively established by capitalizing on those marketing communications options best suited to eliciting a particular consumer response or establishing a particular type of brand association. As part of the highly successful "Drivers Wanted" campaign, VW has used television to introduce a story line that they continued and embellished on their Web site.

- *Versatility* refers to the extent to which a marketing communications option is robust and works for different groups of consumers. With any integrated communication program, some consumers will already have encountered other marketing contacts for the brand, whereas other consumers will not have had any prior exposure.

- *Cost.* Evaluations of marketing communications on all of these criteria must be weighed against their cost to arrive at the most effective and efficient program.

SUMMARY

Health care organizations and personnel must have skills in communicating effectively to their clients and stakeholders. Communications will be most meaningful when they are planned with a clear audience in mind and knowledge of the audience's media habits and responses to various appeals and themes. Successful communication involves understanding the nine elements in communication: sender, encoding, message, media, decoding, receiver, response, noise, and feedback. Health care organizations also need to understand the different levels of audience response, from awareness to knowledge to liking to preference to convictions to purchase.

Developing effective marketing communications involves eight steps: (1) identifying the target audience, (2) determining the communication objectives, (3) designing the communications, (4) selecting the communication channels, (5) estimating the total marketing communications budget, (6) deciding on the media mix, (7) measuring the results, and (8) managing integrated communications. Each of these steps encompasses various activities and tools.

The health care organization has to decide on the best mix to make of the communications tools of advertising, sales promotion, public relations and publicity, events and experiences, personal selling and direct marketing. The organization must constantly reevaluate the mix by using measures of communication tool impact on awareness, interest, knowledge, preference, and purchase. The organization should strive to manage, through time, a well-integrated marketing communications program.

DISCUSSION QUESTIONS

1. Many physicians think that "marketing" is another word for advertising or sales. They can react negatively to all three words in the context of health care. How would you open the mind of a physician concerning the value and use of different promotion strategies in health care?

2. A pediatric patient has tragically died at a medical center due to an administrative mistake. As the director of public relations for the medical center, what recommendations do you have for how the hospital should handle this crisis?

3. Hospital media advertising spending in Boston had traditionally been low compared with other markets. From 2005 to 2006, however, it jumped 68 percent. Assume that you are a Boston hospital marketing director, and the hospital CEO wants to know if your hospital should significantly increase its media spending. What questions would you want answered before you provided your recommendation?

4. Medical device companies, pharmaceutical companies, and health information systems companies all spend heavily on trade shows to reach prospective customers. Research the major trade shows for these three market segments and analyze the target markets, the advantages, the disadvantages, and the best practices for exhibiting with these trade shows.

CHAPTER

14

PERSONAL MARKETING COMMUNICATIONS: WORD-OF-MOUTH, SALES, AND DIRECT MARKETING

LEARNING OBJECTIVES

In this chapter, we will address the following questions:

1. When are personal marketing communications most effective?

2. What is word-of-mouth marketing and how can it be used by health care marketers?

3. How does the sales force operate in different health care markets, and what are the major sales-force decisions that must be made?

4. What are the steps involved in effective personal selling?

5. How are the latest electronic, interactive direct-marketing tools being used in health care?

OPENING EXAMPLE

GSK Develops a Campaign to Sell the Public on the "Value of Medicine" and the Positive Role of the Pharmaceutical Industry   In 1997, the pharmaceutical industry seemed to be held in high esteem. The annual Harris Interactive industry reputation poll put pharma in the top echelon of U.S. industries: 79 percent thought that pharma was "doing a good job of serving customers." Then the numbers started to change. Seven years later, in 2004, only 44 percent thought pharma was doing a good job. The pharmaceutical industry was now in the lower echelon of twenty-five industries, alongside tobacco, oil, and managed care companies. What happened?

There had been an explosion of innovative new product development in the 1990s—instead of the prior average of fifteen new blockbuster drugs a year, an average of thirty new drugs were released annually. This explosion, however, came at a great cost. Although seniors reaped the major benefits, they had to pay for these medications without the advantage of a Medicare prescription drug benefit. Further, managed care plans experienced dramatic growth in the cost of their pharmaceutical benefits, which grew to be more expensive than primary care. On the international scene, pharmaceutical companies were vilified for placing life-saving drugs (like those to treat HIV infections) out of financial reach of the countries most in need. While these events unfolded, the pharmaceutical industry, as a whole, provided no response to the decline in its reputation. Instead, its industry trade association, the Pharmaceutical Manufacturing Association (PhRMA), was focused on shaping legislation in the United States to maintain payment levels and allow direct-to-consumer (DTC) advertising (which began in 1997). Internationally, the industry concentrated on preserving intellectual property rights so poor countries could not make cheaper versions of patented medications. As a result, the public came to believe that pharmaceutical companies were insensitive profiteers.

To change this industry image, in 2004, Mike Pucci, vice president for external advocacy at British-based pharmaceutical giant GSK, developed and led an initiative called "The Value of Medicine." The Value of Medicine program features three basic themes: (1) how today's miracle drugs finance tomorrow's cures, (2) the risks of developing medicines and how R&D costs drive retail prices, and (3) acknowledging and expressing concern for the obstacles many patients face in obtaining the drugs they need.

To communicate the Value of Medicine message, GSK developed strategies to work with the national media using television commercials, forged an alliance with WebMD to develop an on-line presence, and used public relations tools.

The most innovative and personal marketing strategy was training the large GSK sales force as community ambassadors to emphasize the impact of chronic diseases on costs. For example, they make clear to Rotary Clubs, church groups, town hall meetings, and others that 80 percent of health care dollars are used to fight five chronic disease categories: heart, diabetes, allergy and asthma, cancer, and mental illness. Efforts placed on preventing these particular diseases will have a significant effect on lowering health care costs. Further, they explain that evolving technologies will lead pharmaceutical companies to better medicines that will further reduce the costs of these diseases and slow their progression. Finally, the salespeople informed their audiences that GSK and other drug companies had free or low-cost prescription assistance programs and targeted local media and governments in key states to raise awareness about these efforts.

In addition, over the course of a year GSK employees, including trained regional medical scientists, delivered fifteen thousand presentations to grassroots audiences. These scientists targeted physicians and provided grand rounds programs to illustrate the connection between pharma R&D and physicians' clinical research. Pfizer and Eli Lilly, along with a number of other companies, consulted with GSK to develop similar initiatives.

The Value of Medicines marketing program reached two million people and was successful. There were two hundred thousand visits to the pharma forum on WebMD in the three months after launch. The pharmaceutical companies also had seven million consumers qualify for prescription drug assistance, for whom the industry donated $10 million a day in free medicines. Harris poll respondents who thought that the pharma industry did a good job serving consumers increased from 44 percent in 2004 to 56 percent in 2005 and to 61 percent in 2006. Internationally, pharma's image improved after many firms agreed to furnish developing countries with critical expensive medications free or at below cost.

Marketing communications are increasingly seen as an interactive dialogue between the company and it customers. Organizations must ask not only "How can we reach our customers?" but also "How can our customers reach us?" This chapter examines how organizations personalize their marketing communications for more impact. We begin by describing personal communication channels. Next, we examine word-of-mouth marketing. We then consider personal selling, and finally we discuss direct marketing.

OVERVIEW: PERSONAL COMMUNICATION CHANNELS

Personal communication channels involve two or more persons communicating directly with each other face-to-face, person-to-audience, over the telephone, or through e-mail or the Internet. Personal communication channels derive their effectiveness through individualized presentation and immediate feedback.

A further distinction can be drawn among advocate, expert, and social communication channels. *Advocate channels* consist of company salespeople contacting buyers in the target market. *Expert channels* consist of independent experts making statements to target buyers. *Social channels* consist of neighbors, friends, family members, and associates talking to target buyers. The importance of social channels is evidenced by a study of seven thousand consumers in seven European countries, which found that 60 percent of respondents said they were influenced to use a new brand by family and friends.[1]

A study by Burson-Marsteller and Roper Starch Worldwide found that, on average, one influential person's off-line word of mouth tends to affect the buying attitudes of two other people. That circle of influence, however, jumps to eight on-line, due to the power of electronic word of mouth.

On-line visitors increasingly create product information, not just consume it. They join internet interest groups to share information, so that "word of web" is joining "word of mouth" as an important buying influence. Words about good companies and products travel fast; words about bad companies and products travel even faster. As one marketer noted, "you don't need to reach two million people to let them know about a new product—you just need to reach the right two thousand people in the right way and they will help you reach two million."[2]

Personal influence carries particular weight in two situations. One is with products that are expensive, risky, or purchased infrequently. The other is a situation in which the product suggests something about the user's status or taste. In both cases, buyers will consult others for information or to avoid embarrassment. Instant messaging and independent sites to gather consumer reviews are becoming increasingly important sources for collecting market information. Field Note 14.1 presents an example of these principles.

FIELD NOTE 14.1.

Sweet Talk: Using Text Messaging to Better Manage Diabetes For insulin-dependent diabetic patients to adequately control their disease and prevent complications, they must test their blood sugars at regular times and adjust their medication accordingly. Previous clinical studies have shown that intensive treatment is effective only with close supervision by physicians.

Victoria Franklin and Stephen Greene, of the University of Dundee in Scotland, have developed "Sweet Talk," a mobile phone program that sends text messages to patients reminding them of the treatment goals they have set themselves. Sweet Talk also allows the patients to send questions to their doctors. Sweet Talk was tested for over eighteen months with teenage patients receiving both conventional and intensive diabetes treatment. A control group received conventional treatment and no text messages.

The group that received text messaging had a significantly higher "self-efficacy" score on a questionnaire that measures the effectiveness of treatment. In the group receiving intensive treatment the level of glucose control, measured by hemoglobin HbA1c, went down 14 percent more compared to the group that did not receive the text messages. Even a 10 percent decrease is associated with fewer complications such as eye and kidney problems. This finding suggests that text messaging may be a tool for improving health care outcomes and reducing costs.

Source: "A Text a Day . . .," *The Economist*, Mar. 25, 2006, p. 84.

WORD-OF-MOUTH MARKETING

People often ask others—friends, relatives, professionals—for a personal recommendation for a doctor, hospital, or health insurance agent, or a business recommendation for a health information system, a consultant, or an advertising agency. If they have confidence in the recommendation, they normally act on the referral. In such cases, the recommender has potentially benefited the service provider as well as the service seeker.

The Word of Mouth Marketing Association (WOMA) defines *word of mouth* as "The act of consumers providing information to other consumers." *Word-of-mouth marketing* is "giving people a reason to talk about your products and services, and making it easier for that conversation to take place. It is the art and science of building active, mutually beneficial consumer-to-consumer and consumer-to-marketer communications."[3] Word-of-mouth marketing is not only about *creating* word of mouth; it is also about making it work within a marketing objective by encouraging and facilitating it.

Organizations can attempt to make their customers happier by listening to them, making it easier for them to tell their friends, and making certain that influential individuals know about the good qualities of a product or service. Word-of-mouth marketing empowers people to share their experiences.

Word of mouth must not be faked by hiring and paying people who pretend they are objective. Attempting to fake word of mouth is unethical and can create a backlash, damage the brand, and tarnish the corporate reputation. Word-of-mouth marketing must be based on actual customer satisfaction, two-way dialogue, and transparent communications. The basic elements are:

- Educating people about your products and services
- Identifying people most likely to share their opinions
- Providing tools that make it easier to share information
- Studying how, where, and when opinions are being shared
- Listening and responding to supporters, detractors, and neutrals

The importance of word-of-mouth marketing in health care is highlighted in the survey results summarized in Field Note 14.2.

FIELD NOTE 14.2.

Consumer Choice Survey of Providers and Payers Suppose you HAD TO CHOOSE between two health plans. The first one is strongly recommended to you by friends and family, but the second one is rated much higher in quality by independent experts who evaluate plans. If the two plans cost the same, which would you be more likely to choose?

52%	Plan recommended by friends
43%	Plan highly rated by experts
5%	Don't know
100%	

Suppose you HAD TO CHOOSE between two different hospitals. The first one is the hospital you and your family have used for many years without any problems, but the second hospital is rated much higher in quality by the experts. Which hospital would you be more likely to choose?

72%	Hospital that is familiar
25%	Hospital that is rated higher
3%	Don't know
100%	

Suppose you HAD TO CHOOSE between two surgeons at a hospital. The first surgeon has treated your family for a long time, without any problems, but his ratings aren't as high as those of other surgeons at the hospital. The second surgeon's ratings are much higher, but no one you know personally has ever been one of his patients. Which surgeon would you be more likely to choose?

76%	Surgeon seen before, but not well rated
20%	Surgeon not seen before, but rated higher
4%	Don't know
100%	

Source: "Kaiser Family Foundation/Harvard University National Survey of Americans' Views on Consumer Protection in Managed Care" (#1356), The Henry J. Kaiser Family Foundation and Harvard University, Jan. 1998.

Types of Word-of-Mouth Marketing

Word-of-mouth marketing encompasses a range of techniques that encourage and help people to talk to each other about products and services. The following are common types of word-of-mouth marketing:

- *Buzz marketing:* Using high-profile entertainment or news to get people to talk about your brand

- *Viral marketing:* Creating entertaining or informative messages that are designed to be passed along in an exponential fashion, often electronically on the Internet or by e-mail

- *Community marketing:* Forming or supporting niche communities that are likely to share interests about the brand (such as user groups, fan clubs, and discussion forums) and providing tools, content, and information to foster those communities

- *Grassroots marketing:* Organizing and motivating volunteers to engage in personal or local outreach

- *Evangelist marketing:* Cultivating evangelists, advocates, or volunteers who are encouraged to take a leadership role in actively spreading the word on your behalf

- *Product seeding:* Placing the right product into the right hands at the right time; for example, providing information or samples to influential individuals

- *Influencer marketing:* Identifying key communities and opinion leaders who are likely to talk about products and have the ability to influence the opinions of others

- *Cause marketing:* Supporting social causes to earn respect and support from people who feel strongly about the cause

- *Conversation creation:* Producing interesting or fun advertising, emails, catch phrases, entertainment, or promotions designed to start word-of-mouth activity

- *Brand blogging:* Creating blogs, in the spirit of open, transparent communications and sharing information of value that may interest the blog community

- *Referral programs:* Creating tools that enable satisfied customers to refer their friends

Many of the activities in this list can be classified as *guerilla marketing*, which is creating one-to-one communication methods that do not use such traditional media as print, radio, or television. Popular international examples include corporate sponsorships of city animal models, like cows in Chicago, lions in Singapore, and moose in Toronto. An example in the health care arena would be holding a snowman contest to promote a cough and cold treatment product.

Service providers clearly have a strong interest in building referral sources. The two chief benefits of developing referrals using word-of-mouth are:

■ *Word-of-mouth sources are convincing:* Word of mouth is the only promotion method that is of consumers, by consumers, and for consumers. Not only are satisfied customers repeat buyers, but they are also walking, talking billboards for your business.

■ *Word-of-mouth sources are low cost:* Keeping in touch with satisfied customers costs the business relatively little. The business might reciprocate by referring business to the referrer or giving the referrer enhanced service, a discount, or a small gift.

Communication researchers are moving toward a social-structure view of interpersonal communication.[4] They see society as consisting of *cliques* — small groups whose members share similar characteristics and interact frequently. Although the closeness of clique members facilitates effective communication, it also insulates the clique from new ideas. The challenge is to create more system openness so that cliques exchange information with others in the society. This openness is helped by people who function as liaisons and bridges. A *liaison* is a person who connects two or more cliques without belonging to either. A *bridge* is a person who belongs to one clique and is linked to a person in another clique.

In many cases, the "buzz" of word-of-mouth communications can be managed.[5] Michael Cafferky has identified four kinds of people whom companies try to reach in order to stimulate word of mouth referrals.[6] A person can simultaneously fit into one or more of the following categories:

■ *Opinion leaders* are people who are widely respected within defined social groups, such as physicians who are well-known in a particular disease or treatment category. They have a large relevant social network, high source credibility, and a high propensity to talk.

■ *Marketing mavens* are people who spend a lot of time learning the best buys (values) in the marketplace. Most neighborhoods or families seem to have one particular person who fits this description.

■ *Influentials* are people who are socially and politically active; they try to know what is going on and influence the course of events.

■ *Product enthusiasts* are people who are known experts in a product category, such as medical technology experts and health insurance brokers.

Companies can take several steps to stimulate personal influence channels to work on their behalf:

- *Identify influential individuals and companies and devote extra effort to them*. In health care, influencers might be physicians at academic medical centers, health care industry analysts and journalists, selected policy makers, and a sampling of early adopters.[7]

- *Create opinion leaders by supplying certain people with the product on attractive terms*. Pharmaceutical and medical device companies actively build networks of key opinion leaders (KOLs) to give their products credibility and have them speak on their behalf. These KOLs can receive free or heavily discounted products. A major recent concern in the United States has been pharmaceutical company provision of free injectable drugs to high-volume physician customers. These physicians, in turn, bill payers (including the federal government) for these samples. This practice is illegal. A more ethical and legal tactic in this category is offering discounted products, such as diagnostic devices or information systems, to providers who agree to provide a demonstration site for the company.

- *Work through community influentials such as local media personalities and leaders of service and civics organizations*. A radio DJ's promises of easy weight loss during sleep prompted consumers to spend money on Body Solutions Evening Weight Loss Formula.

- *Develop advertising that has high "conversation value."* Incorporate buzz-worthy features into product design. Some ad slogans become part of the cultural vernacular, such as Alka-Seltzer's "plop, plop, fizz, fizz" television commercial that played on the sound of the tablets landing in a glass of water.

- *Develop word-of-mouth referral channels to build business*. Professionals will often encourage clients to recommend their services. Weight Watchers found that word-of-mouth referrals stemming from a relationship with someone in the program had a huge impact on their business.[8]

- *Establish an electronic forum*. Med Help International is a nonprofit organization dedicated to helping patients find high-quality, timely medical information. It accomplishes this goal by offering on-line question-and-answer medical specialty forums in which patients can ask questions of leading physicians and other health care professionals.

- *Use viral marketing*. Internet marketers can use *viral marketing* as a form of word of mouth, or "word of mouse," to draw attention to their sites.[9] Viral marketing involves encouraging customers to pass company-developed products, services, or information from user to user.

Marketers must be careful in reaching out to consumers. One survey found that roughly 80 percent of the sample of consumers was very annoyed by pop-up ads, spam, and telemarketing.[10] The key is to get the permission of interested consumers who say that they are willing to receive information on certain subjects and receive certain types of communications.[11]

Word of Mouth: Buzz Marketing

Marketers' growing interest in word of mouth, buzz, and viral marketing has led to a number of new theories and ideas. Research has suggested that buzz evolves according to basic principles that may seem counter-intuitive.[12] For example, many marketers believe that only exciting, new products can generate buzz. In reality, staid products, such as prescription drugs, can also benefit from effectively structured buzz. A second assumption is that buzz happens randomly. In many cases, however, buzz is the result of a carefully planned and executed marketing strategy. An organization's customers may seem like the best place to originate a buzz campaign, but often a high-energy, grassroots market niche may be the best place to start. Marketers also may assume that heavy media advertising spending or an orchestrated publicity campaign is needed to generate buzz. In fact, groups of individuals who are genuinely strong product advocates often can be more effective in generating sales through buzz. Unplanned media publicity can actually be a by-product of this group action.

Another buzz marketing model offered by Malcolm Gladwell claims that three factors work to ignite public interest in an idea.[13] He calls the first "The Law of the Few." Three types of people help spread an idea like an epidemic. First are mavens, people who are very knowledgeable about a topic. Second are connectors, people who know and communicate with a great number of other people. Third are salesmen, those who possess great natural persuasive power. Any idea that catches the interest of mavens, connectors, and salesmen is likely to be broadcast far and wide.

A second factor is "Stickiness." An idea must be expressed so that it motivates people to act. Otherwise, "The Law of the Few" will not lead to a self-sustaining buzz epidemic. The third factor, the "Power of Context," will control whether those spreading an idea are able to organize groups and communities around it.

Word of Mouth: Marketing Strategies

Positive word-of-mouth marketing strategies involve finding ways to support satisfied customers and making it easier for them to talk to their friends. Methods include one or more of the following:

1. Encouraging communications

   - Developing tools to make telling a friend easier
   - Creating forums and feedback tools
   - Working with social networks

2. Giving people something to talk about

   - Providing information that can be shared or forwarded

- Developing advertising, stunts, and other publicity that encourages conversation
- Working with product development to build WOM elements into products

3. Creating communities and connecting people
   - Creating user groups and fan clubs
   - Supporting independent groups that form around your product
   - Hosting discussions and message boards about your products
   - Enabling grassroots organizations such as local meetings and other real-world participation

4. Working with influential communities
   - Finding people who are likely to respond to your message
   - Identifying people who are able to influence your target customers
   - Informing these individuals about what you do and encouraging them to spread the word
   - Making good-faith efforts to support issues and causes that are important to these individuals

5. Creating evangelist or advocate programs
   - Providing recognition and tools to active advocates
   - Recruiting new advocates, teaching them about the benefits of your products, and encouraging them to talk about them

6. Researching and listening to customer feedback
   - Tracking on-line and off-line conversations by supporters, detractors, and neutrals
   - Listening and responding to both positive and negative conversations

7. Engaging in transparent conversation
   - Encouraging two-way conversations with interested parties
   - Creating blogs and other tools to share information
   - Participating openly in on-line blogs and discussions

8. Co-creation and information sharing
   - Involving consumers in marketing and creative decisions (by providing feedback on creative campaigns, allowing them to create commercials, and so forth)
   - Letting customers "behind the curtain" have first access to information and content[14]

Field Note 14.3 illustrates the application of these concepts in a health care setting.

FIELD NOTE 14.3.

***BzzAgent* Health Care Marketing**   BzzAgent is a Boston company started in 2002 by Dave Balter, who was inspired in part by the book *Butterfly Economics* by Paul Omerod. The book's thesis is that the rate of global communications is rapidly accelerating and is affecting the world economy. Individual people are the change agents in this phenomenon. Balter decided to form an innovative company to harness individual communications and leverage word-of-mouth marketing for clients. BzzAgent has conducted word-of-mouth campaigns with 150 client companies in a variety of industries including health care products and services.

BzzAgents are individuals who volunteer to work on client campaigns. They apply through the Company's Web site and are invited to participate in certain BzzCampaigns based on their interests and demographic attributes. The steps in a BzzCampaign are as follows:

1. *BzzCampaign goes live:* The Central Hive launches a BzzCampaign. An eligible Agent sees it under "BzzCampaigns you can join" on the Agent's My BzzHome page.

2. *BzzAgent signs up:* The Agent clicks on the available BzzCampaign and learns more about it by going through Campaign Camp. At the end of Campaign Camp, the Agent decides whether to participate.

3. *BzzAgent receives BzzKit in the mail:* After the Agent signs up for the BzzCampaign, the BzzKit arrives in the mail a week or two later. Inside the kit are a product sample and a BzzGuide, the custom guide created to help Agents create honest word of mouth about the product or service.

4. *BzzAgent gets to know the BzzGuide and product:* The Agent learns more about the product or service and is able to form his or her own opinion about it.

5. *BzzAgent performs BzzActivity:* If the agent sincerely believes in the worth of the product, the BzzGuide provides a list of BzzActivities to help spread honest word of mouth. These activities make it easier for the Agent to spread honest buzz.

6. *BzzAgent reports BzzActivity:* Each time the Agent spreads Bzz, he or she returns to BzzAgent.com and files a BzzReport, a short report about the "who," "what," "when," and "how" of the buzz they created.

7. *The BzzReport is reviewed:* A BzzAgent Communications Developer reviews the BzzReport and provides helpful and personalized feedback. If the BzzReport is approved, the Agent is awarded BzzPoints.

8. *BzzAgent redeems BzzPoints for BzzRewards:* After submitting a number of BzzReports, Agents redeem their accumulated BzzPoints for BzzRewards of their choice.

The typical campaign runs ten weeks and costs upwards of $100,000. The Company provides its clients with detailed measures of campaign activity including Net Promoter Score and return-on-investment data. The Net Promoter Score was developed by Frederick Reicheld at Bain & Company. Reicheld conducted research on customer loyalty and growth that matched consumer survey responses with their actual repeat purchase behavior and referral patterns. He found that the question "How likely is it that you would recommend [company or product X] to a friend or colleague?" has the highest statistical correlation with profitable growth. Reicheld identified a single metric to measure this relationship: the Net Promoter Score. For BzzAgent, the Net Promoter Score = Percent of Agents who are Promoters minus percent of Agents who are Detractors. BzzAgent uses this score as a key measure of campaign effectiveness. The median net promoter score for all industries is 16, and the median score resulting from BuzzCampaigns is 38. The score for a recent campaign for an over-the-counter drug was 48.

One of the Company's more complex campaigns was for a client that wanted consumers to donate stem cells and umbilical cord blood. This campaign focused on talking to a small, qualified target market—pregnant women—about a relatively controversial subject, stem cell banking. BzzAgents in the campaign had to encounter the right person at the right time, and these women were more often found in birthing classes, hospitals, and physician offices. Although this campaign experienced much slower word of mouth, the metrics indicated that it was successful.

DESIGNING THE SALES FORCE

The oldest form of direct marketing is the sales call. U.S. firms spend over *a trillion* dollars annually on sales forces and sales-force materials—more than they spend on any other promotional method. Nearly 12 percent of the total workforce works full-time in sales occupations, in nonprofit as well as for-profit organizations. Most health product companies, and an increasing number of health service organizations, rely on a professional sales force to locate prospects, convert them into customers, and foster their loyalty to the business. Once the company decides on an approach, it can use either a direct or a contractual sales force. A *direct (company) sales force* consists of full- or part-time paid employees who work exclusively for the company. This sales force includes inside sales personnel who conduct business from the office using the telephone and receive visits from prospective buyers, and field sales personnel who travel and visit customers. A *contractual sales force* consists of manufacturers' representatives (reps), sales agents, and brokers, who either represent the company exclusively or represent a portfolio of noncompeting companies. For example, several prominent companies that provide contract pharmaceutical sales-force services are

Ventiv, Innovex, and PDI. Contract sales compensation can be based on a retainer plus sales commission or 100 percent commission.

Even large pharmaceutical companies will occasionally use a contractual sales force. Additionally, many organizations such as health insurance companies have alliances with independent, direct-selling insurance agents, brokers, and "producers" who supplement their employed sales force. Further, hospitals and medical research institutes often employ fundraisers to contact donors and solicit donations, and a number of hospitals employ salespeople to sell administrative and other services to physicians.

Although a sales force can be a very cost-effective strategy for selling high-margin products and services, organizations are sensitive to the high and rising costs (salaries, commissions, bonuses, travel expenses, and benefits) of maintaining these personnel. Suppose a sales call averages a cost of $400; if closing a sale may require four calls, the total cost can add up to $1,600. Not surprisingly, companies are trying to increase the productivity of the sales force through better selection, training, supervision, motivation, and compensation.

Sales positions can be categorized into six different types that range from low to high complexity and skill.[15] A salesperson may fit into one or more of the following categories:

- *Deliverer:* A salesperson whose major task is the delivery of a product. Some reps simply replenish inventories, such as operating room sutures in hospital supply rooms.

- *Order taker:* A salesperson who acts predominantly as an inside order taker (the salesperson in the customer service department for a medical device company) or outside order taker (the over-the-counter medication salesperson calling on the pharmacy or supermarket manager).

- *Missionary:* A salesperson who is not expected or permitted to take an order but whose major task is to build goodwill or educate the actual or potential user; for example, the medical "detailer" who calls on a physician practice representing a pharmaceutical house.

- *Technician:* A salesperson with a high level of technical knowledge; for example, a former hospital chief financial officer who is primarily a technical consultant in selling hospital financial information systems.

- *Demand creator:* A salesperson who relies on creative methods for selling tangible products, such as weight loss and nutritional products, or intangibles, such as health insurance or fitness services.

- *Solution vendor:* A salesperson whose expertise is solving a customer's problem, often employing such company products and services as computer and communications systems.

It is important to note that although sales personnel serve as the company's personal link *to* the customers, they are also the conduit of information *from* and *about* the customer. Because of this dual function, the company needs to carefully consider its sales-force design—namely, the development of sales-force objectives, strategy, structure, size, and compensation.

Sales-Force Objectives and Strategy

Companies need to define the specific objectives they want their sales force to achieve. For example, a company might want its sales representatives to spend 80 percent of their time with current customers and 20 percent with prospects or 85 percent of their time on established products and 15 percent on new products.

The specific allocation scheme depends on the offerings and customers. Regardless of the selling context, however, salespeople will have one or more of the following specific tasks to perform:

- *Prospecting:* Identifying qualified potential customers

- *Targeting:* Deciding how to allocate their time among prospects and customers to maximize sales

- *Communicating:* Communicating information about the company's products and services and listening in order to uncover customer needs

- *Selling:* Approaching, presenting, answering objections, and closing sales

- *Servicing:* Providing account management services to customers—consulting on problems, rendering technical assistance, arranging financing, and expediting delivery

- *Information gathering:* Conducting market research, gathering competitive intelligence, and reporting this information to the organization

- *Allocating:* Deciding which customers will get scarce products during product shortages

Although these tasks have traditionally been individual efforts, selling increasingly calls for teamwork requiring the participation of other personnel, such as *top management*, who provide support especially when national accounts or major sales are at stake; *technical people*, who supply specialized information and service to the customer before, during, or after product purchase; *customer service representatives*, who provide installation, maintenance, and other services; and an *office staff,* who furnish analytical reports, expedite orders, and provide general administrative services.

In order to succeed, sales representatives need analytical marketing skills; these skills are especially important at the higher levels of sales management. Further, marketing managers believe that sales forces will be more effective in selling in the long run if they understand the firm's strategic marketing plan.

Sales-Force Structure

The company's organizational design and strategy will determine the sales-force structure. For example, if the company sells one product line to one end-using industry with customers in many locations, it would use a territorial sales-force structure. If the company sells many products to many types of customers, it might need a product or market sales-force structure. If geographical coverage needs to be broad, then a more complex structure may be needed.

For example, although orthopedic implant industry leader Synthes has a single sales force, its major competitors in the U.S. manage four types of sales forces: (1) a strategic market sales force composed of technical, applications, and quality engineers and service personnel assigned to major accounts; (2) a geographic sales force calling on hundreds of customers in different territories; (3) a distributor sales force calling on and coaching distributors; and (4) an inside sales force doing telemarketing and taking orders via phone and fax.

Companies typically provide major accounts with a special strategic account management team, consisting of cross-functional personnel who are permanently assigned to them and may even maintain offices at the customer's facility. These clients are called key accounts, national accounts, global accounts, or house accounts.

Sales-Force Size

After the organization determines the sales-force strategy and structure, it is ready to consider sales-force size based on the number of customers it wants to reach. One widely used method is the five-step *workload approach*:

1. Group customers into size classes according to annual sales volume
2. Establish call frequencies, or the number of calls to be made per year on each account in a size class
3. Multiply the number of accounts in each size class by the call frequency to arrive at the total sales call workload
4. Determine the average number of calls sales reps can make per year
5. Divide the total annual calls required by the average annual calls made by a rep to see how many sales reps are needed

Suppose the organization estimates that there are one thousand "A" accounts and two thousand "B" accounts. "A" accounts require thirty-six calls a year, and "B" accounts require twelve calls a year. The organization needs a sales force that can make sixty thousand sales calls a year. If the average rep can make a thousand calls a year, then the company would need sixty full-time sales representatives.

Sales-Force Compensation

To attract top-quality sales reps, the organization needs an attractive compensation package. The four components of sales-force compensation are a fixed amount, a variable amount, expense allowances, and benefits. The fixed amount, a salary, is intended to satisfy the reps' need for some stability. The variable amount, which might include commissions, bonus, or profit sharing, is intended to stimulate and reward greater effort. Expense allowances enable sales reps to meet the costs of travel, lodging, dining, and entertaining. Benefits, such as paid vacations and pension fund matching, provide security and job satisfaction.

Fixed compensation receives more emphasis in jobs with a high ratio of non-selling to selling duties and in jobs in which the selling task is technically complex and involves teamwork. Variable compensation receives more emphasis in jobs in which sales are cyclical or depend on individual initiative. Fixed and variable compensation give rise to three basic types of compensation plans—straight salary, straight commission, and combination salary and commission.

Straight-salary plans provide sales reps with a secure income, make them more willing to perform non-selling activities, and give them less incentive to overstock customers. These plans are easy to administer, and they lower turnover. Straight-commission plans attract higher performers, provide more motivation, require less supervision, and control selling costs. Combination plans feature the benefits of both plans while reducing their disadvantages.

Such plans allow companies to link the variable portion of a salesperson's pay to a wide variety of strategic goals. Some see a new trend toward de-emphasizing volume measures in favor of factors such as gross profitability, customer satisfaction, and customer retention. For example, compensation plans at U.S. Surgical Corporation, which had long emphasized sales revenue quotas, were reworked in the mid-1990s to focus on customer satisfaction measures.

Another example highlights the need to integrate sales-force compensation with the overall company goals. Many independent brokers who worked with managed care plans received commissions based on the number of people they enrolled. This practice led to recruitment of many people who could not get insurance elsewhere because of their health status. Further, these members tend to shop the lowest prices, resulting in costly account turnovers. Realizing that this compensation method was dysfunctional, managed care plans changed the payment method, linking it not only to initial signup but also to renewals. The result was a more favorable mix of clients.

A further concern for sales-force compensation is aligning incentives among sales personnel from different parts of the company in order to drive total sales for the company. For instance, in Canada, GE sales personnel will be "made whole" on their incentive compensation if one needs to reduce price so that both can make a sale.

Managing the Sales Force

In addition to establishing a productive compensation scheme, effective sales-force management entails paying close attention to recruiting and selecting, training, supervising, motivating and evaluating representatives.

Recruiting and Selecting Representatives. At the heart of a successful sales force is the selection of effective representatives. One survey revealed that the top 27 percent of the sales force brought in over 52 percent of the sales. Further, the average annual turnover rate for salespeople across all industries is nearly 20 percent. Turnover leads to lost sales and additional costs of finding and training replacements, and it is often a strain on existing salespeople to pick up the slack. Further, such turnover disrupts longstanding customer relationships.

A marketing approach to hiring salespeople is to ask customers what traits they prefer in a salesperson. Although most customers want honest, reliable, knowledgeable, and helpful reps, determining what traits will actually lead to sales success is a challenge. However, numerous studies have shown little correlation between sales performance and a rep's background and experience, current status, lifestyle, attitudes, personality, and skills. More effective predictors have been composite tests, particularly those conducted at assessment centers where the working environment is simulated.[16] Field Note 14.4 provides some insight into sales rep issues for the medical device sector.

FIELD NOTE 14.4.

Working as a Medical Device Sales Representative The demand for medical device salespeople has been strong due to the demographic-driven health care needs of baby boomers and advances in medical technology. By the year 2007, the U.S. Department of Labor expects employment in medical sales to increase 24 percent higher than employment in other sales professions; and the Bureau of Labor Statistics cites projected growth for medical sales to be 111 percent from 2006 to 2010. The field has relatively high salaries that emanate from the high-margin products sold, and selling in this market segment demands an intellectual ability that requires not only knowledge of the products and the relevant science but also what the competition offers.

Medical device sales are procedure-driven, meaning some reps work with surgeons, talking them through procedures and demonstrating medical instrumentation. If the medical tool is determined to be beneficial, the physician gets the hospital to purchase the equipment and the reps get a commission of up to 15 percent—a significant amount, when products are often more than $100,000. A standard compensation package—a base salary of $70,000 plus commission—can total about $120,000 a year for reps. According to David Hartman, a twelve-year veteran of the medical sales trade, "There are people in medical sales who make a lot more than that."[17]

Former college and professional athletes often make the best medical device sales reps. These individuals are self-starters, disciplined, and achievement driven. Having a strong physical capacity is part of their identity. They must also possess an engineering and artistic sensibility.

A typical day in the life of medical sales rep shows how much endurance and energy are needed for this job.

4:30 AM: Wake up and exercise—the only time available during the rep's day to build the needed strength and endurance.

5:30 AM: Commute to the hospital operating room to set up equipment and instrumentation for the first procedure of the day. Pray for a good traffic report.

6:45 AM: Setup complete. Surgeons do not accommodate tardiness.

7:00 AM–3:00 PM: Instruct, coach, and supervise surgeons in using highly technical medical devices. Be ready and willing to say, "Stop, doctor. Put that down. Do not do that," forcefully but with tact.

3:00 PM–5:30 PM: Prospect for new physician customers in the hospital. Attempt to identify and engage the most appropriate qualified prospects. Paging an unfamiliar, busy surgeon in the hospital is very risky—but if the rep can deliver value immediately, the risk can be justified.

5:30 PM–10:00 PM: Entertain and build relationships with surgeons through dinners or attending a ball game or a charity benefit. Commute home and prepare for a similar day tomorrow.

Source: Conversation with Joseph Rafferty, director of contracts, Synthes Spine, Nov. 8, 2006.

Once management develops selection criteria, the next step is to recruit applicants by soliciting names from current sales reps, using industry recruiters, placing ads on-line and in print publications, and contacting colleges and university career centers. Selection procedures can vary from a single informal interview to prolonged testing and interviewing.

Training and Supervising Sales Representatives. Today's customers expect sales reps to have deep product knowledge, to add ideas to improve the customer's operations, and to be efficient and reliable. This expectation requires companies to make a much higher investment in sales training. The median training period is twenty-eight weeks in industrial products companies, twelve weeks in service companies, and four weeks in consumer products companies. Training time varies with the complexity of the selling task and the type of person recruited into the sales organization. Training often involves a variety of methods: live, in-person training can include simulations, role playing, and sensitivity training, whereas self-paced methods involve audio and video tapes, CD-ROMs and DVDs, and web-based distance learning.

Training is particularly rigorous for existing reps when a new product is launched. For example, when a new drug is coming to market, the company will gather in one location all sales reps who will be responsible for its promotion. Over several days, the firm then conducts an intensive educational program that includes relevant anatomy, physiology, mechanism of action of the product, and analysis of competitors in the same and similar treatment categories. The training is thus designed to help these reps understand the new product, be able to explain its science to health care professionals, and differentiate it from its competitors—all with a friendly and helpful demeanor. Clearly, this sales position requires a special kind of person. Consider the following example.

FOR EXAMPLE

U.S. Surgical Corporation has been world-renowned for its intensive sales training. Sales reps are subjected to regular rounds of training and daily testing. Educating medical salespeople is critical because reps need "medical school" training in order to train physicians in the use of their equipment; they also require specialized training in sale techniques as well as product and industry knowledge. Reps receive training in anatomy, physiology, medical data, statistics, and technical training through suturing foam stomachs and bowels. They coach their physician clients in the operating room, talk physicians through medical procedures, and demonstrate instrumentation.

Companies vary in how closely they supervise sales reps. Reps paid mostly on commission generally receive less supervision. Those who are salaried and must cover definite accounts are likely to receive substantial supervision.

Sales Rep Productivity. How many calls should a company make on a particular account each year? Some research has suggested that sales reps are spending too much time selling to smaller, less profitable accounts when they should be focusing more of their efforts on larger, more profitable ones. Companies often specify how much time reps should spend prospecting for new accounts and set up prospecting standards. For example, broadening the customer base by prospecting can be very time-consuming and far less profitable for the rep and the organization; some companies therefore rely on a missionary sales force to open new accounts.

FIELD NOTE 14.5.

Virtual Reality Technology Supports Pharmaceutical Sales Cephalon, a pharmaceutical company specializing in drugs to treat and manage neurological diseases, sleep disorders, cancer, pain, and addiction, hired a Philadelphia video-production company to help its sales force use video iPods to support physician prospecting. The consultants, Hall Media Productions, developed sixty short segments promoting Vivitrol, a drug used to fight alcohol dependence. The segments include real-life testimonials by people who have used the drug.

To help pitch Cephalon's alertness drug, Provigil, Hall Media created a 3-D virtual-reality simulator that simulates the effects of sleepiness. By putting on the virtual-reality goggles and earphones, a viewer gets a first-hand look at the disastrous effect a sleepy fork-lift driver can have on a stack of boxes in a warehouse. Physicians, who are hard-pressed to make time for sales reps, have been receptive.

Studies have shown that the best sales reps are those who know how to manage their time effectively. One planning tool, *time-and-duty analysis*, helps reps understand how they spend their time and how they might increase their productivity. Sales reps spend time planning, traveling, waiting, actually selling, and in administrative tasks (report writing and billing, attending sales meetings, and talking to others in the company about production, delivery, billing, sales performance, and other matters). With so many duties, it is no wonder that actual face-to-face selling time amounts to as little as 29 percent of a rep's total working time!

Companies are constantly seeking ways to improve sales-force productivity. These may include training sales representatives in the use of "phone power," simplifying administrative tasks such as record keeping, and using the computer and the Internet to develop call and routing plans, supply customer and competitive information, and automate the order preparation process. For example, pharmaceutical reps can now electronically batch and send sales encounter reports from their tablet personal computers, instead of filing paper reports documenting each physician contact.

To reduce the time demands on their outside sales force, many companies have increased the size and responsibilities of their inside sales force. There are three types of inside salespeople. *Technical support people* provide technical information and answers to customers' questions. *Sales assistants* provide clerical backup for the outside salespersons by confirming appointments, checking credit, following up on deliveries, and answering customers' questions. *Telemarketers* find new leads and qualify and sell to them.

Motivating Sales Representatives. Motivating sales representatives is difficult because of their stressful work environment. Reps usually work alone during irregular hours, often away from home. They confront aggressive, competing sales reps; have an inferior status relative to the buyer; often do not have the authority to do what is necessary to win an account; and sometimes lose large orders they have worked hard to obtain. Most marketing managers believe that the higher the salesperson's motivation, the greater the effort and the resulting performance, rewards, and satisfaction.

To increase motivation, marketers reinforce intrinsic and extrinsic rewards of all types. One study measuring the importance of different rewards found that the reward with the highest value was pay, followed by promotion, personal growth, and sense of accomplishment.[18] The least-valued rewards were liking and respect, security, and recognition. The researchers also found that the importance of motivators varied with demographic characteristics: financial rewards were more valued by older, longer-tenured people and those who had large families. Rewards such as recognition and sense of accomplishment were more valued by young salespeople who were unmarried or had small families and usually more formal education.

Many companies set annual sales quotas based on dollar sales, unit volume, margin, selling effort or activity, and product type, with compensation often tied to degree of quota fulfillment. Sales quotas are often developed from the annual marketing plan. The organization first prepares a sales forecast that becomes the basis for planning production, workforce size, and financial requirements. Management then establishes quotas for regions and territories, which typically add up to more than the total sales forecast in order to encourage managers and salespeople to perform at their best levels. If they fail to make their quotas, the company nevertheless might still reach its sales forecast. It is important, however, to set the quotas at realistic levels; if they are set too high, sales reps may not attempt to achieve even attainable goals. This situation has occurred with some pharmaceutical products.

Each area sales manager divides the area's quota to arrive at an individual quota for each sales rep. A common approach to individual quotas is to set the individual rep's quota at least equal to the person's past year sales plus some fraction of the difference between territory sales potential and past-year sales.

As mentioned earlier, it is also important to note that some companies sell multiple products lines to the same customer segment and have a separate sales force for each. In such firms, the marketing department must structure bonus incentives to foster cooperation among these reps.

Evaluating Sales Representatives. We have been describing the *feed-forward* aspects of sales supervision—how management communicates what the sales reps should be doing and motivates them to do it. Good feed-forward requires good *feedback*, which means getting regular information *from* reps to evaluate performance. Information about reps can come from sales reports and through personal observation, customer-initiated communication, company-initiated customer surveys, and conversations with other sales representatives. Many companies require representatives to develop an annual territory marketing plan for developing new accounts and increasing business from existing accounts. This report casts sales reps into the role of market managers and profit centers. Sales managers study these plans, make suggestions, and use them to develop sales quotas.

Sales reps complete call reports, expense reports, new-business reports, lost-business reports, and reports on local business and economic conditions. These reports provide raw data from which sales managers can extract key indicators of sales performance, such as

- Average number of sales calls per salesperson per day
- Average sales call time per contact
- Average revenue per sales call
- Average cost per sales call
- Entertainment cost per sales call
- Percentage of orders per hundred sales calls
- Number of new customers per period
- Number of lost customers per period
- Sales-force cost as a percentage of total sales

The sales force's reports, along with other observations, supply the basic information used in conducting evaluations. One type of evaluation compares current performance to past performance and to overall company averages on key indicators. These comparisons help management pinpoint specific areas for improvement. For example, if a rep's average gross profit per customer is lower than the company's average, that rep could be concentrating on the wrong customers or not spending enough time with each customer. Evaluations can also assess the rep's knowledge of the firm, products, customers, competitors, territory, and responsibilities; relevant personality characteristics; and any problems in motivation or compliance.

Principles of Personal Selling

Personal selling is an ancient art that has spawned many principles. Effective salespersons have more than instinct; they are trained in methods of analysis and customer management. Today's companies spend hundreds of millions of dollars each year to train salespeople in the art of selling. One reason for this training is to overcome the negative connotations often connected with selling. When asked to think of a word associated with selling, many people say "pushy," "deceptive," "unethical," or "greedy." Although there are a plethora of different sales training methods and philosophies, one of the most effective training approaches is to train salespeople to not only focus on *customer* needs while using a consultative approach but to also to behave and seem *not* like a salesperson.

Most sales training programs agree on the major steps involved in any effective sales process. We next discuss these steps and their applications to health care selling.

Prospecting and Qualifying. The first step in selling is to identify appropriate prospects. More organizations are relying on their marketing departments to attract and qualify leads so that the salespeople can focus their selling time doing what they can do best. Marketing managers and their sales forces should come to a mutual understanding of the definition of a "qualified" lead; failure to do so often results in sales' ignoring the leads forwarded by marketing. This practice wastes the time, effort, and expense of the marketing department, and the sales team is likely to overlook at least some leads that are worth pursuing.[19]

Preapproach. The salesperson needs to learn as much as possible about the prospect organization, including what it needs, who is involved in the purchase decision, and its buyers' personal characteristics and buying styles. The salesperson can consult standard sources such as Moody's, Standard & Poor's, Dun & Bradstreet, acquaintances, and others to learn about prospects, but ideally the organization's marketing department should be providing the sales team with all the information that it needs on the target market, the environment, the competition, and other market information.

Presentation and Demonstration. The salesperson now tells the product "story" to the buyer. Sales strategies include the AIDA formula of gaining *attention*, holding *interest*, arousing *desire*, and obtaining *action*. The salesperson could also use a *features, advantages, benefits*, and *value* approach (FABV). Too often, salespeople follow a product orientation by emphasizing product features. A customer orientation places the focus on the customer's needs and value proposition instead of on the product.

Overcoming Objections. Customers typically pose objections during the presentation or when asked for the order. *Psychological resistance* includes resistance to interference, or preference for established supply sources or brands, apathy, reluctance to give up something, unpleasant associations created by the sales rep, predetermined ideas, dislike of making decisions, and innate reluctance to spend money. *Logical resistance* consists of objections to the price, delivery schedule, or certain product or company characteristics. To handle these objections, the salesperson maintains a positive approach, asks the buyer to clarify the objection, questions the buyer in a way that the buyer has to answer his or her own objection, denies the validity of the objection, or turns the objection into a reason for buying. It is important for the sales reps to communicate the objections they encounter to the marketing department so that the company's products and services can be improved and the firm can anticipate and develop strategies to address customer concerns.

Closing. Some salespeople do not get to this stage or do not do it well. Sales reps need to know how to recognize closing signs from the buyer, including physical cues, statements or comments, and questions. There are a number of hackneyed closing lines taught in some sales training courses (such as "Would you prefer delivery this week or next week?"), but a more effective closing is to have a thorough understanding of the customer's need for the product or service being sold. This information should be gathered during the course of questioning that takes place throughout the sales process. The salesperson should identify areas of prospective customer pain or gain through questioning and then propose a solution. The questioning includes the prospect's assessment of when a solution would need to be in place to alleviate the pain or to reap the gain: "When is the *latest* you would want to implement this solution?" Following the anti–sales stereotype approach, this question does not pressure the prospect to make an immediate buying decision but allows him or her to determine the timing of the close, to feel in control of the sales process, and to be more likely to buy.

Follow-up and Maintenance. To ensure customer satisfaction, repeat business, and referrals, the salesperson should confirm all necessary details on delivery time, purchase terms, and other matters that are important to the customer. The salesperson should also schedule a follow-up call when the initial order is received to assess proper installation, instruction, and servicing. This visit or call will detect any problems, assure the buyer of the salesperson's interest, and reduce any buyer's regret that might have arisen. Finally, the salesperson should develop a maintenance and growth plan for the account.

Negotiation

Marketing is concerned with exchange activities and the manner in which the terms of exchange are established. In *routinized exchange*, the terms are established by administered programs of pricing and distribution. In *negotiated exchange*, price and other terms are set through bargaining behavior, in which two or more parties negotiate binding agreements. In addition to price, some other issues to be negotiated are contract completion time; quality of goods and services offered; purchase volume; responsibility for financing, risk taking, promotion, and title; and product safety.

The most important rule in successful negotiating is that a concession is never provided without another concession being granted in return. For example, if the customer asks for a discount on the selling price, the salesperson should counter with a request for faster payment, later delivery, a longer service agreement, or some other attribute that provides the seller with comparable or perceived value. If the salesperson grants the request from the buyer for a lower price without negotiating a concession of his own, then the buyer may decide to further test the salesperson with another concession or ask for an even lower price.[20]

Relationship Marketing

The principles of personal selling and negotiation we have described are largely transaction-oriented, intended to close a specific sale. In many cases, however, the organization wants to build a long-term supplier-customer relationship by demonstrating that it has the capabilities to serve the account's needs in a superior way. Because today's customers are large and often global, they prefer suppliers who can sell and deliver a coordinated set of products and services to many places, quickly solve problems that arise in different locations, and work closely with customer teams to improve products and processes. Salespeople working with key customers must do more than call when they think customers might be ready to place orders; they should call or visit at other times, take a personal interest in customers, and make useful suggestions about their business.

When a relationship marketing program is properly implemented, the organization will begin to focus as much on managing its customers as on managing its products. At the same time, companies should realize that although there is a strong and warranted move toward relationship marketing, it is not effective in all situations. Ultimately, companies must judge which segments and which specific customers will respond profitably to relationship marketing.

HEALTH CARE SALES TO HOSPITALS AND PHYSICIANS

To understand health care sales that target hospitals and physicians, it is important to distinguish among three general categories of products: medical supplies and devices, pharmaceuticals, and capital equipment. Medical supplies such as bandages, tongue depressors, and syringes are usually funded by operating budgets and, in general, are a less complex sale. Typically, a budget for such items is developed by forecasting the number of procedures using the items and multiplying by the cost of the supply. Medical supply and device sales are usually driven by group purchasing agreements that give selected companies the *opportunity* to sell to hospitals or physician groups; they do not necessarily translate into sales. Sales professionals need to know not only who to contact but also the client's revenue cycle. For example, federal government clients have fiscal years that start October 1, whereas many hospitals begin their accounting on January 1.

In selling pharmaceuticals to hospitals, sales managers must realize that although new drugs are continually coming to market, the pharmacy budget cannot always be adjusted to accommodate the extra costs. It is therefore crucial for the pharmaceutical salesperson to know what the organization is empowered to purchase, the process for obtaining approval, and how the hospital will get paid by *its* customers. The process in hospitals (and managed care plans) for approving purchase of pharmaceuticals involves a group of physicians, pharmacists, and administrators called the Pharmacy and Therapeutics (P&T) Committee. This committee will assess the medication's cost and benefit as well as any comparative advantage to competing drugs.

For pharmaceutical sales to individual physicians or group practices, the focus is on educating the physicians who write prescriptions. The key to understanding effective pharmaceutical and medical device calls to physicians is understanding that they have one or both of the following value propositions:

1. Will the product help me take better care of my patients?
2. Will the product create more time for me by eliminating wasted effort or making me more efficient at what I do?

Using the first value proposition, the sales rep could, for example, educate the physician about the drug's superior performance treating patients with certain illnesses. Employing the second concept, the rep could state that the drug is as effective as its competitors, but because it has fewer side effects patients' phone calls about symptoms will be reduced.

As physicians are pressured to maximize the number of patients they see, their ability to spend time with sales reps has diminished. There are virtually no more thirty-minute sales calls. Research by Scott Levin consulting firm shows the average length of a sales rep visit has fallen from four minutes in 1998 to just ninety seconds today—with thirty-second hallway visits being commonplace.[21] To meet the challenge, pharma companies spend time preparing interesting and convincing visual presentations for the sales rep to use in person or to leave with physicians for them to view on their own time. Pharmaceutical companies also hire physically appealing and personable sales reps to make the visit more enjoyable.

Physician calls are a good opportunity to employ relationship marketing techniques. For example, it may be more effective to spend a few seconds on the product and a few minutes inquiring about the physician's family or recent vacation. We should stress that relationship marketing is not a gratuitous activity but must reflect a genuine personal interest in others. For this reason, selection of sales-force staff is especially critical.

For capital equipment sales—items such as MRI machines—the buying cycle is dramatically longer than for devices or pharmaceuticals. Such capital equipment companies as General Electric, Siemens, and Toshiba require an in-depth understanding of the organization's long-term strategies, its decision makers, its reimbursement structure, and its stakeholders. See Field Note 14.6 for factors associated with effective health care sales.

FIELD NOTE 14.6.

A Prescription for Effective Health Care Sales   Based on Miller Heiman research and insights from its industry experts, here are several key steps health care sales professionals should take to improve their effectiveness:

1. *Research the institutions.* Understand the funding mechanism of the organization and how the dollars flow. Get coaching about how to read financial statements and what organizations desire from a return-on-investment perspective.

2. *Complete a win/loss analysis on all deals.* Interview your customer to determine why they bought and your prospect to learn why they did not buy. Pay particular attention to what administration says. Use this language in your selling efforts going forward.

3. *In existing accounts, develop a strategy to retain and grow the business.* Communicate every six months with the administration to show that you understand their business and organizational issues and how you are helping them to achieve their objectives.

4. *Pay attention to what successful salespeople in your organization are doing.* Who are they calling on? What do they say to move the sale forward? How have they enhanced their credibility? What language do they use when communicating with their customers? Ask them to coach you.

5. *Understand your customers.* This is very different from pushing products. You may have the greatest product in the world, but without a keen understanding of how an organization makes its buying decisions, who in the organization makes the decisions, and when they make them, you're probably wasting your time.

6. *Speak the right language.* Executives may not speak "Clinicalese"—and even if they do, that is not the language they use every day to discuss their needs and their challenges. What language do they speak in administration? Successful salespeople will make the effort to find out before making a presentation. If you don't understand the executives' issues challenges and concerns (that is, if you don't speak the C-suite language), consider finding someone in your organization who does.

7. *Identify coaches.* Speaking the right language, grasping the complexities of a budget, or identifying an organization's decision-makers and their concerns may not come easy. Selling to health care organizations is complex, it involves long sales cycles, and it involves a broad cast of characters.

Source: Seven Steps to Better Healthcare Sales. Reno, Nev.: Miller Heiman, 2006. Reprinted with permission.

Pharmaceutical Sales Challenges

Pharmaceutical companies spend an average of $31.9 million annually on sales for each blockbuster primary care drug they market and $25.3 million annually selling each specialty pharmaceutical product marketed These figures translate to $150,000 per primary care rep annually and $330,000 per specialty drug rep spent on salary, travel, and technology, not including the funds for promotional materials and samples. The overall average field force budget in the industry is nearly $875 million, with top-spending organizations committing more than $1 billion to sales budgets. In 2004, the number of world-wide pharmaceutical sales reps surpassed one hundred thousand for the first time.[22] The top forty pharma companies have doubled the size of their sales forces in the past five years, according to InPharm, but prescribing has increased only 15 percent in the same period.

Since that time, several changes in the industry have affected the need for this many salespersons:

- Fewer new products are coming to market.

- Many companies used "mirrored sales forces." This type of selling involves numerous reps promoting the same medications. The reps may come from different divisions of the same company or may be from different companies who have agreed to comarket the product. Although message reinforcement is sometimes helpful, this practice often leads to "overkill" and confusion.

- Many companies found using a contract sales force to be a cost-effective strategy.

- Many customers, particularly academic medical centers, limit or no longer permit sales calls. Data presented at eyeonpharma's 2004 Sales Force Effectiveness Congress revealed that 70 percent of U.S. physicians are actively implementing policies to restrict sales rep access. For example, starting in 2007, the Henry Ford Health System in Detroit requires all pharmaceutical and medical product salespeople to make an appointment before calling on physicians and pay $100 for a certificate that documents they have taken training in appropriate ethical marketing behavior. The University of Michigan Medical System, whose vendor contact rules are even stricter than those at Henry Ford, started to ban samples in 2002.

As a result of these changes, many companies are now reducing their sales forces and stressing other methods of customer contact. For example, in 2005, Wyeth announced it would cut its sales force by as much as 30 percent; in 2006 Pfizer revealed it would cut its eleven-thousand-person team by 20 percent. Further, these changes have resulted in only 43 percent of rep calls leading to face-to-face meetings with physicians.

Free samples have become the hard currency of prescription drug marketing since 2003, when the pharmaceutical industry agreed to clean up its act and rein the most aggressive sales practices with a self-imposed code of conduct. A bill pending in the New Jersey Legislature would limit gifts to doctors, not including samples, to $100. At least nine other states are considering similar legislation. The American Medical Association is contemplating a rather draconian recommendation that bans sales reps in medical offices and gratuities of all kinds, including free samples, continuing education programs, and research grants. The AMA stated goal is to avoid any appearance that marketing has any role in prescription decision making by physicians.

Hospital Sales Departments

As far back as 1986, Gaston Memorial Hospital in Gastonia, North Carolina, has had a sales department based on the consumer packaged goods organizational model. This department targeted employers and physicians to sell them hospital services such as inpatient case management, laundry, occupational medicine, and health promotion services.

Most hospitals today, however, do not perceive a need to organize and manage a sales department; rather, they may have "network development" departments that target physicians for referrals. Most of these departments evolved from hospital efforts in the mid-1990s to purchase physician practices. The typical hospital soon discovered that owning physician practices resulted in financial losses, and the practice acquisition strategy was replaced with a strategy to increase patient referrals and admissions from surrounding physician practices. Unlike most salespeople, hospital network development representatives are usually not accountable for meeting territory-based sales quotas nor do they receive compensation based on sales performance.

Novant Health in Winston-Salem, North Carolina, is an exception. Bob Seehausen, the senior vice president of business development and sales for this four-hospital system, has focused the sales function on meeting the needs of physicians. For a fee, Novant offers products and services to physicians and mid-level providers that include services used daily for patient care, business processes that enhance revenue and improve operational efficiencies, negotiating and contracting with managed care plans on their behalf, credentialing, and access to group supply purchasing and lab testing.

DIRECT MARKETING

Direct marketing is using channels to reach and deliver goods and services to customers without using middlemen. These channels include direct mail, catalogs, telemarketing, kiosks, Web sites, television and radio ads, and mobile devices. Direct marketers seek a measurable response—typically a customer order, in which case it is sometimes called *direct-order marketing*. Today, many direct marketers use direct marketing to build a long-term relationship with the customer by sending birthday cards, informational materials, or small premiums to strengthen bonds over time. Many business marketers have shifted resources into direct mail and telemarketing and away from field sales as the costs of building and managing a sales force have increased.

The extraordinary growth of direct marketing is the result of many factors. Market "demassification" has resulted in an ever-increasing number of market niches. Ordering or reordering medical supplies through the Web is now commonplace. The growth of next-day delivery via FedEx, Airborne, and UPS has made ordering fast and easy. Despite the growth of the Internet, e-mail, mobile phones, and fax machines, which has made product selection and ordering much simpler, some find direct mail is more effective than on-line marketing. According to Philadelphia-area marketing executives polled at a 2006 seminar hosted by W. A. Wilde Co. (a direct-marketing fulfillment company), 50 percent cited traditional mail as the most successful marketing tool, with web-related marketing cited as the second most successful and e-mail marketing ranked third.

The Benefits of Direct Marketing

Direct marketing benefits customers by allowing them to learn about available products and services without tying up time in meeting with salespeople. Sellers also benefit. Direct marketers can buy a mailing list containing the names of almost any market segment; for example, diabetics, overweight people, or hospital chief financial officers. They can also customize and personalize their messages, build a continuous relationship with each customer, reach the most interested prospects at the right time, test alternative media and messages in search of the most cost-effective approach, shield the offer and strategy from competitors, and measure responses to their campaigns to decide which have been the most profitable.

Major Channels for Direct Marketing

Personal or face-to-face selling is a form of direct marketing, but direct marketers can also use a number of the other channels we mentioned earlier to reach individual prospects and customers. Much of the direct marketing in health care is business-to-business (B2B), but research institutions like St. Jude Children's Medical Center use television and other media to solicit donations from consumers (business-to-consumer or B2 C).

According to a 2006 Government Accountability Office (GAO) study, 94 percent of the $4.2 billion spent on direct-to-consumer (DTC) advertising in 2005 was for broadcast and print advertisements. The U.S. Food and Drug Administration (FDA) is responsible for establishing criteria for ads for drugs and devices, including a statement of major side effects and a contact source for more information (such as the company's toll-free phone number, referral to physicians, Web site, or even a print ad in a specific magazine). Because of the proliferation of these messages, the FDA does not have the time or resources to sufficiently monitor or regulate them. For example, in 2006, the agency issued only two warnings.[23] That this method is effective is highlighted by a 2005 study that showed significant increases in physician prescribing for patients who made brand-specific requests for antidepressants.[24]

Direct Mail

Direct-mail marketing involves sending an offer, announcement, reminder, or other item to a potential customer. Using highly selective mailing lists, direct marketers send out millions of mail pieces each year—letters, flyers, foldouts, and other forms of communication designed to break through the clutter. Direct mail is popular with marketers because it permits target market selectivity, can be personalized, is flexible, and allows early testing and response measurement. Although the cost per thousand people reached is higher than for mass media, those who are reached are much more qualified prospects. Examples include the following: a physician who is new to a community announces the opening of and information about her practice; a hospital sends an annual report to members of the community documenting the quality of care and new clinical programs; a pharmacy informs the community that on Wednesdays, prescription drugs will be 20 percent off usual prices.

Direct marketers must decide on their objectives, target markets, prospects, and offer elements. To measure effectiveness, they must also determine the means of testing the campaign and measures of its success.

Objectives. Although a typical campaign's success is judged by the order response rate (2 percent is normally considered good), direct mail can achieve other objectives such as producing sales leads, strengthening customer relationships, informing and educating customers, reminding customers of offers, and reinforcing customer purchase decisions.

Target markets and prospects. To identify the characteristics of potential customers who are most able, willing, and ready to buy, direct marketers usually apply the R-F-M formula (*recency, frequency, monetary amount*)—that is, selecting customers according to how much time has passed since their last purchase, how many times they have purchased, and how much they have spent since becoming a customer.

Prospects can also be identified on the basis of such variables as age, sex, income, education, previous mail-order purchases, occasions, and consumer lifestyle. Dun & Bradstreet operates information services that provide a wealth of data that can be used to select appropriate prospects.

Offer elements. Nash sees the offer strategy as consisting of five elements—the *product*, the *offer*, the *medium*, the *distribution method*, and the *creative strategy*.[25] All of these elements can be tested. In addition, the marketer has to decide on five components of the mailing itself: the outside envelope, sales letter, circular, reply form, and reply envelope. Direct mail can be followed up by e-mail, a less expensive and intrusive—but more passive—approach than telemarketing.

Testing elements. One of the great advantages of direct marketing is the ability to test, under real marketplace conditions, different elements of an offer strategy, such as products, product features, copy platform, mailer type, envelope, prices, or mailing lists. Response rates typically understate a campaign's overall long-term impact. As mentioned previously, although only 2 percent of targeted consumers may actually buy as a result of the campaign, organizations should also measure the impact of direct marketing on awareness, intention to buy, and word of mouth.

Measuring campaign success: lifetime value. By adding up the planned campaign costs, the direct marketer can calculate in advance the needed breakeven response rate (net of returned merchandise and bad debts). Even when a specific campaign fails to break even in the short run, it can be worthwhile if the expected profit on all future purchases is considered. For an average customer, one would calculate the longevity, annual expenditure, and gross margin, minus the cost of customer acquisition and maintenance (discounted for the opportunity cost of money) (see Field Note 14.7).

FIELD NOTE 14.7.

Siemens "Stop Worrying" Direct Mail Promotion Works   Siemens Integrated Service Management provides hospitals with service contracts for diagnostic and biomedical equipment. Their market research indicated that hospital administrators were concerned with the internal versus external costs of equipment maintenance, fear of unplanned system downtime, compliance with Joint Commission accreditation standards, and problems with managing different service contracts for various pieces of equipment. In response, Siemens created a direct-mail piece that was designed to address these issues and to cut through the direct mail clutter.

The "Stop Worrying" campaign consisted of a seven-inch-by-seven-inch cardboard box, two inches deep, that was mailed to hospital administrator prospects. The outside of the box was printed with only the words "Stop Worrying." Inside the box was a ten-panel graphic insert entitled "Stop worrying. Start believing." The insert covered each of the four issues, had a customer testimonial, and included a call to action for a free service assessment.

The most interesting element of this direct mail promotion was the enclosed "worry stone" and its explanation. The smooth ceramic, dark green, oblong stone, embedded in a foam rubber mat, was accompanied by the following explanation: "Otherwise known as a 'pocket tranquilizer' . . . some people believe that rubbing the smooth surface of the stone puts pressure on nerves within the thumb that may release endorphins, the brain's natural relaxants." Regardless of the stone's powers, Siemens management judged this promotion a success, as it generated requests for service assessments that exceeded their promotion objectives.

Telemarketing

Telemarketing is the use of the telephone and call centers to attract prospects, sell to existing customers, and provide service by taking orders and answering questions. Companies use call centers for *inbound telemarketing* (receiving calls from customers) and *outbound telemarketing* (initiating calls to prospects and customers). Telemarketing includes:

- *Telesales:* Taking orders from catalogs or ads and also doing outbound calling to cross-sell the company's other products, upgrade orders, introduce new products, open new accounts, and reactivate former accounts

- *Telecoverage:* Calling customers to maintain and nurture key account relationships and give more attention to neglected accounts

- *Teleprospecting:* Generating and qualifying new leads for closure by another sales channel

- *Customer service and technical support:* Answering service and technical questions

Effective telemarketing depends on choosing the right telemarketers, training them well, and providing performance incentives. Although telemarketing is a major direct-marketing tool and helps to replace more expensive field sales calls, both consumers and businesses can find it intrusive. The Federal Trade Commission established a consumer National Do Not Call registry (at www.ftc.gov) in October 2003, and more than 105 million consumers have already signed up to prevent telemarketers from calling them at home. Only political organizations, charities, telephone surveyors, or companies with existing relationships with consumers are exempt.

Telemarketing is increasingly being used by hospitals. UCLA Medical Center uses in-bound telemarketing to let patients set appointments with physicians, and referring physicians can call to have instant consults with specialists. Visitors to the Emory Healthcare Web site who have a health question can click a button and receive an immediate outbound phone call from a nurse. Also, pharmaceutical benefit management (PBM) companies allow patients to renew medications by phone.

Other Media for Direct-Response Marketing

Direct marketers use all the major media to make direct offers to potential buyers.

Newspapers and magazines carry abundant print ads offering announcements of new physicians joining a practice, the content and location for a seminar on LASIK eye surgery, and other health care goods and services that individuals can order by dialing a toll-free number.

Direct-response media advertising, often through thirty- and sixty-minute television infomercials, attempts to combine the sell of commercials with the draw of educational information and entertainment. These shows often resemble documentaries and include testimonials plus a toll-free number for getting further information or making a charitable contribution. Longer direct-response formats include the Jerry Lewis Muscular Dystrophy Labor Day Telethon. This twenty-one-and-a-half-hour, star-studded television variety show was first broadcast in 1966; it simultaneously entertains, informs, and raises funds for the service and research programs of the Muscular Dystrophy Association. The Children's Miracle Network is a national alliance of premier children's hospitals that annually treat seventeen million patients for a wide range of diseases and injuries. The Children's Miracle Network Radiothon is a partnership of radio stations and hospitals that come together to raise funds and awareness for the benefit of children's health.

Interactive Marketing

The newest channels for direct marketing are electronic. The Internet provides marketers and consumers with opportunities for much greater interaction and individualization. Companies in the past would send standard media—magazines, newsletters, ads—without any individualization or opportunity for interaction. Today these companies can send customized content that consumers themselves can further individualize. For example, Mayo Clinic publishes *Housecall*, a free weekly e-newsletter that provides the latest health information from Mayo Clinic physicians. While signing up for this service, the Web site instructs individuals to "Select the health topics that you want to appear on your personalized page" from a list that appears below the request.

The exchange process in the age of information, however, has become increasingly customer-initiated and customer-controlled. Even after marketers enter the exchange process, customers define the rules of engagement, and they can insulate themselves with the help of agents and intermediaries. Customers define what information they need, what offerings interest them, and what prices they are willing to pay.[26] Health care organizations need to monitor blogs for any content that might affect them. For example, pharmaceutical companies may want to monitor these sources for any revelations of medication side effects or complaints about the company. In 2007 the American Medical Association set up a blog site for physicians to trade information, including adverse drug reactions.

Benefits of Interactive Marketing. Since it is highly accountable and its effects can be easily tracked, interactive marketing offers many unique benefits.[27] Marketers can buy ads on sites that are relevant to their offerings and customers and can place advertising based on contextual keywords from on-line search companies like Google. In that way, the Web can be used to reach people when they have actually started the buying process. The University of North Carolina–Chapel Hill, School of Public Health Executive Program tested a large number of keywords that it purchased using Google AdWords. It also varied the sponsorship ads by time of day and day of the week. The program was able to markedly increase its applications through analyzing the most effective words and placement times. The business model of WebMD is based on selling ads to companies who know that their potential customers (including physicians) will search the site seeking health care information.

Designing an Attractive Web Site. A key challenge is designing a Web site that is attractive on first viewing and interesting enough to encourage repeat visits. Rayport and Jaworski have proposed that in order to be effective, marketers consider the following seven design elements, which they call the 7Cs:[28]

- *Context:* Layout and design
- *Content:* Text, pictures, sound, and video the site contains
- *Community:* How the site enables user-to-user communication

- *Customization:* The site's ability to tailor itself to different users or to allow users to personalize the site

- *Communication:* How the site enables site-to-user, user-to-site, or two-way communication

- *Connection:* The degree to which the site is linked to other sites

- *Commerce:* The site's capabilities to enable commercial transactions

To motivate visitors to return to the site, organizations need to pay special attention to context and content factors and also embrace another C—constant change.[29]

Visitors will judge a site's performance on its ease of use and its physical attractiveness. Ease of use chiefly consists of three attributes: (1) the site downloads quickly, (2) the first page is easy to understand, and (3) the visitor can easily navigate to other pages that open quickly. Physical attractiveness is determined by the following factors: (1) the individual pages are clean looking and not overly crammed with content, (2) the type faces and font sizes are all very readable, and (3) the site makes good use of color and sound. Certain types of health care content aid in attracting first-time visitors and bringing them back again, namely, (1) deep information with links to related sites, (2) changing news of interest, and (3) changing free offers to visitors, such as mailings, coupons, or opportunities to join clinical trials.

Placing Ads and Promotion On-line

A company has to decide which forms of internet advertising will be most cost-effective in achieving its advertising objectives. *Banner ads* are small rectangular boxes containing text and perhaps a picture, which companies pay to place on relevant sites. The larger the audience reached, the more the placement will cost.

Many companies get their names on the Internet by sponsoring special content on Web sites that carry news, health information, and so on. *Sponsorships* are best placed in well-targeted sites where they can offer relevant information or service. The sponsor pays for showing the content and in turn receives acknowledgment as the supporter of that particular service on the Web site. A *microsite* is a limited area on the Web managed and paid for by an external advertiser. Microsites are particularly relevant for companies selling low-interest products such as health insurance. The insurance company could create a microsite on a hospital Web site, offering advice for setting up a health savings account (HSA) and at the same time offering a good insurance deal.

Interstitials are advertisements, often with video or animation, that pop-up between changes on a Web site. Ads for Johnson & Johnson's Tylenol headache reliever pop up on brokers' Web sites whenever the stock market falls by one hundred points or more. Because consumers have found many of the pop-ads to be intrusive or infected with viruses and spyware, many computer users have installed software to block these ads.

The hottest growth area has been that of *search-related ads*.[30] Thirty-five percent of all searches are for products or services. Search terms are used as a proxy for the consumer's consumption interests, and relevant links to product or service offerings are listed alongside the search results from Google, MSN, and Yahoo. Advertisers pay only if people click on the links. The cost per click depends on how high the link is ranked and the popularity of the keyword searched. Average click-through is about 2 percent, much more than comparable on-line ads.[31] For example, Brigham and Women's Hospital was interested in attracting patients for a new neurological procedure, but the condition helped by the procedure was not common. The budget to promote this procedure was also small. The Hospital was successful in using Google AdWords to reach patients in the local Boston market as well as globally. A newer trend, *content-target advertising*, links ads not to keywords but to the content of Web pages.

E-Marketing Guidelines. If a company does an e-mail campaign correctly, it can not only build customer relationships but also reap additional profits. Here are some important guidelines followed by pioneering e-mail marketers:[32]

- *Give the customer a reason to respond*. Organizations should offer powerful incentives for reading e-mail pitches and on-line ads, such as special health topic white papers, survey research results, or access to the organization's database archive of health information.

- *Personalize the e-mail content*. *HealthLeaders*, a traditional, monthly health care management newsprint magazine, also sends customized content e-mails directly to customers' offices each week. Customers who agree to receive the newsletter select from topics listed on an interest profile.

- *Offer something the customer could not get via direct mail*. Because e-mail campaigns can be carried out quickly, they can offer time-sensitive information. For example, *Modern Healthcare* magazine sends frequent e-alerts with breaking health care management news.

- *Make it easy for customers to unsubscribe*. On-line customers should have a positive exit experience. According to a Burston-Marsteller and Roper Starch Worldwide study, the top 10 percent of Web users who communicate much more often on-line typically share their views by e-mail with eleven friends when satisfied but contact seventeen friends when they are dissatisfied.[33]

Organizations that use on-line marketing tools will face many challenges in expanding the public's use of e-commerce. For example, customers must feel that the information they supply is confidential and will not be sold to others. Organizations must encourage communication by inviting questions, suggestions, and even complaints via e-mail. Some sites even include a call-me button (like Emory

Healthcare)—the customer clicks on it and his or her phone rings: it's a call from a customer representative, ready to answer a question.

Smart on-line marketers, such as Yale New-Haven Medical Center, respond quickly to inquiries by sending out newsletters, special products, or promotion offers based on purchase histories, reminders of service requirements or warranty renewals, or announcements of special events. Yale New-Haven uses small, provocative, inexpensive banner newspaper ads to attract consumer attention. When consumers call the phone number on the ad or click on the Web site for more information on the advertised health topic, Yale New-Haven asks for permission to send them future supplemental information by e-mail.

Direct marketing must be integrated with other communication and channel activities.

Podcasting: Extending E-Mail Marketing. More than 12 percent of internet users have downloaded a podcast over the past year, according to a 2007 report from the Pew Internet & American Life Project, a significant jump from the 7 percent of users who reported use in the research agency's February-April 2006 report. Existing marketing—particularly e-mail, which can provide a direct link to the podcast content—is an ideal way to spread the word about the new effort. Field Note 14.8 provides some insights into the potential for using podcasts.

FIELD NOTE 14.8.

Podcasts Lisa Wehr, founder and CEO of on-line marketing company Oneupweb, provides some insight and advice for those looking to start or improve their podcasting efforts. Here is what she had to say when interviewed by *BtoBOnline*.

BtoBOnline.com: Why should marketers consider doing a corporate podcast?

Wehr: Podcasts let you build a one-on-one relationship by connecting with listeners and putting out a message that has an emotional aspect to it. Listeners hear a voice and associate that voice with your company, which is a great way to get them coming back again and again.

BtoBOnline.com: How do you select the right "voice" for your podcast?

Wehr: Particularly in the B2B market, it's important for listeners to hear your message from upper-level management. It lends the message more integrity and comes off as less of a marketing spiel. Business customers want to hear about news and new products direct from the horse's mouth.

BtoBOnline.com: How often should marketers create new podcasts and how long should they be?

Wehr: The true value of podcasting is to build an audience. To do that, you need relationship and frequency. The listener needs to feel a connection to you or your company, while the podcasts have to be frequent enough to maintain an audience. This usually means a one-off podcast is going to provide very little value. You should try to introduce a new podcast once a week or once a month. As for length, we did a study of podcasters in the B2B space. We concluded that there is a wide range of length, but boiled down that most people did fifteen minute podcasts, which makes sense. The average commute is thirty minutes, so if you can stay in the fifteen minute to twenty minute range, you're good.

BtoBOnline.com: How should marketers use e-mail to promote their podcasts?

Wehr: Any good marketer knows that teasing the audience a bit with information that's in the podcast is a good idea. You can pull out quotes or information that's contained in the podcast and put it into your normal e-mail communications. Also, with each new podcast, you should be doing a summary [of the podcast] and placing it on your site so search engines can pick it up. You should also refer to previous podcasts in current podcasts since a lot of people might come in midstream and you want them to be going back and listening to your existing content.

Source: K. J. Bannan, "Why e-mail marketers should consider pod-casting." *BtoB.com.* Crain Communications, Inc. [http://ctstage.sv.publicus.com/apps/pbcs.dll/article?AID = /20061221/FREE/612210701&SearchID = 73281453687741]. Dec. 21, 2006.

SUMMARY

Health care organizations are relying on more than the standard mass communication tools of advertising, sales promotion, and public relations to get their messages to the public, especially to specific target groups. People are exchanging word-of-mouth opinion all the time on organizations, products, and services. Marketers are developing new ways to create a favorable buzz about their organizations and services. In addition, hospitals and commercial health care organizations use sales forces to find leads, make contacts and presentations, and secure business. Sales forces are an expensive marketing tool and must be designed and managed carefully. Decisions must be made about sales-force objectives, strategy, structure, size, and compensation. The organization must recruit and select sales reps, then train, motivate, and evaluate their work. Sales rep training consists of mastering the steps of prospecting and qualifying, approaching prospects, presenting and demonstrating, overcoming objections, negotiating, closing the sale, and following up and maintaining the relationship.

Health care organizations are also making increased use of direct marketing, namely direct mail, telemarketing, and interactive on-line marketing (Web site, e-mail, blogs, podcasts, and so on). Direct marketing provides an opportunity to test different elements of an intended communication to find the elements that are the most cost-effective. As a result, direct marketing can more easily meet the need to measure the financial impact of different communications.

DISCUSSION QUESTIONS

1. You are on the brand management team for Cialis, the Eli Lilly erectile dysfunction drug, and the team is interested in exploring a word-of-mouth marketing strategy to increase sales. Outline a recommendation for this strategy, including the basis of the recommendation, the steps for implementation, and the metrics that will be used to evaluate its effectiveness.

2. Compiling names, addresses, phone numbers, and other consumer information in databases is vital for direct marketing, but health care information, confidentiality, and privacy are protected by regulation. How can health care marketers gather and use information to build relationships with consumers in this environment?

3. A salesperson for a surgical device company can often be found supervising its use and coaching a surgeon for hours in an operating room. Conversely, pharmaceutical sales reps spend much of their time in physician office waiting rooms hoping to see a doctor for a few minutes of conversation while they drop off drug samples or lunch. Critique these two different sales models. Which one delivers more value to physicians and the company?

4. Web 2.0 refers to a second-generation of web-based communities and hosted services. Examples include weblogs, social networking communities such as MySpace, video-sharing portals like YouTube, podcasts, and RSS feeds that allow both downloading and uploading of content. What are the different ways a pharmacy chain, a chiropractor, and a health and fitness club could use Web 2.0 to reach their personal marketing communications goals?

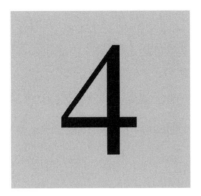
IMPLEMENTING AND CONTROLLING THE MARKETING EFFORT

CHAPTER

15

ORGANIZING, IMPLEMENTING, AND CONTROLLING MARKETING

LEARNING OBJECTIVES

In this chapter, we will address the following questions:

1. How can a health care organization set up its marketing department and what tasks should it address?

2. How can the marketing group help the rest of the organization to become patient-centered?

3. What steps will ensure a successful implementation of the marketing plans and campaigns?

4. What controls and tools can the organization use to ensure that it is moving efficiently toward its goals?

OPENING EXAMPLE

Rush Medical College Carries Out Strategic Planning   Rush Medical College has been around for 170 years, longer than any other health care institution in Chicago. Its hospital, Presbyterian St. Luke's, has origins dating as far back as 1864. Rush University Medical Center, as it was renamed in 2003, is an academic institution comprising a 613-bed hospital serving adults and children, the 61-bed Johnston R. Bowman Health Center, several affiliated hospitals in the greater metropolitan area, and Rush University.

During the 1980s, when other area hospitals started marketing programs, Rush relied on its excellent reputation to attract patients. The "marketing department" had no strategic plan to guide activities; it served principally as an on-demand communications resource for departments. By 2002, this benign neglect took its toll when patient volume continued to decrease and Rush fell from first to fourth place in consumer surveys.

Enter Christine Malcolm, senior vice president of strategic planning, marketing, and program development, and Michele Flanagin, associate vice president of strategic and program development. The newly hired pair was charged with doing something never before done at Rush—planning, marketing, and strategic assessments, as well as providing strategic vision and management for new business initiatives and programs.

"It was basic blocking and tackling," says Flanagin, who has since been promoted to vice president of strategic planning, marketing, and program development. "We didn't do anything innovative. It was just new for Rush."

Starting from zero, Flanagin and Malcolm built a strong business case, using tightly constructed financial models to convince the board and administration that Rush could not increase admissions without strategic planning and marketing. "Rush was not performing well financially, and the leadership had to fight its instinct to cut budgets. Marketing is riskier," Flanagin says.

Convinced, the board took the leap of faith with Flanagin and Malcolm, and the pair launched a "quick-start" strategic planning retreat with 150 senior leaders and physicians. During the retreat, key services were identified and a basic strategic outline was developed. "It got everyone to agree to 'do' something," Flanagin says. "The physicians in particular were so hungry for planning and marketing leadership, they wanted to do anything to help."

An advertising agency was hired in December 2002 and spent six months on the marketing planning process, conducting interviews and focus groups, creating a positioning platform, and developing a budget for the fiscal year starting July 2003. An October deadline was set for rolling out a comprehensive advertising campaign, complete with television and radio commercials, billboards, transit signs, newspaper ads, a redesigned Web site, and a series of brochures.

During the planning process, it became obvious that something else needed to change—Rush's name. The organization had been known as Rush-Presbyterian-St. Luke's

Medical Center since 1969. Driven by the marketing research, the board voted to change the institution's name to Rush University Medical Center. The decision would be announced in September, just before the campaign was scheduled to begin in October 2003.

All the pieces were in place: research conducted, plans made, budgets approved, advertising creative strategy developed, deadlines established. The communications staff now had four months before the campaign's launch to shift from an internally focused model to an externally focused one, introduce the medical center's new name, and build all the necessary marketing tools—including new recruitment materials, a new community newsletter, a redesigned Web site, and assessment tools—from the ground up.

Sara Stern, associate vice president of marketing communications, was charged with coordinating the effort. She started by assessing the roles and responsibilities of the fifteen in-house staff members, determining which activities needed to stop, and restructuring the department to focus on the immediate marketing needs for a redesigned Web site, a new referral and consultation guide for physicians, and the ad campaign. The creative part, Web site and community newsletter were all outsourced. Stern says the team approach helped ensure that the campaign's message was the same across all media. "Everything had the look and feel of the new branding effort, including ads for six different service lines, seven radio ads in Spanish and English, signage, HR recruitment . . . even the call center."

A major component of the marketing program was to reconnect with neglected primary care physicians and referring physicians in the area. In addition to the development of the new referral and consultation guide, Rush developed a primary care directory for specialty physicians. New tool kits were designed to help physicians coordinate their marketing efforts with the medical center's new look and feel. Also, a new staff member was hired to develop physician relationships and create more links with community hospitals.

Rush launched the campaign in October 2003, using television, radio, newspapers, billboards, and transit signs. The first wave of the broadcast-dominant campaign lasted six weeks and targeted women aged thirty-five to sixty-four. To grab attention, the first flight of TV ads featured sixty-second spots; subsequent spots were thirty seconds. Ads ran on six stations, including network, public broadcasting, and cable, with a 99-percent reach and 10.5 frequency for all adults. Radio ads ran on the top twelve stations (English and Spanish) with strong female demographics. Moderate-size newspaper ads were alternated between the *Chicago Tribune* and the *Chicago Sun-Times* in the business, news, and lifestyle sections.

"The ad tag line, 'It's how medicine should be,' communicates to the public Rush's special approach to care and the level of expertise [clinicians] bring to patients," Stern says. "The ads distinguish Rush from other hospitals and reflect what audience research had found: that Rush caregivers share a uniquely collaborative approach to patient care, that research and innovation benefit patients, and that the quality of the nursing care is superb . . ."

The redesigned Web site had a strong visual tie-in with the advertising campaign. The new site debuted the same day the ads began and featured many improvements for the approximately seventy-five thousand visitors who access the site each month. Improvements included a greatly enhanced physician directory, comprehensive health information in both English and Spanish, better site navigation, a database of clinical research trials, and extensive information about Rush's programs and services.

According to Marie Mahoney, director of internet communications, it cost $53,000 to redesign the Web site to match the marketing and improve basic functionality. An additional $1,106,000 in 2004 and $900,000 in 2005 were allocated in the marketing and information technology support budgets to purchase software, increase staff and training, and continue improving online content management, marketing, and referral tools.

All the hard work paid off. In the weeks following the launch, Rush saw call volume to its physician referral line nearly double. There was a fivefold increase in queries to the "Find a Doctor" section of the Web site. Queries rose from a pre-launch level of less than five thousand per month to almost twenty-five thousand per month a year later. There also was a 20 percent increase in first-time visitors to the Web site.

The campaign also narrowed the consumer preference gap. Rush went from fourth to third place in top-of-mind awareness in the sixteen weeks following the launch. This preference is translating to an overall upward trend in inpatient admissions and outpatient visits. Admissions rose 2.3 percent from the prior year and outpatient volume grew 10 percent. In addition, clinical program growth in top service lines is strong, with a better-than-average payer mix.

The 2003 campaign also marked a return to profitability for Rush after a period of losses. Rush reported a profit of $6.5 million, which is an improvement of almost $20 million from the previous year. In addition, hospital operating revenues increased 9 percent. *Source:* B. Long, "Market Share Is Not Sustained by Reputation Alone," Strategic Health Care Communications. [http://www.strategichealthcare.com/pubs/shcm/f2_MarketShare_print.php]. Published by permission of the publisher, Health Care Communications.

In this final chapter, we will examine how organizations can get more productivity from their marketing activities by properly organizing, implementing, and controlling marketing plans and activities.

OVERVIEW: ORGANIZING FOR MARKETING

The role and scope of marketing vary greatly in different types of health care organizations, such as pharmaceutical firms, medical device and equipment companies, and health care service organizations such as hospitals.

For instance, the critical role that marketing plays in the pharmaceutical industry requires marketers to participate at every step of the development process:

identifying opportunity areas; gathering information from physicians and consumers to aid in decisions about dosage, pill size, packaging, naming, advertising, and sampling; and conducting post-launch monitoring programs to monitor effectiveness and competitive positioning. Marketing also must prepare salespeople to make their case in recommending the use of new drugs by different types of physicians and acceptance on formularies in hospitals and by pharmaceutical benefit management companies (PBMs).

Marketing played an important, but quantitatively smaller, role in health care service businesses such as hospitals, nursing homes, and non-profit organizations. In the past, these firms only used public relations (PR) staff to promote and protect the organization's reputation. The PR staff supplied positive stories to news media and sought to prevent broadcast or publication of negative stories about their organization. Because hospitals were at full capacity in the 1970s, they did not see much of a need for marketing. After that time, however, some urban areas were becoming crowded with competitors as a result of hospital expansions and the emergence of alternative care sites such as ambulatory care centers and outpatient surgicenters. When this competition caused some hospitals to close whole floors, they engaged marketing consultants and hired a marketing director to manage market research and advertising. A few appointed a marketing vice-president who would sit with other senior executives and participate in the hospital planning and strategy sessions. Hospitals began to think more strategically about their position in the local market; they became aware that their institution was actually a brand, whether or not they actively shaped it. They therefore needed to develop a clearer mission and vision, one that they could communicate to their target markets. Hospitals began to recognize the need for market segmentation, targeting, and positioning as well as better in-hospital service, advertising, community relations, and promotional events.

Today, marketing is a well-established function in most health care service organizations. The size of the marketing department, its budget, and its activities depend on many factors, including the organizational size, finances, and competitive position in the local area. Although the following sections describe the marketing department in hospitals, the principles are equally applicable to other health care organizations.

The Tasks of the Marketing Vice President

A hospital that decides to hire a marketing vice president (MVP) must first establish a job description to facilitate the search for the right person; the following characteristics will help set the expectations for that post. The MVP must:

- Help the hospital better define its position and brand in the community
- Provide data on changing consumer and patient demographics and identify new opportunities
- Monitor the activities of competitors, medical associations, and government regulators

- Develop metrics for measuring the results of marketing expenditures
- Be available to help individual hospital departments needing marketing assistance

In searching for the right person to take the position of MVP, there are two contending philosophies. One is to seek a person who has worked in brand management in a well-known, fast-moving consumer goods company and can bring fresh marketing ideas and practices to an otherwise staid organization. This tactic is likely to lead to the hospital's thinking of marketing as primarily a communication and advertising function. At many hospitals, the marketing department basically consists of a director of communications with people reporting on publications, direct mail, internet, graphic design and outreach/events.

The other approach is to hire a person who has medical experience or has worked in a professional organization, a high-tech firm, a bank, or a public utility. An example of this practice is the Brigham and Women's Hospital's marketing department, whose organization chart is shown in Figure 15.1.

What Are the Characteristics of an Effective Marketing Department?

In order to achieve marketing excellence, marketing managers must think more holistically and less departmentally. To succeed in this fashion, they must get to know the medical staff and the heads of various departments, be available as advisors on marketplace problems, and be able to supply customer and competitive data and insight to others on the staff. Further, marketers must take some responsibility for identifying new services that will contribute to the hospital's growth and help the hospital define its brand and communicate it to the public.

Marketers bring to a hospital not only traditional skills, such as marketing research, advertising, sales management, pricing, and setting up distribution channels, but also some new ones, such as:

- Database marketing and data-mining
- Contact center management and telemarketing

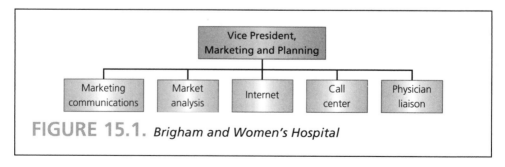

FIGURE 15.1. *Brigham and Women's Hospital*

Note: The MVP has "planning" in the title as well as marketing, and there is a separate position for market analysis. Some hospitals add other reporting positions, such as patient service and new opportunity development.

- Public relations marketing (including event and sponsorship marketing)
- Brand building and brand asset management
- Experiential marketing
- Integrated marketing communications
- Profitability analysis by segment, customer, channel

HELPING THE HOSPITAL BECOME PATIENT-ORIENTED

One of the major challenges of a hospital is to gain and instill in the staff a better understanding of patients and their needs. A Cincinnati friend told one of the authors that although he can choose better-known and larger hospitals, he prefers a particular smaller one because its personal attention is superior. The nurses at that hospital are chosen because of their deeply felt humanity and because they are happy in their work. He has not found such caring in most other hospitals that he has experienced; those others are more oriented to serving the needs of the physicians or other staff members than to serving the needs of the patients.

Ultimately, the quality of medical care will depend on the CEO and his or her interest in making the hospital customer satisfied. Consider what the late Bernard J. Lachner—former CEO of the Evanston Hospital, now Evanston Northwestern Healthcare in Evanston, Illinois—told one of the authors: "When the physician, house staff, nurse, waiter, X-ray or emergency room, personnel or admitting clerk is rude, or the maid bumps the bed while cleaning, the parking lot attendant is less than helpful when the lot is full, the cafeteria turns away visitors, the pharmacy has limited hours for outpatients—all of this suggest that hospitals operate for their own convenience and not that of the patient, his family and friends."

Many hospitals are adopting a drive to improve their service level and performance. The task is to build a consumer-oriented culture. To accomplish this goal, a CEO must:

- *Convince other senior managers of the need to become customer-focused.* The CEO must convince physicians, nursing staff, maintenance, and others of the benefits of making patients as comfortable as possible during their hospital stays. Patients perceive quality care as much from their service experience as from the technical component of care.

- *Exemplify the behavior that the CEO wants others to emulate.* The CEO needs to personally exemplify a strong patient concern by dropping in on patients, inviting discussions with nurses about their problems, making it easy for visitors to be comfortable, and investing in improvements in the facilities' aesthetics and appeal.

- *Get outside help and guidance.* Engage the services of a consulting firm that has firsthand experience in helping hospitals improve their service quality, customer orientation, and image.

- *Develop an improved information system on patient data and satisfaction.* Install a system for gathering information on patient satisfactions and dissatisfactions.

- *Change the organization's incentive and reward system.* Develop a system of incentives to reward the right behavior. Set up occasions to honor those staff members who are high performers in patient care.

- *Develop in-house training programs.* Make sure that staff in all patient-related departments are trained in handling patient concerns and providing compassionate care.

- *Empower the employees.* Progressive organizations encourage and reward their employees for coming up with new ideas to improve patient care and empower them to settle complaints quickly.

MARKETING IMPLEMENTATION

The marketing staff must not only develop marketing plans but also carry them out to a successful conclusion. The most brilliant marketing plan counts for little if it is not implemented properly. Consider the following example: After a local hospital learned that patients were not receiving good service from any of the neighboring hospitals, the CEO decided to make excellent customer service its major strategic initiative. When this strategy failed, a postmortem revealed a number of implementation failures: physicians were overworked, nurses were in short supply, nurse call systems were not working well, and the hospital continued to focus most of its attention on cost containment and current profitability. In short, the hospital had failed to make the changes required to carry out its strategic plan.

Plans address the *what* and *why* of marketing activities. Implementation addresses the *who*, *where*, *when*, and *how*. As another example, a hospital administrator decided to build a new medical specialty in plastic surgery. To translate this initiative into specific activities and people assignments, the human resources department must compile a list of the best potential department heads for plastic surgery to attract to the hospital; senior management must decide how much they would pay for a leading plastic surgeon; the facilities department needs to assign operating room capacity to support the new service; and the marketing department must decide on how to announce and promote this new service once it is ready to be launched.

Thomas Bonoma identified four sets of skills for implementing marketing programs:

1. *Diagnostic skills.* When marketing programs do not fulfill expectations, is it the result of poor strategy or poor implementation? If implementation, what went wrong?

2. *Identification of organization level.* Implementation problems can occur in three levels: the marketing function, the marketing program, and the marketing policy level.

3. *Implementation skills.* To implement programs successfully, marketers need broad business skills: *allocating skills* for budgeting resources, *organizing skills* to develop an effective organization, and *interaction skills* to motivate others to get things done.

4. *Evaluation skills.* Marketers need monitoring skills to track and evaluate marketing actions.[1]

In order for health care organizations to make their marketing operations more efficient, they need answers to such questions as, What are the results from our advertising campaign on measures of reach, frequency and impact? Has the campaign increased consumer awareness, knowledge, interest, preference, and even admissions for this hospital? Have health event programs drawn a sufficient number of the right kind of potential customers? Have the field salespeople been improving their negotiation results with pharmaceutical firms and health maintenance organizations? In each case, the organization needs to establish appropriate metrics for measuring the results of marketing actions.

EVALUATION AND CONTROL

In spite of the need to monitor and control marketing activities, many organizations have inadequate control procedures. A private study of a cross-section of organizations in different industries revealed these findings:

- Smaller organizations do a poorer job of setting clear objectives and establishing systems to measure performance.

- Fewer than half the organizations studied knew their individual products' profitability. About one-third had no regular review procedures for spotting and eliminating underperforming products and services.

- Almost half of the organizations failed to compare their prices with those of the competition, analyze their costs, analyze the causes of customer dissatisfaction, conduct formal evaluations of advertising effectiveness, or review their sales force's call reports.

- Many organizations take four to eight weeks to develop control reports, which by that time are no longer timely and are occasionally inaccurate.

To remedy these problems, an organization needs four types of marketing control: annual-plan control, profitability control, efficiency control, and strategic control.

Annual-Plan Control

This activity aims to ensure that the organization achieves the sales, profits, and other goals established in its annual plan. The heart of annual-plan control is management by objectives. Four steps are involved: set monthly or quarterly goals; monitor marketplace performance; determine the causes of serious performance deviations;

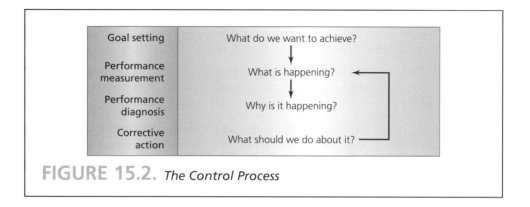

FIGURE 15.2. *The Control Process*

and take corrective action to close the gaps between goals and performance (see Figure 15.2).

This control model applies to all levels of the organization. Top management sets annual sales and profit goals that become specific goals for lower levels of management. Each product manager is committed to attaining specified levels of sales and costs; each sales representative is committed to specific goals. Each period, top management reviews and interprets the individual and consolidated results.

Efficiency Control

Suppose a profitability analysis reveals that the organization is achieving poor sales or profits in certain products, services, territories, or markets. Are there more efficient ways to manage the sales force, advertising, sales promotion, and distribution in connection with these marketing entities?

Some organizations have established a *marketing controller* position to improve marketing efficiency. Marketing controllers work in the institution's controller's office but specialize in the marketing side of the business. They examine adherence to sales and profit plans, help prepare marketing budgets, measure the efficiency of promotions, analyze media production costs, evaluate customer and geographic profitability, and educate marketing personnel on the financial costs of marketing activities.[2]

Sales-Force Efficiency. Sales managers need to monitor the following key indicators of efficiency in their territories:

- Average number of calls per salesperson per day
- Average sales call time per contact
- Average revenue or results per sales call
- Average cost per sales call
- Entertainment cost per sales call
- Sales-force cost as a percentage of total sales

Advertising Efficiency. Many managers believe it is almost impossible to measure the financial return on their advertising dollars. Nevertheless, they should keep track of at least the following statistics:

- Advertising cost per thousand target customers reached by media vehicle
- Percentage of audience who noted, saw, recalled, or recognized each ad
- Consumer opinions on the ad's content and effectiveness
- Before-and-after measures of attitude toward the organization or its service
- Number of inquiries stimulated by the ad
- Cost per inquiry

Hospital management can take a number of steps to improve advertising efficiency, including doing a better job of positioning the hospital, defining objectives, pretesting messages, using computer technology to guide the selection of media, looking for better media buys, and doing posttesting.

Sales-Promotion Efficiency. Sales promotion includes dozens of devices for stimulating buyer interest and product trial. To improve sales-promotion efficiency, management should record the costs and sales impact of each promotion and monitor the following statistics:

- Number of persons attending health care events
- Number of inquiries resulting from an event
- Display costs per sales dollar

The marketer can analyze the results of different promotions and advise the organization on the most cost-effective types to use.

Distribution Efficiency. Management needs to search for distribution economies in providing ambulatory care sites, by monitoring

- Number of patient cases at each ambulatory care site
- Profit or loss from operating each ambulatory care site
- Number of patient referrals to the main hospital

This information will help a hospital know, for instance, whether it needs to add or close down ambulatory care units.

Strategic Control

From time to time organizations need to undertake a critical review of overall marketing goals and effectiveness. Each organization should periodically reassess its strategic approach to the marketplace through marketing effectiveness reviews, marketing audits, and marketing weaknesses reviews.

The Marketing Effectiveness Review. An organization's or department's marketing effectiveness is reflected in the degree to which it exhibits the five major attributes of a marketing orientation: *customer philosophy, integrated marketing organization, adequate marketing information, strategic orientation,* and *operational efficiency* (see Field Note 15.1). Most organizations and departments receive scores in the fair-to-good range.[3]

FIELD NOTE 15.1.

Marketing Effectiveness Review Instrument Check one answer to each question.

Customer Philosophy

A. Does management recognize the importance of designing the company to serve the needs and wants of chosen markets?

   0 Management primarily thinks in terms of selling current and new products to whoever will buy them.

   1 Management thinks in terms of serving a wide range of markets and needs with equal effectiveness.

   2 Management thinks in terms of serving the needs and wants of well-defined markets and market segments chosen for their long-run growth and profit potential for the company.

B. Does management develop different offerings and marketing plans for different segments of the market?

   0 No.

   1 Somewhat.

   2 To a large extent.

C. Does management take a whole marketing system view (suppliers, channels, competitors, customers, environment) in planning its business?

   0 No. Management concentrates on selling and servicing its immediate customers.

   1 Somewhat. Management takes a long view of its channels although the bulk of its effort goes to selling and servicing the immediate customers.

   2 Yes. Management takes a whole marketing systems view, recognizing the threats and opportunities created for the company by changes in any part of the system.

Integrated Marketing Organization

D. Is there high-level marketing integration and control of the major marketing functions?

   0   No. Sales and other marketing functions are not integrated at the top and there is some unproductive conflict.

   1   Somewhat. There is formal integration and control of the major marketing functions but less than satisfactory coordination and cooperation.

   2   Yes. The major marketing functions are effectively integrated.

E. Does marketing management work well with management in research, manufacturing, purchasing, logistics, and finance?

   0   No. There are complaints that marketing is unreasonable in the demands and costs it places on other departments.

   1   Somewhat. The relations are amicable although each department pretty much acts to serve its own interests.

   2   Yes. The departments cooperate effectively and resolve issues in the best interest of the company as a whole.

F. How well organized is the new-product development process?

   0   The system is ill-defined and poorly handled.

   1   The system formally exists but lacks sophistication.

   2   The system is well-structured and operates on teamwork principles.

Adequate Marketing Information

G. When were the latest marketing research studies of customers, buying influences, channels, and competitors conducted?

   0   > 3 years ago.

   1   1 to 3 years ago.

   2   < 1 year ago.

H. How well does management know the sales potential and profitability of different market segments, customers, territories, products, channels, and order sizes?

   0   Not at all.

   1   Somewhat.

   2   Very well.

I. What effort is expended to measure and improve the cost-effectiveness of different marketing expenditures?

0 Little or no effort.

1 Some effort.

2 Substantial effort.

Strategic Orientation

J. What is the extent of formal marketing planning?

   0 Management conducts little or no formal marketing planning.

   1 Management develops an annual marketing plan.

   2 Management develops a detailed annual marketing plan and a strategic long-range plan that is updated annually.

K. How impressive is the current marketing strategy?

   0 The current strategy is not clear.

   1 The current strategy is clear and represents a continuation of traditional strategy.

   2 The current strategy is clear, innovative, data-based, and well reasoned.

L. What is the extent of contingency thinking and planning?

   0 Management does little or no contingency thinking.

   1 Management does some contingency thinking but little formal contingency planning.

   2 Management formally identifies the most important contingencies and develops contingency plans.

Operational Efficiency

M. How well is the marketing strategy communicated and implemented?

   0 Poorly.

   1 Fairly.

   2 Successfully.

N. Is management doing an effective job with its marketing resources?

   0 No. The marketing resources are inadequate for the job to be done.

   1 Somewhat. The marketing resources are adequate but they are not employed optimally.

   2 Yes. The marketing resources are adequate and are employed efficiently.

O. Does management show a good capacity to react quickly and effectively to on-the-spot developments?

   0 No. Sales and market information is not very current and management reaction time is slow.

1 Somewhat. Management receives fairly up-to-date sales and market information; management reaction time varies.

2 Yes. Management has installed systems yielding highly current information and
fast reaction time.

Total Score

The instrument is used in the following way. The appropriate answer is checked for
each question. The scores are added—the total will be somewhere between 0 and
30. The following scale shows the level of marketing effectiveness:

0–5 = None	11–15 = Fair	21–25 = Very good
6–10 = Poor	16–20 = Good	26–30 = Superior

Source: P. Kotler, "From Sales Obsession to Marketing Effectiveness," *Harvard Business
Review*, Nov.–Dec. 1977, pp. 67–75. Copyright © 1977 by the President and Fellows of
Harvard College; all rights reserved. *Note:* Question G was modified from the original.

The Marketing Audit. Organizations that discover weaknesses should undertake a *marketing audit*.[4] A marketing audit is a comprehensive, systematic, independent, and periodic examination of an organization's or business unit's marketing environment, objectives, strategies, and activities, with a view to determining problem areas and opportunities and recommending a plan of action to improve the organization's marketing performance.

A marketing audit has four characteristics:

- *Comprehensive:* The marketing audit covers the major marketing activities of a business, not just a few trouble spots. It would be called a functional audit if it covered only the sales force, pricing, or some other marketing activity. Although functional audits are useful, they sometimes mislead management. Excessive sales-force turnover, for example, could be a symptom not of poor sales-force training or compensation but of poor customer service and promotion. A comprehensive marketing audit is usually more effective in locating the real source of problems.

- *Systematic:* The marketing audit is an orderly examination of the organization's marketing objectives, strategies, and plans; marketing systems; and specific activities. The audit indicates the most-needed improvements, which are then incorporated into a corrective action plan involving both short-run and long-run steps to improve overall effectiveness.

- *Independent:* A marketing audit can be conducted in several ways. The best audits come from outside consultants who have the necessary objectivity, broad experience, and familiarity with the industry being audited, and undivided time and attention to give to the audit.

TABLE 15.1. **Major Weaknesses in Marketing Organizations and Corrective Measures**

Deadly Sins	Signs	Solutions
1. The Company Is Not Sufficiently Market Focused and Customer Driven	■ Poor identification of market segments. ■ Insufficient prioritization of market segments. ■ No market segment managers. ■ Most employees think that it is the job of marketing and sales to serve the customers. ■ There is no training program to create a customer culture. ■ There are no incentives to treat the customer especially well.	■ Adopt more advanced techniques in segmentation, such as benefit segmentation, value segmentation, and loyalty segmentation. ■ Prioritize the most important segments. ■ Specialize the sales force. ■ Develop a clear hierarchy of company values with customers at the top. ■ Engage in activities that will produce more "customer consciousness" in employees and the company's agents. ■ Make it easy for customers to reach the company by phone, fax, or e-mail with inquiries, suggestions, and complaints—and respond quickly.
2. The Company Does Not Fully Understand Its Target Customers	■ Your last study of customers was done three years ago. ■ Customers are not buying your product at the expected rate; competitor's products are selling better. ■ There is a high level of customer returns and complaints.	■ Do more sophisticated consumer research. ■ Use more analytical techniques. ■ Establish customer and dealer panels. ■ Install customer relationship marketing software and do data mining.

3. The Company Needs to Better Define and Monitor Its Competitors	- Your company over-focuses on its near competitors and misses distant competitors and disruptive technologies. - Customers are not buying your product at the expected rate; competitor's products are selling better.	- Establish a person or office for competitive intelligence. - Hire away people from competitors. - Watch every new technology that might hurt the company. - Prepare offerings similar to your competitors'.
4. The Company Has Not Properly Managed Its Relationships with Its Stakeholders	- Your employees are not happy. - You have not attracted the best suppliers. - You don't have the best distributors and your dealers are unhappy. - Your investors are not happy.	- Move from zero-sum thinking to positive-sum thinking. - Manage employees better. - Manage supplier relations better. - Manage distributors and dealers better. - Manage investors better.
5. The Company Is Not Good at Finding New Opportunities	- Your company has not identified any exciting new opportunities in recent years. - The new ideas that your company has launched have largely failed.	- Set up a system for stimulating the flow of new ideas from your partners. - Use creativity systems for generating new ideas.
6. The Company's Marketing Planning Process is Deficient	- Your marketing plan format does not carry the right components or logic. - Your plans lack a means for simulating the financial implications of alternative strategies. - Your plans lack contingency planning.	- Establish a standard plan format including situational analysis, SWOT, major issues, objectives, strategy, tactics, budgets, and controls. - Ask marketers what changes they would make if they were given 20 percent more budget or 20 percent less budget. - Run an annual marketing awards program with prizes going to the best plans and performance.

(Table 15.1 continued)

Deadly Sins	Signs	Solutions
7. The Company's Product and Service Policies Need Tightening	▪ The company has too many products and many are losing money. ▪ The company is giving away too many services free. ▪ The company is poor at cross-selling its products and services.	▪ The company needs to establish a system for tracking weak products and fixing or eliminating them. ▪ The company should offer and price services at different levels. ▪ The company should improve its processes for cross-selling and up-selling.
8. The Company's Brand-Building and Communication Skills Are Weak	▪ Your target market does not know much about your company. ▪ Your brand is not seen as distinctive as and better than other brands. ▪ Your company allocates its budget to the same marketing tools in approximately the same amounts each year. ▪ You do little evaluation of the ROI impact of your different promotional programs.	▪ Improve your brand-building strategies and your measurement of results. ▪ Shift money into those marketing instruments that show increasing effectiveness. ▪ Develop a financial mindset in the marketers and require them to estimate the ROI impact in advance of their spending requests.

9. The Company Is Not Well Organized to Carry On Effective and Efficient Marketing	▪ The head of marketing does not seem to be very effective. ▪ The staff lacks some marketing skills needed in the twenty-first century. ▪ There are bad vibes between marketing/sales and the other departments.	▪ Appoint a stronger leader of the marketing department. ▪ Build new skills in the marketing department. ▪ Improve marketing's relations with the other departments.
10. The Company Has Not Made Maximum Use of Technology	▪ The company has made minimal use of the Internet. ▪ The company's sales automation system is outdated. ▪ The company has not introduced any market automation. ▪ The marketing group lacks decision-support models. ▪ The marketing group needs to develop marketing dashboards.	▪ Make more use of the Internet. ▪ Improve the sales automation system. ▪ Apply market automation to routine marketing decisions. ▪ Develop some formal marketing decision models. ▪ Develop marketing dashboards.

Source: P. Kotler and K. Keller, *Marketing Management*, 12th ed. Upper Saddle River, N.J.: Prentice-Hall, 2006, p. 725.

- *Periodic:* Typically, marketing audits are initiated only after sales or profits have turned down, morale has fallen, and other problems have occurred. Organizations are thrown into a crisis partly because they failed to review their marketing operations during good times. A periodic marketing audit can benefit organizations in good health as well as those in trouble.

The Marketing Weaknesses Review. Organizations can rate their performance in relation to the best marketing practices of high-performing competitors. The major weaknesses found in marketing organizations along with the appropriate corrective actions are shown in Table 15.1.

SUMMARY

Marketing organizations are found in pharmaceutical medical device and equipment companies, as well as health care service organizations such as hospitals. Their role and scope differ greatly between and within separate companies.

Marketing organizations are effective when they set clear objectives, strategies, and plans, and develop sufficient metrics and marketing controls to gauge their performance. Marketers are most effective when they work closely with other departments to help set courses and solve problems.

A brilliant strategic marketing plan counts for little if it is not implemented properly and monitored carefully. Implementing marketing plans calls for skills in recognizing and diagnosing a problem, assessing the organization level where the problem exists, evaluating the results, correcting errors, and redirecting efforts in more productive directions.

The marketing department must monitor and control marketing activities through efficiency control and strategic control instruments. The former refers to finding ways to increase the efficiency of the sales force, advertising, sales promotion, and distribution. The latter entails a periodic reassessment of the organization and its strategic approach to the marketplace, using the tools of the marketing audit and marketing excellence reviews.

DISCUSSION QUESTIONS

1. Complete the instrument in Field Note 15.1 in any way that totals to a score of 11. If you are an external consultant, how would you use these answers to make specific improvement suggestions to your client? (Assume the company is in whatever industry sector you like as you formulate your answer.)

2. Your hospital wants to start a new "men's health" product line. As vice president of marketing, how would you organize the marketing function for this new program? What obstacles might you face? Who would you need to get involved to make the program a success? How would you evaluate its success or failure (in both economic and noneconomic terms) after it has been rolled out?

GLOSSARY

Key to Definition Sources
[1] Adopted or adapted from the Blue Cross/Blue Shield Association
[http://www.bcbs.com/coverage/glossary/]
[2] DOD Glossary of Health Care Terminology
[3] Adopted or adapted from Centers for Medicare and Medicaid Services (CMS) glossary
[http://www.cms.hhs.gov/apps/glossary/default.asp?Letter=ALL&Language=English]
[4] Adopted or adapted from the American Marketing Association Dictionary of Marketing Terms
[http://www.marketingpower.com/mg-dictionary.php]
[5] World Health Organization
[6] Institute of Medicine, National Academy of Sciences
[7] National Cancer Institute [http://plan2005.cancer.gov/glossary.html]

A

Access. A person's ability to obtain affordable medical care on a timely basis.[1]

Accreditation. An evaluative process in which a health care organization undergoes an examination of its policies, procedures, and performance by an external entity (*accrediting body*) to ensure that it is meeting predetermined criteria. These standards are set by private, nationally recognized groups such as the National Committee for Quality Assurance (NCQA) and the Joint Commission.[3]

Actuaries. Professionals who perform the mathematical analysis necessary for setting insurance premium rates.[1]

Acute illness. A health care incident in which the patient is treated for a single episode of a suddenly occurring event for a short period of time, usually less than thirty days, and from which the patient can be expected to return to his or her normal or previous state and level of activity.[2]

Activities of daily living (ADLs). A basic measure of individual functioning, including getting in and out of bed, dressing, bathing, eating, and using the bathroom. ADLs are used to evaluate benefits for long-term care and disability benefits as well as clinical care plans.[3]

Administrative services only (ASO). An arrangement whereby a self-insured entity contracts with a third party administrator (TPA) to administer its health plan.[3]

Admission. The act of placing an individual under treatment or observation in a hospital, skilled nursing facility, or other institution for a stay that is normally at least overnight.[2]

Advance directive (health care). A written document stating a person's desires regarding medical care or designating who else is empowered to make decisions if that person loses the ability to make them independently. It may include a Living Will and a Durable Power of Attorney for health care.[3]

Adverse event. Any harm a patient suffers that is caused by factors other than the patient's underlying condition.[1]

Adverse selection. The tendency of people who have a greater-than-average likelihood of loss to seek health care coverage to a greater extent than individuals who have an average or less-than-average likelihood of loss.[1]

Advertising. The use of a variety of media to bring a product or service to the attention of current and/or potential customers.

Agent. *See* Broker

Alternative delivery systems. Health care delivery modes that provide a substitute for traditional fee-for-service by integrating financing controls with patient care services. Any service that was based on a payment structure other than fee-for-service medicine used to be considered "alternative." However, today's rapidly changing health care environment, with the growth of HMOs, PPOs, and other managed care entities, has made the "alternative" more like the norm.[2]

Ambulatory care. The examination, diagnosis, and treatment of all categories of patients who do not require an overnight stay in a health care facility. *See* Outpatient[2]

Ambulatory care facility. A medical care center that provides a wide range of health care services, including preventive care, acute care, surgery, and outpatient care, in a centralized place and does not keep patients overnight. Also known as a medical clinic.[3]

Ambulatory surgical center. A place other than a hospital that does outpatient surgery.[3]

America's Health Insurance Plans (AHIP). Association of many private health insurance plans in the United States. Formerly known as Health Insurance Association of America, or HIAA.

American College of Health Care Executives (ACHE). A professional association that devotes itself to such activities as continuing education and fellowship certification.[3]

American Dental Association (ADA). A professional organization for dentists.[3]

American Hospital Association (AHA). A health care industry association that represents the concerns of hospitals.[3]

American Marketing Association (AMA). A professional association for individuals and organizations involved in the practice, teaching, and study of marketing worldwide.[4]

American Medical Association (AMA). A professional organization for physicians. The AMA also holds copyright to and maintains the Current Procedural Terminology (CPT) medical code set.[3]

American National Standards Institute (ANSI). An organization that accredits various standards-setting committees and monitors their compliance with the open rule-making process that they must follow to qualify for ANSI accreditation. HIPAA prescribes that the standards mandated under it be developed by ANSI-accredited bodies whenever practical.[3]

Ancillary services. Health care-related services other than those performed directly by a patient's treating physician. Examples include diagnostic X-rays and laboratory services; home health services; and physical, speech, and occupational therapies.[3]

Annual and lifetime maximum benefit amounts. Maximum dollar amounts set by insurance companies that limit the total amount the plan must pay for all health care services provided to a subscriber per year or in the subscriber's lifetime.[1]

Antitrust laws. Legislation designed to protect commerce from unlawful restraint of trade, price discrimination, price fixing, reduced competition, and monopolies. *See also* Sherman Antitrust Act, Clayton Act, and Federal Trade Commission Act[1]

At-risk. Term used to describe a provider organization that bears the insurance risk associated with the health care it delivers or arranges to deliver.[1]

Attending physician. The medical doctor who is normally responsible for overall patient care during an episode of illness and is expected to certify and recertify the medical necessity of services rendered.[3]

Authorization. A health plan's system of approving payment of benefits for services that satisfy the plan's requirements for coverage.[1]

B

Baby boomers. The segment of the population born between 1946 and 1964.

Balance billing. The practice of a provider invoicing a patient for charges not paid by the insurance plan, even if those charges are above the plan's fee schedule or are considered medically unnecessary. Health plans generally prohibit providers from balance billing except for allowed co-pays, coinsurance, and deductibles. Such prohibition against balance billing may even extend to the plan's failure to pay at all (for example, because of bankruptcy) and may be a contractually required provision under state law.[2]

Behavioral health care. Mental health and chemical dependency (or substance abuse) services.[1]

Benchmark. A target used as a reference to raise the standard of care. While the relative reference point will vary, in many instances an appropriate aim would be results that appear in the top 10 percent of all providers for more than a year.[3]

Beneficiary. A person who receives benefits under an insurance plan. *See* Benefits[3]

Benefit design. The process an insurance company uses to determine which benefits or level of benefits will be offered to its members, the degree to which members will be expected to share the costs of such benefits, and how a member can access medical care through the health plan.[1]

Benefits. The money or services an insurance policy must provide under terms of a contract with the beneficiary or entity that pays premiums.[3]

Biologicals. Usually a drug or vaccine made from a live product and used medically to diagnose, prevent, or treat a medical condition.[3]

Blue Cross and Blue Shield Association. A trade association that represents the common interests of Blue Cross and Blue Shield health plans, including brand protection, franchise grants and maintenance, research and coordination of national accounts.[3]

Board-certified. A physician who has special training and has passed an advanced exam in a particular area of medicine. Both primary care doctors and specialists may be board-certified.[3]

Brand. A name, number, term, sign, symbol, design, or combination of these elements that an organization uses to identify one or more products.[1]

Broker. A salesperson who has obtained a state license to sell and service contracts of multiple health plans or insurers, and who is ordinarily considered to be an agent of the buyer, not the health plan or insurer.[1]

Bundling. The process of combining into one payment the charges for various medical services rendered during one health care encounter or global episode of treatment. Bundling often combines the payment from physician and hospital services into one reimbursement. Also known as package pricing.[2]

Business-to-business marketing (B2B). A process that involves delivering valued products and services to other entities within the same value chain and often involves larger quantities than consumers would require.[4]

Business-to-consumer marketing (B2C). A process that involves delivering valued products and services to the end user or purchaser.[4]

C

Capitation. A prepaid fee arrangement on a per-person (member) basis set by advanced agreement rather than on the actual cost of separate episodes of care and services delivered. It is usually expressed in units of per member per month (PMPM) payments and may vary by such factors as age, sex, and benefit plan of the enrolled member.[2]

Carrier. A private company that adjudicates and pays physician bills.[3]

Carve-out. The separation of a medical service (or a group of services) from the basic set of benefits in some way, paid or provided in a manner separate from the underlying insurance product.[1]

Case management. A method of managing the provision of health care to members with catastrophic or high-cost medical conditions. The goal is to coordinate the care so as to both improve continuity and quality of care as well as lower costs.[2]

Case mix. The distribution of patients into categories reflecting differences in severity of illness or resource consumption.[3]

Centers for Disease Control and Prevention (CDC). A federal organization that tracks diseases, issues intervention recommendations about treatment of epidemics, and recommends appropriate immunization schedules.[3]

Certificate of need (CON). The requirement that a health care organization obtain permission from a government-appointed agency before making changes. It generally applies to facilities or facility-based services and is frequently based on a certain dollar threshold.[2]

Centers for Medicare and Medicaid Services (CMS). The branch of the Department of Health and Human Services that administers the Medicare and Medicaid programs.

Channel. *See* Marketing channel

Claim. Any request for payment for services rendered for care and treatment of a beneficiary.[2]

Clayton Act. A federal act that forbids certain actions believed to lead to monopolies, including (1) charging different prices to different purchasers of the same product without justifying the price difference and (2) giving a distributor the right to sell a product only if the distributor agrees not to sell competitors' products. The Clayton Act applies to insurance companies only to the extent that state laws do not regulate such activities. *See also* Antitrust laws[1]

Clinic. A health treatment facility staffed by physicians or registered nurses or both that is primarily intended to provide urgent and routine ambulatory services.[2]

Clinical integration. A type of operational integration that enables patients to receive a variety of health care services from the same organization or entity, which streamlines administrative processes and increases the potential for the delivery of high-quality health care.[1]

Clinical practice guideline. Utilization and quality management mechanisms derived from research studies that are designed to aid providers in making decisions about the most appropriate course of treatment for a specific clinical case.[1]

Clinical trials. A study in a large population that is the final stage of determining whether a drug or device is effective and safe for approval by the Food and Drug Administration. Clinical trials may also be used to compare different treatments for the same condition to determine which treatment is better, or to test new uses for treatments already in use.[3]

COBRA. *See* Consolidated Omnibus Budget Reconciliation Act[1]

Coinsurance. A method of cost-sharing in a health insurance policy that requires a group member to pay a stated percentage of all remaining eligible medical expenses after the deductible amount has been paid.[1]

Community rating. A pricing method that sets premiums for financing medical care according to the health plan's expected costs of providing medical benefits to the community as a whole rather than to any subgroup within the community. Both low-risk and high-risk classes are factored into the community rating, which spreads the expected medical care costs across the entire community.[1]

Complementary goods/services. Products that are manufactured together, sold together, bought together, or used together that aid or enhance each other's value.[4]

Concurrent review. A type of utilization review that occurs while treatment is in progress and typically applies to services that continue over a period of time.[1]

Consolidated Omnibus Budget Reconciliation Act (COBRA). A federal act that requires each group health plan to allow employees and certain dependents to continue their group coverage for a stated period of time following a qualifying event that causes their loss of group health coverage. Qualifying events include reduced work hours, death or divorce of a covered employee, and termination of employment. The plan may require the beneficiary to pay the full premium plus an administrative fee.[1]

Consumer. The ultimate user of goods, ideas, and services. The term is also often used to refer to buyers or decision makers.[4]

Consumer Price Index (CPI). A measure of the average change in what people pay for a specified set of goods and services during a given time period. In addition to the overall economy's CPI, there is a subset for health care products and services.[3]

Continuum of care. The process of providing for the health needs of populations that includes the entire spectrum of services and products ranging from prevention to the most acute and intensive treatment.[2]

Coordination of benefits (COB). A program that determines which insurance policy will pay first if two plans cover the same benefits. If one of the plans is a Medicare health plan, federal law may decide who pays first.[3]

Co-payment. A specified dollar amount that a member must pay out of pocket for a specified service at the time the service is rendered.[1]

Corporation. An organization that is recognized by the authority of a governmental unit as a legal entity separate from its owners.[1]

Cost. The tangible or intangible price that must be paid to acquire goods or services. The following are some related terms:

> *Direct costs* can be traced to a service, organizational unit, individual provider, or manager.
> *Indirect costs* cannot be traced directly to the unit of production and must be allocated.
> *Fixed costs* do not vary with the number of units the firm produces.
> *Variable costs* change in a constant fashion with all units produced (over a given range of output).
> *Marginal costs* are those incurred for producing *one additional unit* of service.

Cost-effective. A way of relating the cost of care to the achievement of a desired health outcome. The most cost-effective method is the one that achieves the health outcome at the least cost.[2]

Cost sharing. The portion of medical care expenses that the beneficiary pays, like a co-payment, coinsurance, or deductible. *See* Coinsurance; Co-payment; Deductible[3]

Cost shifting. The practice of charging certain groups of patients higher rates to offset lower rates negotiated with, or mandated by, other payers.[2]

Covered service/benefit. All of the medical services a beneficiary may receive at no additional charge, or with an out-of-pocket payment significantly less than the actual charge (subject to deductible amounts). The insurer thus pays the major portion of the charge.[2]

Credentialing. Obtaining and reviewing the documentation of professional providers for such items as education and training, licensure, certifications, evidence of malpractice insurance, and malpractice history. It generally includes both reviewing information provided by the provider as well as verification that the information is correct and complete.[2]

Culture. The institutionalized ways or modes of appropriate behavior. It is the modal or distinctive patterns of behavior of a people, including implicit cultural beliefs, norms, values, and premises that govern conduct. It includes the shared superstitions, myths, folkways, mores, and behavior patterns that are rewarded or punished.[4]

Current Procedural Terminology 4th Edition (CPT-4). A set of five-digit codes issued and copyrighted by the American Medical Association that apply to delivered medical care and are used by professionals to bill for their services.

Custodial care. Nonskilled, personal care, such as help with activities of daily living.[3]

Customer. The actual or prospective purchaser of products or services.[3]

D

Database marketing. Creating a pool of customer information—including demographic, consumer preference, and sales history information—which is used to narrow the focus of an organization's direct-marketing efforts.[3]

Days per thousand. A standard unit of measurement of utilization. It refers to the annualized use of institutional care adjusted for a thousand persons eligible to receive benefits under a health insurance plan.[2]

Decision support system (DSS). A form of information technology that uses databases and decision models to aid clinicians and managers in formulating appropriate judgments.[1]

Deductible. A flat amount a health plan member must pay before the insurer will make any benefit payments.[1]

Demographic data. Characteristics of populations that include, but are not limited to, age, sex, race/ethnicity, and primary language.[3]

Department of Health and Human Services (DHHS). A division of the executive branch of government that administers many of the "social" programs at the federal level dealing with the health and welfare of the citizens of the United States. (It is the "parent" of CMS.)[3]

Diagnosis-related groups (DRG). A classification system that clusters patients according to diagnosis, type of treatment, age, and other relevant criteria. Under the Medicare prospective payment system, hospitals are paid a set fee for treating patients in a single DRG category, regardless of the actual cost of care for the individual.[3]

Direct mail. An advertising medium, usually in print form, that uses a mail service to distribute an organization's sales offers or advertising messages.[1]

Direct marketing. A method that uses one or more media to elicit an immediate and measurable action—such as an inquiry or a purchase—from a customer or prospect. Also known as direct response marketing.[1]

Direct-to-consumer (DTC) advertising. In health care, this term refers to promotional activities directed at the end users of products or services (such as actual or potential patients) as opposed to other decision makers (such as insurance companies or physicians).

Disability. For Social Security purposes, the inability to engage in substantial gainful activity by reason of any medically determinable physical or mental impairment that can be expected to result in death or to last for a continuous period of not less than twelve months. An additional period is necessary to qualify for Medicare.[3]

Discharge planning. A process used to decide what a patient needs for a smooth transfer from one level of care to another. It includes moves from a hospital to a nursing home or to home care.[3]

Disease management. A coordinated system of preventive, diagnostic, and therapeutic measures intended to provide cost-effective, quality health care for a patient population that has, or is at risk for, a specific chronic illness or medical condition. Also known as disease state management.[1]

Disproportionate share hospital. A hospital that cares for a much larger than average share of low-income patients. Under Medicaid, states augment payment to these hospitals. Medicare inpatient hospital payments are also adjusted for this added burden.[3]

Distribution. The activities and systems designed to make products or services available so that consumers can buy them.[3]

Diversification. A means whereby a firm increases its total sales by identifying opportunities to build or acquire businesses that are not directly related to the company's current businesses.[4]

DRG. *See* Diagnosis related group

Dual eligibles. Persons who are entitled to Medicare (Part A and/or Part B) and who are also eligible for Medicaid.[3]

Durable medical equipment (DME). A tangible item ordered by a physician that is not disposable (that is, it is used repeatedly) and is related only to care for a medical condition. Examples include walkers, wheelchairs, and home hospital beds.[2]

E

Early and Periodic Screening, Diagnostic, and Treatment (EPSDT) Services. A Medicaid program for recipients younger than twenty-one that provides screening, vision, hearing, and dental services at intervals that meet recognized standards of medical and dental practices and at other intervals as necessary to determine the existence of physical or mental illnesses or conditions.[1]

Electronic commerce (e-commerce). The use of computer networks to perform business transactions and to facilitate the delivery of health care and nonclinical services.[1]

Electronic data interchange (EDI). The exchange of routine business transactions from one computer to another in a standard format, using standard communications protocols.[3]

Electronic medical record (EMR). A computerized record of a patient's clinical, demographic, and administrative data. Also known as a computer-based patient record.[1]

Eligibility. The process whereby an individual is determined to be qualified for coverage under a particular health insurance plan.[3]

Emergency Medical Treatment and Active Labor Act (EMTALA). Requires any Medicare-participating hospital that operates a hospital emergency department to provide an appropriate medical screening examination to any patient who requests such an examination, regardless of ability to pay. If the hospital determines that the patient has an emergency medical condition, it must either stabilize the patient's condition or arrange for a transfer; however, the hospital may transfer the patient only if the medical benefits of the transfer outweigh the risks or if the patient requests it.[3]

Employee Retirement Income Security Act (ERISA). A broad-reaching law that establishes the rights of pension plan participants, standards for the investment of pension plan assets, and requirements for the disclosure of plan provisions and funding. It is the enabling legislation for companies to establish self-funded health insurance plans that must comply with federal regulations but are exempt from such state regulatory requirements as benefit mandates and contributions to insurance pools.[1]

Encounter. A visit of any type by a health plan member to a provider of care or services.[1]

Encounter report. A statement that supplies clinical and management information about services, provided each time a patient visits a provider.[1]

Enroll. To join a health plan.[3]

Enrollee. One who has joined a health plan.

Enterprise-wide information system. A computerized network that permits physician groups, hospitals, and other facilities and professionals within an organization to function as a single, coordinated unit in arranging access to facilities and resources and treat for patients.[3]

Epidemiology. The study of the patterns, causes, and control of disease in groups of people.[7]

Episode of care. The health care services provided during a certain period of time; for example, during a hospital stay.[3]

EPSDT. *See* Early and Periodic Screening, Diagnostic, and Treatment Services[1]

ERISA. *See* Employee Retirement Income Security Act[1]

Ethics in Patient Referrals Act. A federal act that, along with its amendments, prohibits a physician from referring patients to laboratories, radiology services, diagnostic services, physical therapy services, home health services, pharmacies, occupational therapy services, and suppliers of durable medical equipment in which the physician has a financial interest. Also known as the Stark Laws, after U.S. Representative Fortney "Pete" Stark.[1]

Expense. Funds actually spent or amounts incurred providing goods, rendering services, or carrying out other mission-related activities during a specified period.[3]

Experience rating. A price-setting method under which an insurance company analyzes an individual's or group's recorded health care costs and calculates the premium partly or completely according to that history.[3]

Explanation of benefits (EOB). A statement that is sent to a member or covered insured explaining how and why a claim was or was not paid.[2]

F

Federal Insurance Contribution Act Payroll Tax (FICA). Employers and employees each contribute 1.45 percent of taxable wages, with no limitations, to finance the Medicare Part A Trust Fund.[3]

Federal Register. The official, daily, federal publication of rules, proposed rules, and notices of federal agencies and organizations, as well as executive orders and other presidential documents.[3]

Federal Trade Commission Act. A federal act that established the Federal Trade Commission (FTC) and gave the FTC power to work with the Department of Justice to enforce the Clayton Act. The primary function of the FTC is to regulate unfair competition and deceptive business practices, which are presented broadly in the Act. As a result, the FTC also pursues violators of the Sherman Antitrust Act. *See also* Antitrust laws[1]

Fee schedule. The price determined by a health plan to be acceptable for a procedure or service and that contracted providers and suppliers agree to accept as payment in full. Also known as a fee allowance, fee maximum, or capped fee.[1]

Fee-for-service (FFS) payment system. A benefit payment system in which an insurer reimburses the group member or pays the provider directly for each covered medical expense after the expense has been incurred.[1]

Fiscal intermediary. A private company that pays for the institutional part of health care services, such as hospital care.[3]

Fiscal year. The annual financial planning and reporting cycle of public or private organizations. For example, Medicare uses October 1st through September 30th as its fiscal year, whereas many private insurers use a calendar year.[3]

Focus group interview. An unstructured, informal session in which, typically, six to ten people are led by a moderator who asks questions to guide them into an in-depth discussion of a given topic.[1]

Food and Drug Administration (FDA). A division of the Department of Health and Human Services that, according to its Web site, "is responsible for protecting the public health by assuring the safety, efficacy, and security of human and veterinary drugs, biological products, medical devices, the nation's food supply, cosmetics, and products that emit radiation." The FDA evaluates the safety and efficacy of all drugs and devices before they are allowed to go to market and the safety after they achieve broader use.[3]

Formulary. A list of certain drugs and their proper dosages. In health plans, these drugs are also divided into preference categories, including the patient's financial responsibility for each class. Usually the patient pays the least for generic drugs, more for branded drugs on a preferred list, and most for branded drugs not on the preferred list.[3]

Franchise. The privilege, often exclusive, granted to a distributor or dealer by a brand owner or manufacturer to sell its products within a specified territory.[4]

Fraud and abuse. *Fraud:* To purposely bill for services that were never given or to bill for a service that has a higher reimbursement than the service produced.

Abuse: Payment for items or services that are billed by mistake by providers, but should not be paid. These terms are most often applied to Medicare and Medicaid.[3]

Freedom of Information Act (FOIA). A law that requires the U.S. government to give out certain information to the public when it receives a written request. FOIA applies only to records of the executive branch of the federal government, not to those of the Congress or federal courts, and does not apply to state governments, local governments, or private groups.[3]

Functional status. The patient's ability to perform the activities of daily living (ADLs).[1]

G

Gatekeeper (primary care manager). A primary care physician who is responsible (often financially and also clinically) for delivering care to specific individuals in a managed care organization or other integrated health system. The primary care gatekeeper assists patients throughout the provider network, and patients cannot see specialist physician without a referral from their primary care gatekeeper.[2]

Generic drug. A prescription drug that has the same active-ingredient formula as a brand name drug. Generic drugs usually cost less than brand name drugs and are rated by the Food and Drug Administration (FDA) to be as safe and effective as brand name drugs.[3]

Gross domestic product. The total dollar value of all goods and services produced in a year in a country.[3]

Group health plan. Health insurance that provides coverage to employees, former employees, and/or their families and is supported by an employer or employee organization.[3]

Group model HMO. An HMO that contracts with a multi-specialty group of physicians who are employees of the group practice. Also known as a group practice model HMO.[1]

Guidelines. Expert-developed suggestions to assist practitioners and help patients decide about appropriate health care for specific clinical circumstances.[3]

H

Health. The state of complete physical, mental, and social well-being, not merely the absence of disease or infirmity.[5]

Health care provider. A person who is trained and licensed to deliver health care to patients; for example, physicians, nurses, and therapists.[3]

Health Care Quality Improvement Act (HCQIA). A federal act that exempts hospitals, group practices, and HMOs from certain antitrust provisions as they apply to credentialing and peer review so long as these entities adhere to due process standards that are outlined in the Act.[1]

Health Insurance Portability and Accountability Act of 1996 (HIPAA). A federal law that has two Acts. Act I allows persons to qualify immediately for comparable health insurance coverage when they change their employment relationships. Act II gives HHS the authority to mandate the use of standards for the electronic exchange of health care data; to specify what medical and administrative code sets should be used within those standards; to require the use of national identification systems for health care patients, providers, payers (or plans), and employers (or sponsors); and to specify the types of measures required to protect the security and privacy of personally identifiable health care information.[3]

Health maintenance organization (HMO). A health care plan that delivers comprehensive coordinated services to its members on a prepaid basis.

Health promotion programs. Preventive care programs designed to educate and motivate members to prevent illness and injury and to promote good health through lifestyle choices, such as smoking cessation and dietary changes. Also known as wellness programs.[1]

Health risk assessment (HRA). A process by which a health plan uses information about a plan member's health status, personal and family health history, and health-related behaviors to predict the member's likelihood of experiencing specific illnesses or injuries. Also known as health risk appraisal.[1]

Healthcare Common Procedural Coding System (HCPCS). A federally issued medical code set that identifies health care procedures, equipment, and supplies for claim submission purposes.[3]

Healthcare Financial Management Association (HFMA). An organization of professionals for the improvement of the financial management of health care–related organizations.

Healthcare Effectiveness Data and Information Set (HEDIS). A set of standard quality performance measures for health plans that the National Committee on Quality Assurance (NCQA) issues, monitors, and reports to the public and governmental agencies. Formerly called Healthplan Employer Data and Information Set.[3]

Hold harmless provision. A contract clause that forbids providers or suppliers from seeking compensation from patients if the health plan fails to pay them because of insolvency or for any other reason.[3]

Home health agency. An organization that provides such home care services as skilled nursing care, physical therapy, occupational therapy, speech therapy, and personal care by home health aides.[3]

Home health care. Limited, part-time, or intermittent skilled nursing care and home health aide services, physical therapy, occupational therapy, speech-language therapy, medical social services, durable medical equipment (such as wheelchairs, hospital beds, oxygen, and walkers), medical supplies, and other services.[3]

Hospice. A home or institutional setting where professionals can provide physical care and psychological support to terminally ill patients and their families or significant others.[2]

Hospital. A health treatment facility that is staffed and equipped to provide diagnostic and therapeutic services and has the supporting facilities to deliver inpatient care according to its mission. As hospitals are regulated in each state, the legal definition will vary by locality.[2]

I

Incidence. The frequency of new occurrences of a condition within a defined time interval. The incidence rate is the number of new cases of specific disease divided by the number of people in a population over a specified period of time, usually one year.[3]

Incurred but not reported (IBNR) claims. Claims or benefits that occurred during a particular time period, but that have not yet been reported or submitted to an insurer, so they remain unpaid.[1]

Indemnity health insurance. A plan that pays for services or products only after they are delivered; that is, after some loss has been demonstrated. The opposite is prepaid health insurance.

Independent Practice Association (IPA). An IPA is a corporation formed by physicians who maintain their separate practices but participate in the IPA to secure managed care business. IPAs accept financial risk for their members through capitation or discounted fees.[2]

Individual market. A segment composed of customers not eligible for Medicare or Medicaid who are covered under their own direct contract for health coverage. The opposite is group market.[1]

Information system. An interactive combination of people, computer hardware and software, communications devices, and procedures designed to provide a continuous flow of information to the people who make decisions or perform activities necessary for successful organization operation.[1]

Information technology. The wide range of electronic devices and tools used to acquire, record, store, transfer, or transform data or information.[1]

Informed consent. A legal principle requiring that the patient must be informed of all proposed medical or surgical procedures, the material risks of these procedures, alternative courses of action, and the material risks attendant to the alternatives prior to consenting to the receipt of the recommended treatment.[2]

Inpatient. An individual who is admitted (placed under treatment or observation) to a bed in a medical treatment facility (usually hospital) with the expectation that he or she will remain at least overnight.[2]

Integrated delivery systems (IDS). A seamless consolidation of providers (such as hospitals and physicians) that focuses on the coordination, delivery, and management of care to a defined population. Also called an organized delivery system.[2]

Integrated marketing. A planning process designed to ensure that all brand contacts received by a customer or prospect for a product or service are relevant to that person and consistent over time.[4]

Integration. The unification of two or more previously separate organizations under common ownership or control, or the combination of the business operations of two or more organizations that were previously carried out separately and independently. Horizontal integration refers to the combination of like businesses (such as two hospitals). Vertical integration refers to the combination of businesses that are different, but related (such as a hospital and home care agency).[1]

Intensive care. The constant, complex, detailed health care provided for various acute, life-threatening conditions by specially trained professionals.[2]

Intensive care unit (ICU). A hospital unit in which patients with various acute, life-threatening conditions are closely monitored and provided a high level of technical services that require special training and knowledge. Types of ICUs are the Medical ICU (MICU), Surgical ICU (SICU), Neonatal ICU (NICU) and Pediatric ICU (PICU).[2]

International Classification of Diseases (ICD). A medical code set maintained by the World Health Organization (WHO) that classifies illnesses. Many countries have modified this code set for their own purposes.[3]

Internet. A public, international collection of interconnected computer networks.[1]

Internist. A physician who counsels, diagnoses, and treats adults.[3]

Intranet. An internal (private) computer network, built on web-based technologies and standards that is available only to members of that network.[1]

IPA model HMO. A health maintenance organization that contracts with one or more associations of physicians in independent practice who agree to provide medical services to HMO members.[1]

J

Joint Commission. A private, not-for-profit organization composed of representatives of the American College of Surgeons, American College of Physicians, American Hospital Association, American Medical Association, and American Dental Association, as well as the public, whose purpose is to establish quality standards for the operation of health facilities and services, conduct surveys, and determine accreditation status of medical treatment facilities. Formerly called Joint Commission on Accreditation of Healthcare Organizations, or JCAHO.[2]

Joint venture. A type of partial structural integration in which one or more separate organizations combine resources to achieve a stated objective. The companies share ownership of the venture and responsibility for its operations, but usually maintain separate ownership and control over their operations outside of the joint venture.[1]

L

Length of stay (LOS). The number of days, counted from the day of admission to the day of discharge, that a health plan member is confined to a hospital or other facility for each admission.[1]

Licensure. The granting of permission by an official agency of a state, the District of Columbia, or a commonwealth, territory, or possession of the United States to a person or entity to provide health care independently in a specified discipline in that jurisdiction.[2]

Life cycle. The different stages over time through which a product and/or its market develops.

Long-term care. A variety of services that help people with health or personal needs and activities of daily living over a period of time at home, in the community, or in various types of facilities, including nursing homes and assisted living facilities. The term is the opposite of acute care.[3]

M

Magnetic resonance imaging (MRI). A system that produces images of the body by using a strong magnetic field and computers.[2]

Managed care. The integration of both the financing and delivery of health care within a system that seeks to manage the accessibility, cost, and quality of that care. A single provider or group of providers who manage patients' care by acting as their advocates, monitoring all care, avoiding needless care, and referring patients to economical care sources. Such systems negotiate discount fees with providers and stress keeping people healthy through health promotion and preventive medicine.[2]

Managed care organization (MCO). Integrates the financing and delivery of appropriate health care services to covered individuals by means of arrangements with selected providers to furnish a comprehensive set of health care services to members, explicit criteria for the selection of health care provides, and significant financial incentives for members to use providers and procedures associated with the plan. Managed care plans typically are labeled as HMOs (staff, group, IPA, and mixed models), PPOs, or Point-of-Service plans. Managed care services are reimbursed via a variety of methods including capitation, fee for service, and a combination of the two.[3]

Mandates. State laws that require health insurance companies to provide specified benefits as a condition of doing business in that state.

Market area. A geographical area containing the actual or potential customers of a particular firm or group of firms for specific goods or services.[4]

Market segmentation. The process of dividing the total market for a product or service into smaller, more manageable subsets or groups of customers.[1]

Marketing. The process of planning and executing the conception, pricing, promotion, and distribution of ideas, goods, and services to create exchanges that satisfy individual and organizational objectives.[1]

Marketing channel. A set of institutions necessary to transfer the title to goods and to move those goods from the point of production to the point of consumption that, as such, consists of all the entities and activities in the marketing process. The resulting system is an integrated network of independent firms that obtain the economies and market impacts that could not be obtained by unilateral action. Under this system, the identity of the individual firm and its autonomy of operation remain intact.[4]

Marketing director. The manager who oversees an organization's marketing and sales activities, including advertising, client relations, and enrollment and sales forecasting. Also known as a chief marketing officer.[1]

Marketing mix. The four major marketing elements—product, price, promotion, and distribution (place)—that foster the exchange process.[1]

Marketing research. The function that links the consumer, customer, and public to the marketer through information used to identify and define opportunities and problems; generates, refines, and evaluates actions; monitors performance; and improves understanding of the process. Marketing research specifies the information required to address these issues, designs the method for collecting information, manages and implements the data collection process, analyzes the results, and communicates the findings and their implications.[4]

Marketing strategy. A statement (implicit or explicit) of how a brand or product line will achieve its objectives. The strategy provides decisions and direction regarding variables such as the segmentation of the market, identification of the target market, positioning, marketing mix elements, and expenditures. A marketing strategy is usually an integral part of a business strategy that provides broad direction to all functions.[4]

McCarran-Ferguson Act. A federal act that placed the primary responsibility with the states for regulating health insurance companies and HMOs that service private sector (commercial) plan members.[1]

Medicaid. A joint federal-state government program, established under Title XIX of the Social Security Act of 1965, that provides hospital and medical expense coverage to the low-income population and certain aged and disabled individuals.[1]

Medical expense ratio. For a health plan, the quotient that results from dividing the amount paid on patient care by total revenues. Also called the medical loss ratio.

Medical underwriting. The process that an insurance company uses to decide, based on an individual's or group's medical history, whether or not to accept an application for insurance, whether or not to add a waiting period for preexisting conditions (if state law allows it), and how much to charge the applicant for that insurance.[3]

Medically necessary services. Services or supplies as provided by a physician or other health care provider to identify and treat a member's illness or injury, which, as determined by the payer, are consistent with the symptoms, diagnosis, and treatment of the member's condition; are in accordance with the standards of good medical practice; are not solely for the convenience of the member, member's family, physician, or other health care provider; and are furnished in the least intensive type of medical care setting required by the member's condition.[1]

Medicare. A federal government program established under Title XVIII of the Social Security Act of 1965 for people sixty-five years of age or older, certain younger people with disabilities, and people with end-stage renal disease (permanent kidney failure with dialysis or a transplant, sometimes called ESRD).[3]

Medicare Coverage Advisory Committee (MCAC). A body that advises CMS on whether specific medical items and services are reasonable and necessary under Medicare law. The MCAC is advisory in nature, with the final decision on all issues resting with CMS. The MCAC is used to supplement CMS's internal expertise and to ensure an unbiased and contemporary consideration of "state of the art" technology and science.[3]

Medicare Economic Index. A measure often used in the calculation of the increases in the prevailing charge levels that help to determine allowed charges for physician services. In 1992 and later, this index is considered in connection with the update factor for the physician fee schedule.[3]

Medicare Part A (hospital insurance). Medicare insurance that pays for inpatient hospital stays, care in a skilled nursing facility, hospice care, and some home health care, subject to cost sharing and duration limits.[3]

Medicare Part B (medical insurance). Medicare insurance that helps pay for doctors' services, outpatient hospital care, durable medical equipment, and some medical services that are not covered by Part A.[3]

Medicare Part C (Medicare Advantage). Private health plans that contract with Medicare to provide the benefits of Parts A and B as well as a Medicare supplement. They may also cover prescription drug benefits of a Part D plan. Medicare Advantage plans include HMOs, PPOs, and private fee-for-service plans.

Medicare Part D. A federally subsidized program to provide prescription drugs for Medicare beneficiaries, administered by private companies who also assume the associated risk.

Medicare Payment Advisory Commission (MEDPAC). A group established by Congress in the Balanced Budget Act of 1997 to replace the Prospective Payment Assessment Commission and the Physician Payment Review Commission. MedPAC is directed to provide the Congress with advice and recommendations on policies affecting Medicare.[3]

Medicare supplement. A private medical expense insurance policy that provides reimbursement for out-of-pocket expenses, such as deductibles and coinsurance payments, or benefits for some medical expenses specifically excluded from Medicare coverage. Also called a Medigap policy.[1]

Medicare Trust Funds. Treasury accounts established by the Social Security Act for the receipt of revenues, maintenance of reserves, and disbursement of payments for Medicare parts A and B.[3]

Morbidity rate. The speed of occurrence or proportion of people with a specific disease in a population often distinguished by a particular characteristic (such as sex or location).[3]

Mortality rate. The speed of occurrence or proportion of deaths from a particular cause in a population often distinguished by a particular characteristic (such as sex or location).[3]

Mutual company. A company that is owned by its members or policy owners.[1]

N

National Association of Insurance Commissioners (NAIC). An association of the insurance commissioners of the states and territories that issues guidelines for the administration of insurance products.[3]

National Center for Health Statistics. A federal organization within the CDC that collects, analyzes, and distributes health care statistics.[3]

National Committee for Quality Assurance (NCQA). A private, nonprofit organization that accredits and measures quality of managed care plans. The NCQA also maintains and administers the Healthcare Effectiveness Data and Information Set (HEDIS).[3]

National Drug Code. A list maintained by the Food and Drug Administration that contains codes for drugs that are FDA-approved. The secretary of HHS has adopted this code set as the standard for reporting drugs and biologics in standard transactions.[3]

National Practitioner Data Bank (NPDB). A database, maintained by the federal government, that contains information on physicians and other medical practitioners against whom medical malpractice claims have been settled or other disciplinary actions have been taken.[3]

Network. A group of doctors, hospitals, pharmacies, and other health care experts contracted with a health plan to take care of its members.[3]

Network model HMO. An HMO that contracts with more than one group practice of physicians or specialty groups.[3]

Niche strategy. A plan employed by a firm that specializes in serving particular market segments in order to avoid clashing with the major competitors in the market. "Nichers" pursue market segments that are of sufficient size to be profitable while at the same time are of less interest to the major competitors.[4]

Nosocomial. Pertaining to or originating in a hospital.[1]

Nurse practitioner. A registered nurse who has two or more years of advanced training and has passed a special exam to enable him or her to start, alter, or suspend defined regimens of medical and/or nursing treatment provided to a patient, on either a routine or occasional basis. A nurse practitioner often works with a physician.[1]

Nursing facility. An institution that primarily provides skilled nursing care and related services for the rehabilitation of injured, disabled, or sick persons, or on a regular basis, health-related care services above the level of custodial care to other than mentally retarded individuals.[3]

O

Occupational therapy services. A preventive and restorative treatment process designed to improve physical, psychosocial, and developmental ability; enhance knowledge and skill; and engineer motivation to achieve independence in self care, a vocation, and work.[1]

Open access. A provision specifying that plan members may self-refer to a specialist, either in-network or out-of-network, at full benefit or at a reduced benefit, respectively, without first obtaining a referral from a primary care provider.[1]

Open enrollment period. The period in which an employee may change health plans; usually occurs once per year.[1]

Out-of-pocket costs. Health care costs that the individual must pay; includes deductibles, coinsurance, and co-payments.[3]

Outcome indicators/measures. Evaluations that gauge the extent to which the results of providing health care services succeed in improving or maintaining satisfaction and patient health.

Outliers. Those cases that differ from average expectations by having either unusually long or short lengths of stay or unusually high or low resource consumption. Often used in reference to DRGs.[2]

Outpatient. An individual receiving health care services who does not require admission to a medical treatment facility for an overnight stay (inpatient care).[2]

Outpatient Prospective Payment System. The way that Medicare pays for most outpatient services at hospitals or community mental health centers under Medicare Part B.[3]

Outsourcing. The hiring of external vendors to perform specified functions, such as data and information management activities.[1]

P

P&T committee. *See* Pharmacy and therapeutics committee[1]

Patient. A sick, injured, wounded, or other person requiring medical or dental care or treatment.[3]

Patient acuity. The measurement of the intensity of care required for a patient, ranging from minimal care to intensive care.[2]

Payer. An entity that assumes the financial risk of paying for prevention, diagnosis, and medical treatment.[3]

PBM. *See* Pharmacy benefit management plan[1]

PCP. *See* Primary care physician/provider and Primary care[1]

Peer review. A system in which the appropriateness of health care services delivered by a provider to health plan members is evaluated by a panel of medical professionals.[1]

Pharmacy and therapeutics (P&T) committee. A formally constituted group of health care professionals that develops, updates, and administers the organization's formulary and regularly reviews reports on clinical trials, drug utilization reports, current and proposed therapeutic guidelines, and economic data on drugs. Such committees are most often found in MCOs, PBMs, and hospitals.[1]

Pharmacy benefit management (PBM) plan. A type of managed care specialty service organization that seeks to contain the costs of pharmaceuticals while promoting more efficient and safer drug use. Also known as a prescription benefit management plan.[1]

Physical therapy services. The activities related to evaluation and treatment of patients with neuromusculoskeletal complaints to prevent injury and maintain and/or restore function.[2]

Physician. A licensed professional possessing a degree in medicine (MD) or osteopathy (DO).[2]

Physician assistant. A licensed professional who has successfully completed two or more years of advanced training in an accredited Physician Assistant education program and is granted privileges to determine, start, alter, or suspend regimens of medical care under the supervision of a licensed physician.[2]

Physician-hospital organization (PHO). A joint venture between a hospital and many or all of its admitting physicians whose primary purpose is contract negotiations with MCOs and marketing.[1]

Point-of-service plan (POS). An insurance product, based on an HMO format, that requires the member to select a primary care physician, but allows for opting out of the network (called self-referring) at a substantially reduced benefit.[2]

Positioning. The way in which marketers help consumers, users, buyers, and others view their offerings against competitive brands or types of products.[4]

PPO. *See* Preferred provider organization[1]

Preauthorization. The approval given by a health plan prior to the provision of health care that allows reimbursement for inpatient care, designated outpatient procedures, or specialized care. This approval is based on the determination that the care or procedure being considered is medically necessary, the proposed location for delivery of that care is appropriate, and the site is contracted with the plan. Also called prior authorization and precertification.[2]

Pre-existing condition. In health insurance, a condition for which an individual received a diagnosis or medical care during a specified time period immediately prior to the effective date of coverage.[1]

Preferred provider organization (PPO). A term applied to a variety of direct contractual relationships between health plans and providers, which typically share three characteristics: a negotiated system for payment for services; financial incentives for patients to use contracting providers (usually in the form of reduced co-payments and deductibles, broader coverage of services, or simplified claims processing); and an extensive utilization review program.[2]

Premium. A payment or series of payments made to a health plan by purchasers, and often plan members, for medical benefits.[1]

Prepaid care. Health care services provided to an HMO member in exchange for a fixed, monthly premium paid in advance of the delivery of medical care.[1]

Prevalence. The number of existing cases of a disease or condition in a given population at a specific time.[3]

Preventive services. Health care intended to keep a person healthy or to avoid illness; for example, Pap tests, pelvic exams, flu shots, and screening mammograms.[3]

Price elasticity. A measure of the sensitivity of demand to changes in price. It is formally defined as the percentage change in quantity demanded relative to a given percentage change in price.[4]

Price fixing. An illegal business practice that occurs when two or more independent competitors agree on the prices or fees that they will charge for goods or services.[1]

Pricing. The process of deciding the customer charge for goods or services.

Primary care. The provision of integrated, accessible health care services by clinicians who are accountable for addressing a large majority of personal health care needs, developing a sustained partnership with patients, and practicing in the context of family and community.[6]

Primary data. The information collected specifically for the purpose of the investigation at hand.[4]

Process measures. Health care quality indicators related to the methods and procedures that providers use to furnish service and care.[1]

Product. A bundle of attributes (features, functions, benefits, and uses) capable of exchange or use; usually a mix of tangible and intangible forms. Thus a product may be an idea, a physical entity (a good), or a service, or any combination of the three. It exists for the purpose of exchange in the satisfaction of individual and organizational objectives.[4]

Promotion. The element of the marketing mix that an organization uses (1) to inform consumers about its products, the prices of its products, and how to obtain its products; (2) to persuade consumers to purchase its products; and (3) to remind consumers about the benefits associated with transacting business with the organization.[1]

Promotion mix. The four tools of promotion—advertising, personal selling, sales promotion, and publicity.[1]

Prospective payment system. A method of reimbursement in which payment is made based on a predetermined, fixed amount based on the classification system of that service (for example, DRGs for Medicare inpatient hospital services).[3]

Protected health information. Individually identifiable health data transmitted or maintained in any form or medium, which is held by an entity or its business associate, that is subject to HIPAA compliance.[3]

Provider. Any entity (for example, hospital, skilled nursing facility, home health agency, outpatient physical therapy, comprehensive outpatient rehabilitation facility, end-stage renal disease facility, hospice, physician, non-physician provider, laboratory, supplier) that furnishes medical services to current or prospective patients.[3]

Provider profiling. The collection and analysis of information about the practice patterns of individual providers.[1]

Public relations. The form of communication management that seeks to make use of publicity and other nonpaid forms of promotion and information to influence the feelings, opinions, or beliefs about the company, its products or services, or about the value of the product or service or the activities of the organization to buyers, prospects, or other stakeholders.[4]

Pull strategy. Communications and promotional activities by the marketer to persuade consumers to request specific products or brands from retail channel members.[4]

Push strategy. Communications and promotional activities by the marketer to persuade wholesale and retail channel members to stock and promote specific products.[4]

Q

Quality (of health care). The provision of efficient and effective care to appropriately selected patients at the right time and in an expert manner, consistent with the current state of medical knowledge and patient preferences.

Quality assurance. The process of looking at how well a medical service is provided, including formally reviewing health care given to a person or group of persons, locating problems, correcting the problems, and then checking to see if the corrective action is effective.[3]

Quality improvement organization (QIO). Groups of practicing doctors and other health care experts who are paid by the federal government to check the care provided to Medicare patients, make suggestions for improvement, and, if necessary, recommend sanctions. Formerly called Peer Review Organizations (PROs).[3]

R

Rating. The process of calculating the appropriate premium to charge purchasers, given the degree of risk represented by the individual or group, the expected costs to deliver medical services, and the expected marketability and competitiveness of the health plan.[1]

RBRVS. *See* Resource-based relative value scale

Rebate. A refund on the price of a particular pharmaceutical obtained by a PBM from the pharmaceutical manufacturer, often based on purchase volume.[1]

Referral. An authorization from a health plan-contracted caregiver (usually a primary care provider) approving a patient's receipt of services or products from an entity also contracted with the plan. The purpose is to enhance coordination of care and thus improve quality and lower cost.

Rehabilitation. Services rendered under a physician-directed care plan by nurses and physical, occupational, and speech therapists to restore or maintain physical functioning.[3]

Relative Value Unit (RVU). A system that assigns a rate to health care services by comparing the worth of one services to others or to a standard measure.

Resource-based relative value scale (RBRVS). A uniform, federally issued fee schedule for physicians' services that is derived from the relative values of the sums representing physicians' work, practice expenses net of malpractice expenses, and the cost of professional liability insurance.[3]

Respite care. Temporary or periodic care provided in a nursing home, assisted living residence, or other type of long-term care program so that the usual caregiver can rest or take some time off.[3]

Retrospective review. A type of utilization review that occurs after treatment is completed in order to authorize payment, medical necessity, and appropriateness of care.[1]

Risk-adjustment. The statistical adjustment of outcomes measures to account for factors that are independent of the quality of care provided and beyond the control of the plan or provider, such as the patient's gender and age, the seriousness of the patient's condition, and any other illnesses the patient might have. Also known as case-mix adjustment.[1]

Risk management (RM). A function of planning, organizing, implementing, and directing a comprehensive program of activities to identify, evaluate, and take corrective action against perils that may lead to patient, visitor, or employee injury and property loss or damage with resulting financial loss or legal liability.[2]

S

Sales. Any of a number of activities designed to promote customer purchase of a product or service. Sales can be done in person or over the phone, through e-mail or other communication media. The process generally includes stages such as assessing customer needs, presenting product features and benefits to address those needs, and negotiation on price, delivery, and other elements.[4]

SCHIP. *See* State Children's Health Insurance Program

Screening programs. Preventive care programs designed to determine if a health condition is present even if a person has not experienced symptoms of the problem.[1]

Secondary data. Statistics that are gathered directly from existing sources.

Segmentation. The process of dividing a market into distinct subsets of customers that behave in the same way or have similar needs.[4]

Self-insured. An individual or organization that assumes the financial risk of paying for health care. Also called self-funded.[3]

Senior market. A segment that is composed largely of persons over age sixty-five who are eligible for Medicare benefits.[1]

Sherman Antitrust Act. A federal act that established as national policy the concept of a competitive marketing system by prohibiting companies from attempting to (1) monopolize any part of trade or commerce or (2) engage in contracts, combinations, or conspiracies in restraint of trade. The Act applies to all companies engaged in interstate commerce and to all companies engaged in foreign commerce. *See also* Antitrust laws[1]

Skilled nursing facility (SNF). A licensed facility that primarily provides a high level of care to patients who require medical, nursing, or rehabilitative services but does not provide the level of care or treatment available in a hospital. This level of care requires the daily involvement of skilled nursing or rehabilitation staff who provides such services as intravenous injections, wound care, and physical therapy.[3]

Social health maintenance organization (SHMO). A special type of health plan that provides the full range of Medicare benefits offered by standard Medicare HMOs, plus other services that include the following: prescription drug and chronic care benefits, respite care, and short-term nursing home care; homemaker, personal care services, and medical transportation; eyeglasses, hearing aids, and dental benefits.[3]

Social marketing. A program designed to influence the behavior of a target audience in which the benefits of the behavior are intended by the marketer to accrue primarily to the audience or to the society in general and not to the marketer.[4]

Social Security Administration. The federal agency that, among other things, determines initial entitlement to and eligibility for Medicare benefits.[3]

Specialist. A health care professional whose practice is limited to a certain branch of medicine, specific procedures, certain age categories of patients, specific body systems, or certain types of diseases.[1]

Speech-language therapy. Treatment to regain and strengthen speech and swallowing skills after an illness or injury.[3]

Staff model HMO. An HMO whose physicians are employees of the health plan.[1]

Stakeholders. One of a group of publics who have a substantial interest in a company and about whom the company must be concerned. Key stakeholders include consumers, employees, stockholders, suppliers, and others who have some relationship with the organization.[4]

Standard of care. A diagnostic and treatment process that a clinician should follow for a certain type of patient, illness, or clinical circumstance.[1]

Standards. Authoritative statements of (1) minimum levels of acceptable performance or results, (2) excellent levels of performance or results, or (3) the range of acceptable performance or results.[6]

Stark laws. *See* Ethics in Patient Referrals Act

State Children's Health Insurance Program (SCHIP). A federally subsidized, state-managed program designed to provide health assistance to uninsured, low-income children through either separate initiatives or expanded eligibility under state Medicaid programs.[1]

Stop-loss insurance/coverage. A type of insurance coverage that enables provider organizations or self-funded groups to place a dollar limit on their liability for paying claims and requires the insurer issuing the insurance to reimburse the insured organization for claims paid in excess of a specified yearly maximum.[1]

Strategy. *See* Marketing strategy

Substitute goods/services. Products that look alike, represent the same application of a distinct technology to the provision of a discrete set of customer functions, and have a shared functionality based on the customer's perception of all the ways in which their needs can be satisfied in a given usage or application situation. The attractiveness of a substitute product depends on (1) its initial price, (2) customer switching costs, (3) postpurchase costs of operation, and (4) the additional benefits the customer perceives and values.[4]

Supplier. Any company, person, or agency that provides a medical item or service.[3]

T

Target marketing. The particular segment of a total population on which the retailer focuses its merchandising expertise to satisfy that segment's needs or wants in order to accomplish its profit objectives.[4]

Technology assessment (TA). Health care TA is a multidisciplinary field of policy analysis that studies the medical, social, ethical, and economic implications of the development, diffusion, and use of technologies.[3]

Telemedicine. Various technologies used as part of a coherent, health service information resource management program that captures, displays, stores, and retrieves medical images and data for care of a patient at a site remote from the service provider.[2]

Tertiary care. Services usually provided by a large medical center, requiring sophisticated technology, highly trained specialty professionals, and support facilities for unusual and complex medical problems.

Third-party administrator (TPA). A business associate that performs claims administration and related business functions for a self-insured entity.[3]

Third-party payer. The entity that is financially responsible for paying health claims. The first two parties are the provider and patient.

TPA. *See* Third-party administrator

Triage. The evaluation and classification of the injured or ill for purposes of treatment and evacuation. It consists of sorting patients according to type and seriousness of injury and the establishment of priority for treatment.[2]

Tricare. A Department of Defense regionally managed health care program for active duty and retired members of the uniformed services and their families that combines military health care resources and networks of civilian health care professionals. Formerly known as CHAMPUS (the Civilian Health and Medical Program of the United States).[1]

Tying arrangements. An illegal business practice that occurs when an organization conditions the sale of one product or service on the sale of other products or services.[1]

U

UCR. *See* Usual, customary, or reasonable fee

Unbundling. Separating a procedure into parts and charging for each part rather than using a single code for the entire procedure.[1]

Underwriting. The process of identifying and classifying the risk represented by an individual or group for purposes of setting insurance premium rates.[3]

Upcoding. Using a code for a procedure or diagnosis that is more complex than the actual procedure or diagnosis to gain higher reimbursement for the provider.[3]

UR. *See* Utilization review

Usual, customary, or reasonable. A method of profiling physician fees in an area and reimbursing them on the basis of that profile. Usual fees are what the individual physician most often charges for a particular service. Customary fees are what all similar physicians in the area charge for a given service. Reasonable fees are those that the health plan determines are realistic if no billing information exists for a particular service. For example, one common method is to average a service-specific customary fee and pay physicians the 80th or 90th percentile for that service.

Utilization management (UM). Assessing, controlling, and coordinating the use of medical services to ensure that a patient receives necessary, appropriate, high-quality care in a cost-effective manner.[1]

Utilization review (UR). An evaluation of the medical necessity, appropriateness, and cost-effectiveness of health care services and treatment plans for a given patient using formal, expert-developed criteria.[1]

V

Value. A measure of the contribution to a product's worth by any organization that handles it on its way to the ultimate user. Value added is measured by subtracting the cost of a product (or the cost of ingredients from which it was made) from the price that the organization received for it. For resellers, this means the firm's gross margin; for manufacturing firms, it means the contribution over cost of ingredients. Presumably whatever work that firm did is reflected in the higher price someone is willing to pay for the product, hence that firm's value-added.[4]

Veteran. A person who has served in the U.S military and received an honorable or general discharge.

W

Web site. A specific location on the World Wide Web that provides users access to a group of related text, graphics, and, in some cases, multimedia and interactive files.[1]

Workers' compensation. A state-mandated insurance program that provides benefits for health care costs and lost wages to qualified employees and their dependents if an employee suffers a work-related injury or disease.[1]

World Health Organization (WHO). The directing and coordinating authority for health within the United Nations system. It is responsible for providing leadership on global health matters, shaping the health research agenda, setting norms and standards, articulating evidence-based policy options, providing technical support to countries, and monitoring and assessing health trends.[5]

World Wide Web (www). An internet service that links independently owned databases containing text, pictures, and multimedia elements. Also known as the Web.[1]

NOTES

CHAPTER ONE

1. Zyman, S. *The End of Marketing As We Know It*. New York: HarperBusiness, 1999.
2. Sheth, J. N., and Sisodia, R. S. *4P's of Marketing*. Chicago: American Marketing Association, 2008.

CHAPTER TWO

1. Roemer, M. J. *National Health Systems of the World*, Vol. 1. Oxford University Press, 1991, pp. 3, 4, 31.
2. World Health Organization. *World Health Report 2000*. Geneva, Switzerland: World Health Organization, 2002.
3. Available at www.healthypeople.gov/LHI.
4. Anderson, O. W. *Health Care: Can There Be Equity?* New York: Wiley, 1972.
5. Roemer, M. I. *National Strategies for Health Care Organization*. Ann Arbor, Mich.: Health Administration Press, 1985, p. 36, Fig. 3.3.
6. Anderson, G. F., and others. "It's the Prices, Stupid: Why the United States Is So Different from Other Countries." *Health Affairs*, 2003, *22*, 89–105.
7. Porter, M. *Competitive Strategy*. New York: The Free Press, 1980.
8. See "IHI's Ambition Rises for '07," *Modern Healthcare*, Dec. 18/25, 2006, p. 8.

CHAPTER THREE

1. Statement by James Morgan, quoted in *Modern Healthcare*, Dec. 18/25, 2006, p. 23. Morgan chaired the recent report from the Commonwealth Fund's Commission on a High Performance Health System.
2. McGlynn, E. A. "There Is No Perfect Health System." *Health Affairs*, May/June 2004, *23*(3), 100–102.
3. See M. E. Porter and E. O. Teisberg, *Redefining Health Care: Creating Value-Based Competition on Results* (Boston: Harvard Business School Press, 2006), Chapter 2.
4. Roseleff, F., and Lister, G. In Coopers & Lybrand, *European Healthcare Trends: Towards Managed Care in Europe*, May 1995.
5. Miller, R. M., and Luft, H. S. "HMO Plan Performance Update: An Analysis of the Literature, 1997–2001." *Health Affairs*, 2002, *21*, 63–86.
6. Committee on the Future of Primary Care, Institute of Medicine. *Journal of the American Medical Association*, 1995, *273*, 192.
7. Berwick, D. M. "Payment by Capitation and the Quality of Care." *New England Journal of Medicine*, 1996, *335*, 1227–1231.
8. Datamonitor consulting firm at www.datamonitor.com.
9. Available at http://www.visiongainintelligence.com.
10. *Trends and Indicators in the Changing Health Care Marketplace*. Kaiser Family Foundation, Feb. 2, 2005.
11. "UK Consumer Group Slams Hidden Promotion of Drugs." Reuters, June 26, 2006.

12. Klaber, P. "Drug Ad Rule Perplexes Kiss: Speaker Wonders Why Marketing Costs Dropped from Proposal." *Charleston Gazette*, May 26, 2006.

13. MacDonald, G. J. "Backstory: A Pill They Won't Swallow." *Christian Science Monitor*, Dec. 28, 2005.

14. *Impact of Direct-to-Consumer Advertising on Prescription Drug Spending*. Kaiser Family Foundation, June 2003.

15. Philips, L. "Pharmaceutical Marketing Online: Direct-to-Patient Becomes a Reality." *eMarketer*, Aug. 2006.

16. Scott-Levin data from "Spending Hits a Wall" in *Pharmaceutical Executive*, Sept. 2002.

17. DiMasi, J. A., and others. "The Price of Innovation: New Estimates of Drug Development Costs." *Journal of Health Economics*, 2003, *22*, 151–185.

18. Gilbert, J., and others. "Rebuilding Pharma's Business Model." *Vivo, The Business and Medicine Report*, Nov. 2003.

19. Standard & Poor's, *GICS Sub-Industry Revenue Share*, Sept. 4, 2004.

20. Employee Benefit Research Institute (EBRI). "Fundamentals of Employee Benefit Programs, Part Three, Health Benefits." In *Prescription Drug Plans*, Aug. 19, 2005, pp. 25–34.

21. Atlantic Information Services, Inc. *A Guide to Drug Cost Management Strategies*, 2nd ed., 2004.

22. World POPClock, U.S. Census Bureau, Sept. 1999. [www.census.gov].

23. Moffett, S. "Senior Moment: Fast-Aging Japan Keeps Its Elders on the Job Longer." *Wall Street Journal*, June 15, 2005, p. A1.

24. Washaw, G., Bragg, E., and Shaull, R. "Geriatric Medicine Training and Practice in the United States at the Beginning of the 21st Century." The Association of Geriatric Academic Programs, July 2002.

25. Available at http://blog.fastcompany.com/archives/2004/11/17/the_coming_age_wave.html.

26. Grow, B. "Hispanic Nation." *Business Week*, Mar. 15, 2004, pp. 58–70.

27. Morton, C. C. "At IOM's Invitation, HSPH Researcher Helps Put Health Literacy on National Agenda." *Harvard Public Health NOW*, Feb. 7, 2003. [http://www.hsph.harvard.edu/now/feb7/].

28. See http://www.kron4.com/Global/story.asp?S=1378459.

29. Koss-Feder, L. "Out and About." *Marketing News*, May 25, 1998, pp. 1, 20.

30. "Rural Population and Migration: Overview." Economic Research Service, U.S. Department of Agriculture, 2006. [http://www.ers.usda.gov/Briefing/Population/].

31. Fost, D. "Americans on the Move." *American Demographics Tools Supplement*, Jan.–Feb. 1997, pp. 10–13.

32. Burkhauser, R., and others. "How the Distribution of After-Tax Income Changed Over the 1990s Business Cycle: A Comparison of the United States, Great Britain, Germany and Japan." Working Paper WP 2006–145, University of Michigan Retirement Research Center, Dec. 2006.

33. Fronstin, P. "The Relationship Between Income and Health Insurance: Rethinking the Use of Family Income in the Current Population Survey." *EBRI Notes*, Feb. 2005, *26*(2).

34. Catlin, A., Cowan, C., Heffler, S., and Washington, B., the National Health Expenditure Accounts Team. "National Health Spending in 2005: The Slowdown Continues." *Health Affairs*, 2007, *26*(1), 142–153.

35. Appleby, J. "Health Care Spending Rose at Twice the Rate of Inflation in '05." *USA Today*, Jan. 9, 2007.

36. Rowland, C. "Patients Piling Medical Costs on Credit Cards." *New York Times*, Jan. 22, 2007.

37. Paul, P. "Corporate Responsibility." *American Demographics*, May 2002, pp. 24–25.

38. Wenske, P. "You Too Could Lose $19,000!" *Kansas City Star*, Oct. 31, 1999; "Clearing House Suit Chronology." Associated Press, Jan. 26, 2001.

39. Christensen, C. M., Bohmer, R., and Kenagy, J. "Will Disruptive Innovations Cure Health Care?" *Harvard Business Review*, Sept./Oct. 2000, 102–112.

40. Cohen, D. *Legal Issues on Marketing Decision Making*. Cincinnati: South-Western, 1995.

CHAPTER FOUR

1. Peabody, F. W. "The Care of the Patient." *Journal of the American Medical Association*, 1927, *88*, 877–882.

2. Mendoza-Sassi, R., and Béria, J. U. *Utilización de los Servicios de Salud: Una Revisión Sistemática Sobre los Factores Relacionados* [Health Services Utilization: A Systematic Review of Related Factors]. *Cadernos Saúde Pública*, Aug. 2001, *17*(4), 819–832.

3. Jerant, A. F., and others. "Age-Related Disparities in Cancer Screening: Analysis of 2001 Behavioral Risk Factor Surveillance System Data." *Annals of Family Medicine*, 2004, *2*, 481–487.

4. Doty, H. E., and Weech-Maldonado, R. "Racial/Ethnic Disparities in Adult Preventive Dental Care Use." *Journal of Health Care for the Poor and Underserved*, 2003, *14*, 516–534.

5. Govindarajan, R., and others. "Racial Differences in the Outcome of Patients with Colorectal Carcinoma." *Cancer*, 2003, *97*, 493–498.

6. Goldman, D. P., and McGlynn, E.A. "U.S. Health Care, Facts about Cost, Access, and Quality." RAND Corporation, 2005. [http://www.rand.org/pubs/corporate_pubs/2005/RAND_CP484.1.pdf].

7. Sarmiento, O. L., and others. "Disparities in Routine Physical Examinations Among In-School Adolescents of Differing Latino Origins." *Journal of Adolescent Health*, 2004, *35*, 310–320.

8. Fitzpatrick, R. "Social Status and Mortality" (editorial). *Annals of Internal Medicine*, 2001, *134*, 1001–1003.

9. Van der Meer, J. B., van den Bos, J., and Mackenbach, J. P. "Socioeconomic Differences in the Utilization of Health Services in a Dutch Population: The Contribution of Health Status." *Health Policy*, 1996, *37*, 1–18.

10. Dunlop, S., Coyte, P. C., and McIsaac, W. "Socio-Economic Status and the Utilisation of Physicians' Services: Results from the Canadian National Population Health Survey." *Social Science & Medicine*, 2000, *51*, 123–133.

11. Van der Heyden, J. H., Demarest, S., Tafforeau, J., and Van Oyen, H. "Socio-Economic Differences in the Utilisation of Health Services in Belgium." *Health Policy*, 2003, *65*, 153–165.

12. Croft, P. R., and Rigby, A. S. "Socioeconomic Influences on Back Problems in the Community in Britain." *Journal of Epidemiology and Community Health*, 1994, *48*, 166–170.

13. Mayer, O., Jr, Simon, J., Heidrich, J., Cokkinos, D. V., and De Bacquer, D. "EUROASPIRE II Study Group: Educational Level and Risk Profile of Cardiac Patients in the EUROASPIRE II Substudy." *Journal of Epidemiology and Community Health*, 2004, *58*, 47–52.

14. Huerta, D., Cohen-Feldman, C., and Huerta, M. "Education Level and Origin as Predictors of Hospitalization Among Jewish Adults in Israel: A Population-Based Study." *Harefuah*, 2005, *144*, 407–412.

15. Altinkaynak, S., Ertekin, V., Guraksin, A., and Kilic, A. "Effect of Several Sociodemographic Factors on Measles Immunization in Children of Eastern Turkey." *Public Health*, 2004, *18*, 565–569.

16. Mayer, Simon, Heidrich, Cokkinos, and De Bacquer, 1994.

17. Latza, U., Kohlmann, T., Deck, R., Raspe, H. "Can Health Care Utilization Explain the Association Between Socioeconomic Status and Back Pain?" *Spine*, 2004, *29*, 1561–1566.

18. Davidoff, A., and others. "The Effect of Parents' Insurance Coverage on Access to Care for Low-Income Children." *Inquiry*, 2003, *40*, 254–268.

19. Paine, P., and Wright, M. A. "With Free Health Services, Why Does the Brazilian Working Class Delay in Seeing the Doctor?" *Tropical Doctor*, 1989, *19*, 120–123.

20. Hofstede, G. *Culture's Consequences*, 2nd ed. Thousand Oaks, Calif.: Sage, 2001.

21. Hall, E. T. *Beyond Culture*. New York: Anchor Books/Doubleday, 1976.

22. Schein, E. H. *Organizational Culture and Leadership*, 2nd ed. San Francisco: Jossey-Bass, 1992.

23. Hsairi, M., Fakhfakh, R., Bellaaj, Achour, N. "Knowledge, Attitudes and Behaviours of Women Toward Breast Cancer Screening." *East Mediterranean Health Journal*, 2003, *9*, 87–98.

24. Westin, M., Ahs, A., Brand Persson, K., and Westerling, R. "A Large Portion of Swedish Citizens Refrain from Seeking Medical Care—Lack of Confidence in the Medical Services a Plausible Explanation?" *Health Policy*, 2004, *68*, 333–334.

25. Wong-Kim, E., Sun, A., DeMattos, M.C. "Assessing Cancer Beliefs in a Chinese Immigrant Community." *Cancer Control*, 2003, *10*, 5 Supplement, 22–28.

26. Raspe, H., Matthis, C., Croft, P., and O'Neill, T. *Spine*, 2004, *29*, 1017–1021.

27. Greenspan, A. "Culture Influences Demographic Behavior: Evidence from India." *Asia Pacific Population Policy*, March 1994, 1–4.

28. Dessio, W., Wade, C., Chao, M., Kronenberg, F., Cushman, L. E., and Kalmuss, D. "Religion, Spirituality, and Healthcare Choices of African-American Women: Results of a National Survey." *Ethnicity & Disease*, 2004, *14*, 189–197.

29. Tinkelman, D. G., McClure, D. L., Lehr, T. L., and Scwartz, A. L. "Relationships Between Self-Reported Asthma Utilization and Patient Characteristics." *Journal of Asthma*, 2002, *39*, 729–736.

30. Godfrey-Faussett, P., Kaunda, H., Kamanga, J., van Beers, S., van Cleeff, M., Kumwenda-Phiri, R., and Tihont, V. "Why Do Patients with a Cough Delay Seeking Care at Lukasa Urban Health Centres: A Health Systems Research Approach." *International Journal of Tuberculosis and Lung Disease*, 2002, *6*, 796–805.

31. Shaikh, B. T., and Hatcher, J. "Health Seeking Behaviour and Health Service Utilization in Pakistan: Challenging the Policy Makers." *Journal of Public Health*, 2005, *27*, 49–54.

32. Sisk, J. E., Moskowitz, A. J., Whang, W., Lin, J. D., Fedson, D. S., McBean, A. M., Plouffe, J. F., Cetron, M. S., and Butler, J. C. "Cost-Effectiveness of Vaccination Against Pneumococcal Bacteremia Among Elderly People." *Journal of the American Medical Association*, 1997, *278*, 1333–1339.

33. Tucker, A. W., Haddix, A. C., Bresee, J. S., Holman, R. C., Parashar, U. D., and Glass, R. I. "Cost-Effectiveness Analysis of a Rotavirus Immunization Program for the United States." *Journal of the American Medical Association*, 1998, *279*, 1371–1376.

34. Iskedjian, M., Walker, J. H., and Hemels, M. E. H. "Economic Evaluation of an Extended Acellular Pertussis Vaccine Programme for Adolescents in Ontario, Canada." *Vaccine*, 2004, *22* (31–32), 4215–4227.

35. Duncan, M., Hirota, W. K., and Tsuchida, A. "Prescreening *Versus* Empirical Immunization for Hepatitis A in Patients with Chronic Liver Disease: A Prospective Cost Analysis." *American Journal of Gastroenterology*, 2002, *97*, 1792–1795.

36. Kotler, P., Roberto, N., and Lee, N. *Social Marketing: Improving the Quality of Life*. Thousand Oaks, Calif.: Sage, 2002.

37. Hogan, C., and others. "Medicare Beneficiaries' Costs of Care in the Last Year of Life." *Health Affairs*, 2001, *20*, 188–195.

38. Emanuel, E. J., and Emanuel, L. L. "The Economics of Dying—The Illusion of Cost Savings at the End of Life." *New England Journal of Medicine*, 1994, *330*, 540–544.

39. American Medical Association Committee on Ethical and Judicial Affairs. "Medical Futility in End-of-Life Care: Report of the Council on Ethical and Judicial Affairs." *Journal of the American Medical Association*, 1999, *281*, 937–941.

40. Wennberg, J., and others. "Use of Hospitals, Physician Visits, and Hospice Care During Last Six Months of Life Among Cohorts Loyal to Highly Respected Hospitals in the United States." *British Medical Journal*, 2004, *328*, 607–611.

41. Dranove, D., and Wehner, P. "Physician-Induced Demand for Childbirths." *Journal of Health Economics*, 1994, *13*, 61–73.

42. Delattre, E., and Dormant, B. "Fixed Fees and Physician-Induced Demand: A Panel Data Study on French Physicians." *Health Economics*, 2003, *12*, 741–754.

43. Sørensen, R., and Grytten, J. "Competition and Supplier-Induced Demand in a Health Care System with Fixed Fees." *Health Economics*, 1999, *8*, 497–508.

44. Eisenberg, J. M. *Doctors' Decisions and the Cost of Medical Care*. Ann Arbor, Mich.: Health Administration Press, 1986.

45. Gruber, J., Kim, J., and Mayzlin, D. "Physician Fees and Procedure Intensity: The Case of Cesarean Delivery." *Journal of Health Economics*, 1999, *18*(4), 473–490.

46. Fuchs, V. R. "The Supply of Surgeons and the Demand for Operations." *Journal of Human Resources*, 1978, *13* (Supplement), 35–56.

47. Cromwell, J., and Mitchell, J. B. "Physician-Induced Demand for Surgery." *Journal of Health Economics*, 1986, *5*, 293–313.

48. Hemenway, D., Killen, A., Cashman, S. B., Parks, C. L., and Bicknell, W. J. "Physicians' Responses to Financial Incentives: Evidence from a For-Profit Ambulatory Care Center." *New England Journal of Medicine*, 1990, *322*, 1059–1063.

49. Delattre, E., and Dormont, B. "Fixed Fees and Physician-Induced Demand: A Panel Data Study on French Physicians." *Health Economics*, 2003, *12*(9), 741–754.

50. Noguchi, H., Shimizutani, S., and Masuda, Y. "Physician-Induced Demand for Treatments for Heart Attack Patients in Japan: Evidence from the Tokai Acute Myocardial Study." Economic and Social Research Institute (ESRI), Cabinet Office, Tokyo, Japan. Discussion Paper Series No. 147.

51. Flierman, H. A., and Groenewegen, P. P. "Introducing Fees for Services with Professional Uncertainty." *Health Care Financing Review*, 1992, *14*, 107–115.

52. Jimenez-Martin, S., and others. "An Empirical Analysis of the Demand for Physician Services Across the European Union." Fundacion Centro de Estudios Andaluces (centrA) Documento de Trabajo Serie Economia E2003/455.

53. Rizzo, J. A., and Blumenthal, D. "Is the Target Income Hypothesis an Economic Heresy?" *Medical Care Research and Review*, 1996, *53*, 243–266, 288–293; McGuire, T. G. Commentary [on Rizzo and Blumenthal], *Medical Care Research and Review*, 1996, *53*, 267–273; Reinhardt, U. E. Commentary [on Rizzo and Blumenthal], *Medical Care Research and Review*, 1996, *53*, 274–287.

54. Garrison, L. P. Jr. "Assessment of the Effectiveness of Supply-Side Cost-Containment Measures." *Health Care Financing Review*, Annual Supplement, 1991, 13–20.

55. Dranove, D., and others. "Is Hospital Competition Wasteful?" *RAND Journal of Economics*, 1992, *23*, 247–262.

56. Wennberg, J., and Gittelson, A. "Small Area Variations in Health Care Delivery." *Science*, 1973, *182*, 1102–1108.

57. Fisher, E., and Wennberg, J. E. "Health Care Quality, Geographic Variations, and the Challenge of Supply-Sensitive Care." *Perspectives in Biology and Medicine*, 2003, *46*, 69–79.

58. Wright, J. G. "Physician Enthusiasm as an Explanation for Area Variation in the Utilization of Knee Replacement Surgery." *Medical Care*, 1999, *37*, 946–956.

59. Coyte, P. C., and others. "Physician and Population Determinants of Middle-Ear Surgery in Ontario." *Journal of the American Medical Association*, 2001, *286*, 2128–2135.

60. Muller-Nordhorn, J., and others. "Regional Variation in Medication Following Coronary Events in Germany." *International Journal of Cardiology*, 2005, *102*, 47–53.

61. Gibbs, R. G. J. "Diagnosis and Initial Management of Stroke and Transient Ischemic Attach Across UK Health Regions from 1992–1996." *Stroke*, 2001, *32*, 1085–1090.

62. Detsky, A. S. "Regional Variations in Medical Care." *New England Journal of Medicine*, 1995, *333*, 589–590.

63. Fisher, E. S., and others. "The Implications of Regional Variations in Medicare Spending," Part 1. *Annals of Internal Medicine*, 2003, *138*, 273–287.

CHAPTER FIVE

1. Drucker, P. *Management: Tasks, Responsibilities, and Practices*. New York: Harper and Row, 1973, ch. 7.

2. Levitt, T. "Marketing Myopia." *Harvard Business Review*, July–Aug. 1960.

3. Rayport, J. F., and Jaworski, B. J. *E-Commerce*. New York: McGraw-Hill, 2001, p. 116.

4. Juran, J. M. *Juran on Planning for Quality*. New York: Free Press, 1988.

5. Porter, M. E. *Competitive Advantage: Creating and Sustaining Superior Performance*. New York: Free Press, 1985.

6. Hiebeler, R., Kelly, T. B., and Ketteman, C. *Best Practices: Building Your Business with Customer-Focused Solutions*. New York: Simon & Schuster, 1998.

7. Hammer, M., and Champy, J. *Reengineering the Corporation*. New York: HarperCollins, 2003.

8. Besanko, D., Dranove, D., and Shanley, M. *The Economics of Strategy*. New York: Wiley, 2006.

9. Chandler, A. *Strategy and Structure: Chapters in the History of the American Industrial Enterprise*. Cambridge, Mass.: MIT Press, 1962.

10. Andrews, K. *The Concept of Corporate Strategy*. Homewood, Ill.: Irwin, 1971.

11. Itami, H. *Mobilizing Invisible Assets*. Cambridge, Mass.: Harvard University Press, 1997.

12. Day, G. S., and Montgomery, D. B. "Charting New Directions for Marketing." *Journal of Marketing* (Special Issue 1999), 3–13; Hoffman, D. L. "The Revolution Will Not Be Televised: Introduction to the Special Issue on Marketing Science and the Internet." *Marketing Science*, Winter 2000, 1–3.

13. Ansoff, H. I. "Strategies for Diversification," *Harvard Business Review*, Sept.–Oct. 1957, pp. 1, 123–124. The same matrix can be expanded into nine cells by adding modified products and modified markets. See S. J. Johnson and C. Jones, "How to Organize for New Products," *Harvard Business Review*, May–June 1957, pp. 49–62.

14. Christensen, C. M., Bohmer, R., and Kenagy, J. "Will Disruptive Innovations Cure Health Care?" *Harvard Business Review*, 2000, *78*(5), 102–112.

15. Porter, M. *Competitive Strategy*. New York: Free Press, 1980.

16. The authors are indebted to David Dranove, Ph.D., for his assistance with this section.

17. Porter, *Competitive Strategy*.

18. Treacy, M., and Wiersema, F. *The Discipline of Market Leaders*. Reading, Mass.: Perseus Books, 1995.

19. Ibid.

20. Collins, J. C., and Porras, J. I. *Built to Last: Successful Habits of Visionary Organizations*. New York: HarperBusiness, 1994.

21. Wood, M. B. *The Marketing Plan: A Handbook*. Upper Saddle River, N.J.: Prentice Hall, 2003.

22. Based on Wood, *The Marketing Plan: A Handbook*, Appendix 2.

23. Berry, T., and Wilson, D. *On Target: The Book on Marketing Plans*. Eugene, Ore.: Palo Alto Software, 2000.

CHAPTER SIX

1. Maslow, A. *Motivation and Personality*. New York: Harper & Row, 1954.

2. Herzberg, F. *Work and the Nature of Man*. Cleveland: William Collins, 1966; Thierry, H., and Koopman-Iwerna, A. M. "Motivation and Satisfaction." In P. J. Drenth (ed.), *Handbook of Work and Organizational Psychology*. New York: Wiley, 1984.

3. Proschaska, J., DiClemente, C., and Norcross, J. C. "In Search of How People Change: Applications to Addictive Behavior." *American Psychologist*, 1992, *47*(9), 1102–1114.

4. See note 2 above.

5. Russo, J. E., Meloy, M. G., and Wilks, T. J. "The Distortion of Product Information During Brand Choice." *Journal of Marketing Research*, 1998, *35*, 438–452.

6. Brown, K. R. M. "Health Belief Model." [http://www.tcw.utwente.nl/theorieenoverzicht/Theory%20clusters/Health%20Communication/Health_Belief_Model.doc/]. 1999.

7. National Institutes of Health, National Heart, Lung, and Blood Institute. [http://www.nhlbi.nih.gov/about/nhbpep/]. 2001.

8. National Institutes of Health, National Heart, Lung, and Blood Institute. [http://www.nih.gov/health/hbp-tifl/3.htm]. 2001.

9. Anderson, J. R. *The Architecture of Cognition*. Cambridge, Mass.: Harvard University Press, 1983; Wyer, R. S. Jr., and Srull, T. K. "Person Memory and Judgment." *Psychological Review*, 1989, *96*(1), 58–83.

10. Lynch, J. G. Jr., and Srull, T. K. "Memory and Attentional Factors in Consumer Choice: Concepts and Research Methods." *Journal of Consumer Research*, June 1982, *9*, 18–36; Alba, J. W., Hutchinson, J. W., and Lynch, J. G. Jr. "Memory and Decision Making." In H. H. Kassarjian and T. S. Robertson (eds.), *Handbook of Consumer Theory and Research*. Englewood Cliffs, N.J.: Prentice Hall, 1992.

11. Craik, F. I. M., and Lockhart, R. S. "Levels of Processing: A Framework for Memory Research." *Journal of Verbal Learning and Verbal Behavior*, 1972, *11*, 671–684; Craik, F. I. M., and Tulving, E. "Depth of Processing and the Retention of Words in Episodic Memory." *Journal of Experimental Psychology*, 1975, *104*(3), 268–294; Lockhart, R. S., Craik, F. I. M., and Jacoby, L. "Depth of Processing, Recognition, and Recall." In J. Brown (ed.), *Recall and Recognition*. New York: Wiley, 1976.

12. Shapiro, B., Rangan, V. K., and Sviokla, J., "Staple Yourself to an Order," *Harvard Business Review*, July–Aug. 1992, pp. 113–122. See also C. M. Heilman, D. Bowman, and G. P. Wright, "The Evolution of Brand Preferences and Choice Behaviors of Consumers New to a Market," *Journal of Marketing Research*, May 2000, 139–155.

13. Howard, J. A., and Sheth, J. N. *The Theory of Buyer Behavior*. New York: Wiley, 1969; Engel, J. F., Blackwell, R. D., and Miniard, P. W. *Consumer Behavior*, 8th ed. Fort Worth, Tex.: Dreyden, 1994; Luce, M. F., Bettman, J. R., and Payne, J. W. *Emotional Decisions: Tradeoff Difficulty and Coping in Consumer Choice*. Chicago: University of Chicago Press, 2001.

14. Putsis, W. P. Jr., and Srinivasan, N. "Buying or Just Browsing? The Duration of Purchase Deliberation." *Journal of Marketing Research*, Aug. 1994, 393–402.

15. Stevens, R. J. *Duke Heart Center Advertising Market Research Study*. Durham, N.C.: Health Centric Marketing Services, 2003.

16. Ray, M. L. *Marketing Communication and the Hierarchy of Effects*. Cambridge, Mass.: Marketing Science Institute, Nov. 1973.

17. Narayana, C. L., and Markin, R. J. "Consumer Behavior and Product Performance: An Alternative Conceptualization," *Journal of Marketing*, Oct. 1975, 1–6. See also W. S. DeSarbo and K. Jedidi, "The Spatial Representation of Heterogeneous Consideration Sets," *Marketing Science*, 1995, *14*(3), 326–342; L. G. Cooper and A. Inoue, "Building Market Structures from Consumer Preferences," *Journal of Marketing Research*, Aug. 1996, *33*(3), 293–306.

18. Krech, D., Crutchfield, R. S., and Ballachey, E. L. *Individual in Society*. New York: McGraw-Hill, 1962.

19. Green, P. E., and Wind, Y. *Multiattribute Decisions in Marketing: A Measurement Approach*. Hinsdale, Ill.: Dryden, 1973; McAlister, L. "Choosing Multiple Items from a Product Class." *Journal of Consumer Research*, Dec. 1979, 213–224; Lutz, R. J., "The Role of Attitude Theory in Marketing." In H. H. Kassarjian and T. Robertson (eds.), *Perspectives in Consumer Behavior*. Glenview, Ill.: Scott, Foresman, 1991.

20. Solomon, M. R. *Consumer Behavior: Buying, Having, and Being*. Upper Saddle River, N.J.: Prentice Hall, 2001.

21. Fishbein, M. "Attitudes and Prediction of Behavior." In M. Fishbein (ed.), *Readings in Attitude Theory and Measurement*. Hoboken, N.J.: Wiley, 1967.

22. Bauer, R. A. "Consumer Behavior as Risk Taking." In D. F. Cox (ed.), *Risk Taking and Information Handling in Consumer Behavior*. Boston: Division of Research, Harvard Business School, 1967; Taylor, J. W. "The Role of Risk in Consumer Behavior." *Journal of Marketing*, Apr. 1974, 54–60.

23. La Barbera, P. A., and Mazursky, D. "A Longitudinal Assessment of Consumer Satisfaction/Dissatisfaction: The Dynamic Aspect of the Cognitive Process." *Journal of Marketing Research*, Nov. 1983, 393–404.

24. Webster, F. E. Jr., and Wind, Y. *Organizational Buying Behavior*. Upper Saddle River, N.J.: Prentice Hall, 1972.

25. Collins, M. "Breaking into the Big Leagues." *American Demographics*, Jan. 1996, p. 24.

26. Robinson, P. J., Faris, C. W., and Wind, Y. *Industrial Buying and Creative Marketing*. Boston: Allyn & Bacon, 1967.

27. McQuiston, D. H. "Novelty, Complexity, and Importance as Causal Determinants of Industrial Buyer Behavior." *Journal of Marketing*, Apr. 1989, 66–79; Doyle, P., Woodside, A. G., and Mitchell, P. "Organizational Buying in New Task and Rebuy Situations." *Industrial Marketing Management*, Feb. 1979, 7–11.

28. Ozanne, U. B., and Churchill, G. A. Jr. "Five Dimensions of the Industrial Adoption Process." *Journal of Marketing Research*, Aug. 1971, 322–328.

29. Jackson, D. W. Jr., Keith, J. E., and Burdick, R. K. "Purchasing Agents' Perceptions of Industrial Buying Center Influence: A Situational Approach." *Journal of Marketing*, Fall 1984, 75–83.

30. Webster, F. E. Jr., and Wind, Y. *Organizational Buying Behavior*. Upper Saddle River, N.J.: Prentice Hall, 1972.

31. Ibid.

32. Webster, F. E. Jr., and Wind, Y. "A General Model for Understanding Organizational Buying Behavior." *Journal of Marketing*, Apr. 1972, *36*, 12–19; Webster and Wind, *Organizational Buying Behavior*.

33. Webster, F. E. Jr., and Keller, K. L. "A Roadmap for Branding in Industrial Markets." Working paper, Amos Tuck School of Business, Dartmouth College.

34. Ward, S., and Webster, F. E. Jr. "Organizational Buying Behavior." In T. Robertson and H. H. Kassarjian (eds.), *Handbook of Consumer Behavior*. Upper Saddle River, N.J.: Prentice Hall, 1991.

35. Webster, F. E. Jr., and Wind, Y. *Organizational Buying Behavior*. Upper Saddle River, N.J.: Prentice Hall, 1972.

36. Robinson, P. J., Faris, C. W., and Wind, Y. *Industrial Buying and Creative Marketing*. Boston: Allyn & Bacon, 1967.

37. Grewal, R., Comer, J. M., and Mehta, R. "An Investigation into the Antecedents of Organizational Participation in Business-to-Business Electronic Markets." *Journal of Marketing*, July 2001, *65*, 17–33.

38. Anderson, J. C., Jain, D. C., and Chintagunta, P. K. "A Customer Value Assessment in Business Markets: A State-of-Practice Study." *Journal of Business-to-Business Marketing*, 1993, *1*(1), 3–29.

39. Lehmann, D. R., and O'Shaughnessy, J. "Differences in Attribute Importance for Different Industrial Products." *Journal of Marketing*, Apr. 1974, 36–42.

40. Buvik, A., and John, G. "When Does Vertical Coordination Improve Industrial Purchasing Relationships?" *Journal of Marketing*, Oct. 2000, *64*, 52–64.

41. Rokkan, A. I., Heide, J. B., and Wathne, K. H. "Specific Investment in Marketing Relationships: Expropriation and Bonding Effects." *Journal of Marketing Research*, May 2003, *40*, 210–224.

42. Ghosh, M., and John, G. "Governance Value Analysis and Marketing Strategy." *Journal of Marketing*, 1999, *63* (Special Issue), 131–145.

43. Wathnem, K. H., and Heide, J. B. "Opportunism in Interfirm Relationships: Forms, Outcomes, and Solutions." *Journal of Marketing*, Oct. 2000, *64*, 36–51.

44. Houston, M. B., and Johnson, S. A. "Buyer-Supplier Contracts Versus Joint Ventures: Determinants and Consequences of Transaction Structure." *Journal of Marketing Research*, Feb. 2000, *37*, Feb. 1–15.

CHAPTER SEVEN

1. Kotler, P., and Keller, K. L. *Marketing Management*, 12th ed. Upper Saddle River, N.J.: Prentice Hall, 2006, p. 115.

2. Clancy, K., and Shulman, R. S. *Marketing Myths That Are Killing Business: The Cure for Death Wish Marketing*. New York: McGraw-Hill, 1994.

3. Kotler and Keller, *Marketing Management*, p. 73.

4. Fuld, L. "What Competitive Intelligence Is and Is Not!" [http://fuld.com/Company/CI.html]. Mar. 2007.

5. Peppers, D. "How You Can Help Them." *Fast Company*, Oct.–Nov. 1997, 128–136.

6. Strategy Software. "STRATEGY! Enterprise Top-Ranked Software by Fuld & Co." [http://www.strategy-software.com/indexsol.html]. Mar. 2007

7. Andreasen, A. *Marketing Social Change: Changing Behavior to Promote Health, Social Development, and the Environment*. San Francisco: Jossey-Bass, 1995.

8. Berkman, R. I. *Find It Fast: How to Uncover Expert Information on Any Subject in Print or Online*. New York: HarperCollins, 1997; Galea, C. "Surf City: The Best Places for Business on the Web," *Sales & Marketing Management*, Jan. 1997, 69–73; Curle, D. "Out-of-the-Way Sources of Market Research on the Web," *Online*, Jan.–Feb. 1998, 63–68; Tudor, J. D., "Brewing Up: A Web Approach to Industry Research," *Online*, July–Aug. 1996, 12. For an excellent annotated reference to major secondary sources of business and marketing data, see G. A. Churchill Jr., *Marketing Research: Methodological Foundations*, 7th ed. (Fort Worth, Tex.: Dryden, 1998).

9. Greenbaum, T. L. *The Handbook for Focus Group Research*. New York: Lexington Books, 1993.

10. "Online Focus Groups & Web-Based Surveys." [http://www.e-focusgroups.com/online.html]. Mar. 2007.

11. Greenbaum, T. L. "Online Focus Groups Are No Substitute for the Real Thing." *Quirk's Marketing Research Review*, June 2001.

12. Navarro, F. *The PATH Model—Understanding the Health Care Consumer*. Fontana, Calif.: The PATH Institute, Oct. 2004.

13. Little, J. D. C. "Decision Support Systems for Marketing Managers." *Journal of Marketing*, Summer 1979, *11*.

14. Kotler and Keller, *Marketing Management*, p. 115.

15. Kotler and Keller, *Marketing Management*, p. 116.

16. For further discussion, see G. L. Lilien, P. Kotler, and K. S. Moorthy, *Marketing Models*. Upper Saddle River, N.J.: Prentice Hall, 1992.

17. See www.naics.com and www.census.gov/epcd/naics02.

CHAPTER EIGHT

1. Anderson, J. C., and Narus, J. A. "Capturing the Value of Supplementary Services." *Harvard Business Review*, Jan.–Feb. 1995, 75–83.

2. Blattberg, R., and Deighton, J. "Interactive Marketing: Exploiting the Age of Addressability." *Sloan Management Review*, 1991, *33*(1), 5–14.

3. Zack, I. "Out of the Tube." *Forbes*, Nov. 26, 2001, p. 200.

4. Reda, S. "American Drug Stores Custom-Fits Each Market." *Stores*, Sept. 1994, 22–24.

5. Post, P. "Beyond Brand—The Power of Experience Branding." *ANA/The Advertiser*, Oct.–Nov. 2000.

6. Kane, K. "It's a Small World." *Working Woman*, Oct. 1997, p. 22.

7. Other leading suppliers of geodemographic data are ClusterPlus by Donnelly Marketing Information Services and Acord by C.A.C.I., Inc.

8. Weiss, M. J. "To Be About To Be." *American Demographics*, Sept. 2003, 29–36.

9. *Drug Use in Toronto 2004*. Toronto: Research Group on Drug Use, 2005.

10. "Phillips House Distinctive Services and Amenities." [http://www.massgeneral.org/visitor/phillip_services.htm]. Mar. 2007.

11. White, G. L., and Leung, S. "Middle Market Shrinks as Americans Migrate Toward the Higher End." *Wall Street Journal*, Mar. 29, 2002, pp. A1, A8.

12. Rickard, L. "Gerber Trots Out New Ads Backing Toddler Food Line." *Advertising Age*, Apr. 11, 1994, pp. 1, 48.

13. This classification was adapted from G. H. Brown, "Brand Loyalty: Fact or Fiction?" *Advertising Age*, June 1952–Jan. 1953, a series. See also P. E. Rossi, R. McCulloch, and G. Allenby, "The Value of Purchase History Data in Target Marketing," *Marketing Science*, 1996, *15*(4), 321–340.

14. Walker, C. "How Strong Is Your Brand?" *Marketing Tools*, Jan.–Feb. 1995, 46–53.

15. "The Conversion Model." [www.conversionmodel.com]. May 2007.

16. Robertson, T. S., and Barich, H. "A Successful Approach to Segmenting Industrial Markets." *Planning Forum*, Nov.–Dec. 1992, 5–11.

17. For a market-structure study of the hierarchy of attributes in the coffee market, see D. Jain, F. M. Bass, and Y.-M. Chen, "Estimation of Latent Class Models with Heterogeneous Choice Probabilities: An Application to Market Structuring," *Journal of Marketing Research*, Feb. 1990, 94–101. For an application of means-end chain analysis to global markets, see F. Ter Hofstede, J.-B. E. M. Steenkamp, and M. Wedel, "International Market Segmentation Based on Consumer-Product Relations," *Journal of Marketing Research*, Feb. 1999, 1–17.

18. Macchiette, B., and Abhijit, R. "Sensitive Groups and Social Issues." *Journal of Consumer Marketing*, 1994, *11*(4), 55–64.

19. Ries, A., and Trout, J. *Positioning: The Battle for Your Mind*. New York: Warner Books, 1982.

20. The concept of "points-of-parity" and "points-of-difference" and many of the other ideas and examples in this section were first developed by Northwestern University's Brian Sternthal and further refined in collaboration with Northwestern University's Alice Tybout.

21. Kotler, P., and Keller, K. L. *Marketing Management*, 12th ed. Upper Saddle River, N.J.: Prentice-Hall, 2006.

22. Some of these bases are discussed in D. A. Garvin, "Competing on the Eight Dimensions of Quality," *Harvard Business Review*, Nov.–Dec. 1987, 101–109.

23. Kotler, P. "Design: A Powerful but Neglected Strategic Tool." *Journal of Business Strategy*, Fall 1984, 16–21.

24. Adapted from T. Peters's description in *Thriving on Chaos*. New York: Knopf, 1987, 56–57.

25. Knapp, L. "A Sick Computer?" *Seattle Times*, Jan. 28, 2001, p. D-8.

26. For a similar list, see L. L. Berry and A. Parasuraman, *Marketing Services: Competing Through Quality*. New York: The Free Press, 1991, p. 16.

27. Rayport, J. F., and Jaworski, B. J. *E-Commerce*. New York: McGraw-Hill, 2001, p. 53.

28. Porter, M. E. *Competitive Advantage: Creating and Sustaining Performance*. New York: Free Press, 1985.

29. Rothschild, W. E. *How to Gain (and Maintain) the Competitive Advantage*. New York: McGraw-Hill, 1989, ch. 5.

30. Porter, *Competitive Advantage*, ch. 6.

31. "Business Bubbles." *The Economist*, Oct. 10, 2002.

32. Porter, *Competitive Strategy*, ch. 4; Prabhu, J., and Stewart, D. W. "Signaling Strategies in Competitive Interaction: Building Reputations and Hiding the Truth." *Journal of Marketing Research*, Feb. 2001, *38*, 62–72.

33. Eliashberg, J., and Robertson, T. S. "New Product Preannouncing Behavior: A Market Signaling Study." *Journal of Marketing Research*, Aug. 1988, *25*, 282–292; Calanton, R. J., and Schatzel, K. E. "Strategic Foretelling: Communications—Base Antecedents of a Firm's Propensity to Preannounce." *Journal of Marketing*, Jan. 2000, *64*, 17–30.

34. Kotler, P., and Bloom, P. N. "Strategies for High Market-Share Companies." *Harvard Business Review*, Nov.–Dec. 1975, pp. 63–72. See also Porter, *Competitive Advantage*, 221–226.

35. Buzzell, R. D., and Wiersema, F. D. "Successful Share-Building Strategies." *Harvard Business Review*, Jan.–Feb. 1981, pp. 135–144.

36. Hellofs, L., and Jacobson, R. "Market Share and Customers' Perceptions of Quality: When Can Firms Grow Their Way to Higher Versus Lower Quality?" *Journal of Marketing*, Jan. 1999, *63*, 16–25.

37. Levitt, T. "Innovative Imitation." *Harvard Business Review*, Sept.–Oct. 1966, p. 63. See also S. P. Schnaars, *Managing Imitation Strategies: How Later Entrants Seize Markets from Pioneers.* New York: Free Press, 1994.

38. Uttal, B. "Pitching Computers to Small Businesses." *Fortune*, Apr. 1, 1985, 95–104; Gannes, S. "The Riches in Market Niches." *Fortune*, Apr. 27, 1987, 227–230.

CHAPTER NINE

1. This discussion of product levels is adapted from T. Levitt, "Marketing Success Through Differentiation: Of Anything," *Harvard Business Review*, Jan.–Feb. 1980, 83–91. The first level, core benefit, has been added to Levitt's discussion by the authors.

2. Scalise, D. "The Patient Experience." *Hospitals and Health Networks*, Dec. 2003, pp. 41–47.

3. Boyd, H. W. Jr., and Levy, S. "New Dimensions in Consumer Analysis." *Harvard Business Review*, Nov.–Dec. 1963, pp. 129–140.

4. For some definitions of the features in an appropriate marketing-mix strategy, see P. D. Bennett (ed.), *Dictionary of Marketing Terms.* Chicago: American Marketing Association, 1995; P. E. Murphy and B. M. Enis, "Classifying Products Strategically," *Journal of Marketing*, July 1986, 24–42.

5. U.S. Department of Labor, Bureau of Labor Statistics, Employment Projections. [http://www.bls.gov/emp/home.htm]. Apr. 2007.

6. Shostack, G. L. "Breaking Free from Product Marketing." *Journal of Marketing*, Apr. 1977, 73–80; Berry, L. L. "Services Marketing Is Different." *Business*, May–June 1980, pp. 24–30; Langeard, E., Bateson, J. E. G., Lovelock, C. H., and Eiglier, P. *Services Marketing: New Insights from Consumers and Managers.* Cambridge, Mass.: Marketing Science Institute, 1981; Albrecht, K., and Zemke, R. *Service America! Doing Business in the New Economy.* Homewood, Ill.: Dow Jones-Irwin, 1986; Albrecht, K. *At America's Service.* Homewood, Ill.: Dow Jones-Irwin, 1988; Scheider, B., and Bowen, D. E. *Winning the Service Game.* Boston: Harvard Business School Press, 1995.

7. Booms, B. H., and Bitner, M. J. "Marketing Strategies and Organizational Structures for Service Firms." In J. H. Donnelly and W. R. George (eds.), *Marketing of Services*, pp. 47–51. Chicago: American Marketing Association, 1981.

8. Levitt, T. "Marketing Intangible Products and Product Intangibles." *Harvard Business Review*, May–June 1981, 94–102; Berry, L. L. "Services Marketing Is Different." *Business*, May–June 1980, pp. 24–30.

9. Carbone, L. P., and Haeckel, S. H. "Engineering Customer Experiences." *Marketing Management*, Winter 1994.

10. Lauer, C. S. "Healthcare Quality, Aviation Style." *Modern Healthcare*, Feb. 5, 2007, p. 23.

11. Sasser, W. E. "Match Supply and Demand in Service Industries." *Harvard Business Review*, Nov.–Dec. 1976.

12. Landro, L. "Why Quotas for Nurses Isn't a Cure-All." *Wall Street Journal*, Dec. 13, 2006, p. D8.

13. Bordley, R. "Determining the Appropriate Depth and Breadth of a Firm's Product Portfolio." *Journal of Marketing Research*, Feb. 2003, *40*, 39–53; Boatwright, P., and Nunes, J. C. "Reducing Assortment: An Attribute-Based Approach." *Journal of Marketing*, July 2001, *65*, 50–63.

14. Copland, A. "Talking to Your Boss In His/Her Language: The Marketing/Finance Interface." Presentation made at UNC-Chapel Hill School of Public Health, Chapel Hill, N.C., Aug. 2001.

CHAPTER TEN

1. Booz, Allen & Hamilton. *New Products Management for the 1980s.* New York: Booz, Allen & Hamilton, 1982.

2. "Don't Laugh at Gilded Butterflies." *Economist*, Apr. 24, 2004, pp. 71–73.

3. Deloitte and Touche. "Vision in Manufacturing Study." Deloitte Consulting and Kenan-Flagler Business School, Mar. 6, 1998; Nielsen, A. C. "New Product Introduction—Successful Innovation/Failure: Fragile Boundary." BASES and Ernst & Young Global Client Consulting, June 24, 1999.

4. Cooper, R. G., and Kleinschmidt, E. J. *New Products: The Key Factors in Successes*. Chicago: American Marketing Association, 1990.

5. Hauser, J., and Tellis, G. J. "Research on Innovation: A Review and Agenda for Marketing." Working paper, 2004.

6. Griffin, A. J., and Hauser, J. "The Voice of the Customer." *Marketing Science*, Winter 1993, pp. 1–27.

7. von Hippel, E. "Lead Users: A Source of Novel Product Concepts," *Management Science*, July 1986, 791–805. See also E. von Hippel, *The Sources of Innovation*. New York: Oxford University Press, 1988; R. D. Buzzell, "Learning from Lead Users." In R. D. Buzzell (ed.), *Marketing in an Electronic Age*, pp. 308–317. Cambridge, Mass.: Harvard Business School Press, 1985.

8. "The Ultimate Widget: 3-D 'Printing' May Revolutionize Product Design and Manufacturing." *U.S. News & World Report*, July 20, 1992, p. 55.

9. For additional information about conjoint analysis, see also P. E. Green and V. Srinivasan, "Conjoint Analysis in Marketing: New Developments with Implications for Research and Practice," *Journal of Marketing*, Oct. 1990, pp. 3–19; D. R. Wittnick, M. Vriens, and W. Burhenne, "Commercial Uses of Conjoint Analysis in Europe: Results and Critical Reflections," *International Journal of Research in Marketing*, Jan. 1994, pp. 41–52. For additional technical information on how to perform a conjoint analysis, see B. K Orme, *Getting Started with Conjoint Analysis: Strategies for Product Design and Pricing Research*. American Marketing Association, 2005.

10. Johal S. S., and Williams, H. C. "Decision-Making Methods That Could Be Used to Assess the Value of Medical Devices." Report presented to Multidisciplinary Assessment of Technology Centre for Healthcare, Mar. 2005, p. 46.

11. Hertz, D. B. "Risk Analysis in Capital Investment." *Harvard Business Review*, Jan.–Feb. 1964, pp. 96–106.

12. Hauser, J. "House of Quality." *Harvard Business Review*, May–June 1988, pp. 63–73. Customer-driven engineering is also called "quality function deployment." See L. R. Guinta and N. C. Praizler, *The QFD Book: The Team Approach to Solving Problems and Satisfying Customers through Quality Function Deployment*. New York: AMass.COM, 1993; V. Srinivasan, W. S. Lovejoy, and D. Beach, "Integrated Product Design for Marketability and Manufacturing." *Journal of Marketing Research*, 1997, *34*(1), 154–163.

13. See J.-N. Kapferer, *Strategic Brand Management: New Approaches to Creating and Evaluating Brand Equity*. London: Kogan Page, 1992, 38ff; J. L. Aaker, "Dimensions of Brand Personality," *Journal of Marketing Research*, Aug. 1997, pp. 347–356. For an overview of academic research on branding, see K. L. Keller, "Branding and Brand Equity." In B. Weitz and R. Wensley (eds.), *Handbook of Marketing*. New York: Sage Publications, 2002.

14. Schultz, H., and Schultz, D. *IMC, The Next Generation*. New York: McGraw-Hill, 2004.

15. Aaker, D. *Managing Brand Equity*. New York: Free Press, 1991.

16. Keller, K. L. "The Brand Report Card." *Harvard Business Review*, Jan.–Feb. 2000.

17. Stodghill, R. "The Doctor Is In: A Dose of Compassion Soothes a Merged Hospital." *New York Times*, Jan. 7, 2007, section 3, p. 1.

18. W. T. Robinson and Fornell, C., "Sources of Market Pioneer Advantages in Consumer Goods Industries," *Journal of Marketing Research*, Aug. 1985, pp. 305–317. See also G. L. Urban and others, "Market Share Rewards to Pioneering Brands: An Empirical Analysis and Strategic Implications," *Management Science*, June 1986, pp. 645–659.

19. Kotler, P. "Phasing Out Weak Products." *Harvard Business Review*, Mar.–Apr. 1965, pp. 107–118.

20. See www.ovationpharma.com.

21. Harrigan, K. R. "The Effect of Exit Barriers Upon Strategic Flexibility." *Strategic Management Journal*, 1980, *1*, 165–176.

22. Harrigan, K. R. "Strategies for Declining Industries." *Journal of Business Strategy*, Fall 1980, p. 27.

23. Dhalla, N., and Yuspeh, S. "Forget the PLC Concept." *Harvard Business Review*, Jan.–Feb. 1976, pp. 102–111.

24. Ibid.

CHAPTER ELEVEN

1. "The Price Is Wrong." *The Economist*, May 23, 2002.

2. DoBias, M. "Lifting the Lid Off of Pricing." *Modern Healthcare*, Mar. 20, 2006, pp. 6–7, 16; DoBias, M. "Transparent Pricing." *Modern Healthcare*, Aug. 7, 2006, p. 78.

3. For a thorough, up-to-date review of pricing research, see C. Ofir and R. S. Winer, "Pricing: Economic and Behavioral Models," In B. Weitz and R. Wensley (eds.), *Handbook of Marketing*. London: Sage Publications, 2002.

4. Dickson, P. R., and Sawyer, A. G. "The Price Knowledge and Search of Supermarket Shoppers," *Journal of Marketing*, July 1990, pp. 42–53. For a methodological qualification, however, see H. Estalami, A. Holden, and D. R. Lehmann, "Macro-Economic Determinants of Consumer Price Knowledge: A Meta-Analysis of Four Decades of Research," *International Journal of Research in Marketing*, Dec. 2001, *18*, 341–355.

5. For a different point of view, see C. Janiszewski and D. R. Lichtenstein, "A Range Theory Account of Price Perception," *Journal of Consumer Research*, Mar. 1999, pp. 353–368.

6. Rajendran, K. N., and Tellis, G. J. "Contextual and Temporal Components of Reference Price." *Journal of Marketing*, Jan. 1994, pp. 22–34; Kalyanaram, G., and Winer, R. S. "Empirical Generalizations from Reference Price Research." *Marketing Science*, 1995, *14*(3), pp. G161–G169.

7. Gourville, J. T. "Pennies-a-Day: The Effect of Temporal Reframing on Transaction Evaluation." *Journal of Consumer Research*, Mar. 1998, pp. 395–408.

8. Stiving, M., and Winer, R. S. "An Empirical Analysis of Price Endings with Scanner Data." *Journal of Consumer Research*, June 1997, pp. 57–68.

9. Anderson, E., and Simester, D. "The Role of Price Endings: Why Stores May Sell More at $49 than at $44." Unpublished conference paper, Apr. 2001.

10. Schindler, R. M., and Kirby, P. N. "Patterns of Rightmost Digits Used in Advertised Prices: Implications for Nine-Ending Effects." *Journal of Consumer Research*, Sept. 1997, pp. 192–201.

11. "Japan's Smart Secret Weapon." *Fortune*, Aug. 12, 1991, p. 75.

12. Farris, P. W., and Reibstein, D. J. "How Prices, Expenditures, and Profits Are Linked," *Harvard Business Review*, Nov.–Dec. 1979, pp. 173–184. See also M. Abe, "Price and Advertising Strategy of a National Brand against Its Private-Label Clone: A Signaling Game Approach," *Journal of Business Research*, July 1995, pp. 241–250.

13. Urbany, J. E. "Justifying Profitable Pricing." *Journal of Product and Brand Management*, 2001, 10(3), 141–157.

14. For an interesting discussion of a quantity surcharge, see D. E. Sprott, K. C. Manning, and A. Miyazaki, "Grocery Price Settings and Quantity Surcharges," *Journal of Marketing*, July 2003, *67*, 34–46.

15. Marn, M. V., and Rosiello, R. L. "Managing Price, Gaining Profit." *Harvard Business Review*, Sept.–Oct. 1992, pp. 84–94. See also G. J. Tellis, "Tackling the Retailer Decision Maze: Which Brands to Discount, How Much, When, and Why?" *Marketing Science*, 1995, *14*(3), 271–299; K. L. Ailawadi, S. A. Neslin, and K. Gedeak, "Pursuing the Value-Conscious Consumer: Store Brands Versus National Brand Promotions," *Journal of Marketing*, Jan. 2001, *65*, 71–89.

16. Clancy, K. J. "At What Profit Price?" *Brandweek*, June 23, 1997.

17. Spartos, C. "Sarafem Nation, Renamed Prozac Targets Huge Market: Premenstrual Women." *The Village Voice*, Dec. 6–12, 2000.

18. France, M. "Does Predatory Pricing Make Microsoft a Predator?" *BusinessWeek*, Nov. 23, 1998, pp. 130–132. See also J. P. Guiltinan and G. T. Gundlack, "Aggressive and Predatory Pricing: A Framework for Analysis." *Journal of Advertising*, July 1996, pp. 87–102.

19. For more information on specific types of price discrimination that are illegal, see H. Cheesman, *Contemporary Business Law*. Upper Saddle River, N.J.: Prentice Hall, 1995.

20. For a classic review, see K. B. Monroe, "Buyers' Subjective Perceptions of Price," *Journal of Marketing Research*, Feb. 1973, pp. 70–80. See also Z. J. Zhang, F. Feinberg, and A. Krishna, "Do We Care What Others Get? A Behaviorist Approach to Targeted Promotions," *Journal of Marketing Research*, Aug. 2002, *39*, 277–291.

21. Adapted from R. J. Dolan and H. Simon, "Power Pricers," *Across the Board*, May 1997, pp. 18–19.

22. Ailawadi, K. L., Lehmann, D. R., and Neslin, S. A. "Market Response to a Major Policy Change in the Marketing Mix: Learning from Procter & Gamble's Value Pricing Strategy," *Journal of Marketing*, Jan. 2001, *65*, 44–61.

23. Tarn, D. M., and others. "Physician Communication About the Cost and Acquisition of Newly Prescribed Medications." *American Journal of Managed Care*, 2006, *12*, 657–664.

CHAPTER TWELVE

1. For an insightful summary of academic research on this topic, see E. Anderson and A. T. Coughlan, "Channel Management: Structure, Governance, and Relationship Management." In B. Weitz and R. Wensley (eds.), *Handbook of Marketing*. London: Sage Publications, 2002. See also G. L. Frazier, "Organizing and Managing Channels of Distribution," *Journal of the Academy of Marketing Sciences*, 1999, *27*(2), 226–240.

2. Coughlan, A. T., Anderson, E., Stern, L. W., and El-Ansary, A. I. *Marketing Channels*, 6th ed. Upper Saddle River, N.J.: Prentice Hall, 1996.

3. Kotler, P., and Keller, K. L. *Marketing Management*, 12th ed. Upper Saddle River, N.J.: Prentice-Hall, 2006, p. 473.

4. For additional information on backward channels, see M. Jahre, "Household Waste Collection as a Reverse Channel: A Theoretical Perspective," *International Journal of Physical Distribution and Logistics*, 1995, *25*(2), 39–55; T. L. Pohlen and M. T. Farris II, "Reverse Logistics in Plastics Recycling," *International Journal of Physical Distribution and Logistics*, 1992, *22*(7), 35–37.

5. Bucklin, L. P. *Competition and Evolution in the Distributive Trades*. Upper Saddle River, N.J.: Prentice Hall, 1972. See also Coughlan, Anderson, Stern, and El-Ansary, *Marketing Channels*.

6. Bucklin, L. P. *A Theory of Distribution Channel Structure*. Berkeley, Calif.: Institute of Business and Economic Research, University of California, 1966.

7. For more on relationship marketing and the governance of marketing channels, see J. B. Heide, "Interorganizational Governance in Marketing Channels," *Journal of Marketing*, Jan. 1994, pp. 71–85.

8. Rosenbloom, B. *Marketing Channels: A Management View*, 5th ed. Hinsdale, Ill.: Dryden, 1995.

9. Anderson, E., and Coughlan, A. T. "Channel Management: Structure, Governance, and Relationship Management." In Weitz and Wensley (eds.), *Handbook of Marketing*.

10. For an excellent report on this issue, see H. Sutton, *Rethinking the Company's Selling and Distribution Channels*. New York: The Conference Board, 1986, Research Report No. 885.

11. Note that the terminology used in this section (which is in common use) is counter to that used for integration strategies; that is, *vertical* refers to a marketing channel with one or similar products, while *horizontal* refers to a channel with diverse offerings.

12. Johnston, R., and Lawrence, P. R. "Beyond Vertical Integration: The Rise of the Value-Adding Partnership," *Harvard Business Review*, July–Aug. 1988, pp. 94–101. See also J. A. Siguaw, P. M. Simpson, and T. L. Baker, "Effects of Supplier Market Orientation on Distributor Market Orientation and the Channel Relationship: The Distribution Perspective," *Journal of Marketing*, July 1998, pp. 99–111; N. Narayandas and M. U. Kalwani, "Long-Term Manufacturer—Supplier Relationships: Do They Pay Off for Supplier Firms?" *Journal of Marketing*, Jan. 1995, 1–16; A. Bovik and G. John, "When Does Vertical Coordination Improve Industrial Purchasing Relationships," *Journal of Marketing*, Oct. 2000, *64*, 52–64.

13. Coughlan, A. T., and Stern, L. W. "Marketing Channel Design and Management." In D. Iacobucci (ed.), *Kellogg on Marketing*. New York: Wiley, 2001.

14. This section draws on Stern and El-Ansary, *Marketing Channels*, ch. 6. See also J. D. Hibbard, N. Kumar, and L. W. Stern, "Examining the Impact of Destructive Acts in Marketing Channel Relationships," *Journal of Marketing Research*, Feb. 2001, *38*, 45–61; K. D. Antia and G. L. Frazier, "The Severity of Contract Enforcement in Interfirm Channel Relationships," *Journal of Marketing*, Oct. 2001, *65*, 67–81; J. R. Brown, C. S. Dev, and D.-J. Lee, "Managing Marketing Channel Opportunism: The Efficiency of Alternative Governance Mechanisms," *Journal of Marketing*, Apr. 2001, *64*, 51–65.

CHAPTER THIRTEEN

1. Some of these definitions are adapted from P. D. Bennett (ed.), *Dictionary of Marketing Terms* (Chicago: American Marketing Association, 1995).

2. Alba, J. W., and Hutchinson, J. W. "Dimensions of Consumer Expertise." *Journal of Consumer Research*, Mar. 1987, *13*, 411–453.

3. For an alternate communication model developed specifically for advertising communications, see B. B. Stern, "A Revised Communication Model for Advertising: Multiple Dimensions of the Source, the Message, and the Recipient," *Journal of Advertising*, June 1994, 5–15. For some additional perspectives, see T. Duncan and S. E. Moriarity, "A Communication-Based Marketing Model for Managing Relationships," *Journal of Marketing*, Apr. 1998, pp. 1–13.

4. Vakratsas, D., and Ambler, T. "How Advertising Works: What Do We Really Know." *Journal of Marketing*, Jan. 1999, *63*(1), 26–43.

5. The term *semantic differential* and the tool is described in C. E. Osgood, C. J. Suci, and P. H. Tannenbaum, *The Measurement of Meaning*. Urbana, Ill.: University of Illinois Press, 1957.

6. This section is based on J. R. Rossiter and L. Percy, *Advertising and Promotion Management*, 2nd ed. New York: McGraw-Hill, 1997.

7. Ibid.

8. Hovland, C. I., Lumsdaine, A. A., and Sheffield, F.D. *Experiments on Mass Communication*. Princeton, N.J.: Princeton University Press, 1949.

9. Engel, J. F., Blackwell, R. D., and Minard, P. W. *Consumer Behavior*, 9th ed. Fort Worth, Tex.: Dryden, 2001.

10. Crowley, A. E., and Hoyer, W. D. "An Integrative Framework for Understanding Two-Sided Persuasion." *Journal of Consumer Research*, Mar. 1994, pp. 561–574.

11. Hovland, Lumsdaine, and Sheffield, *Experiments on Mass Communication*, vol. 3, ch. 8; A. Crowley and W. Hoyer, "An Integrative Framework for Understanding Two-Sided Persuasion," *Journal of Consumer Research*, Mar. 1994, 561–574. For an alternative viewpoint, see G. E. Belch, "The Effects of Message Modality on One- and Two-Sided Advertising Messages." In R. P. Bagozzi and A. M. Tybout (eds.), *Advances in Consumer Research*. Ann Arbor, Mich.: Association for Consumer Research, 1983, pp. 21–26.

12. Haugtvedt, C. P., and Wegener, D. T. "Message Order Effects in Persuasion: An Attitude Strength Perspective." *Journal of Consumer Research*, June 1994, 205–218; Unnava, H. R., Burnkrant, R. E., and Erevelles, S. "Effects of Presentation Order and Communication Modality on Recall and Attitude." *Journal of Consumer Research*, Dec. 1994, pp. 481–490.

13. Sternthal, B., and Craig, C. S. *Consumer Behavior: An Information Processing Perspective*. Englewood Cliffs, N.J.: Prentice Hall, 1982, pp. 282–284.

14. Solomon, M. R. *Consumer Behavior*, 6th ed. Upper Saddle River, N.J.: Prentice Hall, 2004.

15. Kelman, H. C., and Hovland, C. I. "Reinstatement of the Communication in Delayed Measurement of Opinion Change." *Journal of Abnormal and Social Psychology*, 1953, *48*, 327–335.

16. Moore, D. J., Mowen, J. C., and Reardon, R. "Multiple Sources in Advertising Appeals: When Product Endorsers Are Paid by the Advertising Sponsor." *Journal of the Academy of Marketing Science*, Summer 1994, pp. 234–243.

17. Osgood, C. E., and Tannenbaum, P. H. "The Principles of Congruity in the Prediction of Attitude Change." *Psychological Review*, 1955, *62*, 42–55.

18. Berry, J., and Keller E. *The Influentials: One American in Ten Tells the Other Nine How to Vote, Where to Eat, and What to Buy*. New York: The Free Press, 2003.

19. *Advertising Ratios and Budgets Report*. Libertyville, Ill.: Schoenfeld & Associates, Inc., 2006, p. 30.

20. Kirmani, A. "The Effect of Perceived Advertising Costs on Brand Perceptions." *Journal of Consumer Research*, Sept. 1990, *17*, 160–171. See also A. Kirmani and P. Wright, "Money Talks: Perceived Advertising Expense and Expected Product Quality," *Journal of Consumer Research*, Dec. 1989, *16*, 344–353.

21. Vakratsas, D., and Ambler, T. "How Advertising Works: What Do We Really Know," *Journal of Marketing*, Jan. 1999, *63*(1), 26–43.

22. Schultz, D. E., Martin, D., and Brown, W. P. *Strategic Advertising Campaigns*. Chicago: Crain Books, 1984, pp. 192–197.

23. Chandy, R., Tellis, G. J., MacInnis, D., and Thaivanich, P. "What to Say When: Advertising Appeals in Evolving Markets." *Journal of Marketing Research*, Nov. 2001, *38*(4); Tellis, G. J., Chandy, R., and Thaivanich, P. "Decomposing the Effects of Direct Advertising: Which Brand Works, When, Where, and How Long?" *Journal of Marketing Research*, Feb. 2000, *37*, 32–46.

24. Weissman, J. S., and others. "Consumers' Reports on the Health Effects of Direct-to-Consumer Drug Advertising." *Health Affairs*, Web Exclusive, Feb. 26, 2003.

25. Schultz, D. E., Martin, D., and Brown, W. P. *Strategic Advertising Campaigns*. Chicago: Crain Books, 1984, p. 340.

26. Betzold, J. "Jaded Riders Are Ever-Tougher Sell." *Advertising Age*, July 9, 2001; McCarthy, M. "Ads Are Here, There, Everywhere." *USA Today*, June 19, 2001; Cheng, K. "Captivating Audiences." *Brandweek*, Nov. 29, 1999; McCarthy, M. "Critics Target 'Omnipresent' Ads." *USA Today*, Apr. 16, 2001.

27. Woltman Elpers, J. L. C. M., Wedel, M., and Pieters, R. G. M. "Why Do Consumers Stop Viewing Television Commercials? Two Experiments on the Influence of Moment-to-Moment Entertainment and Information Value." *Journal of Marketing Research*, Nov. 2003, *40*, 437–453.

28. Palda, K. S. *The Measurement of Cumulative Advertising Effect*. Upper Saddle River, N.J.: Prentice Hall, 1964, p. 87; Montgomery, D. B., and Silk, A. J. "Estimating Dynamic Effects of Market Communications Expenditures." *Management Science*, June 1972, pp. 485–501.

29. From R. C. Blattberg and S. A. Neslin, *Sales Promotion: Concepts, Methods, and Strategies* (Upper Saddle River, N.J.: Prentice Hall, 1990). See also S. Neslin, "Sales Promotion." In Weitz and Wensley, *Handbook of Marketing*, pp. 310–338.

30. Ailawadi, K., Gedenk, K., and Neslin, S. A. "Heterogeneity and Purchase Event Feedback in Choice Models: An Empirical Analysis with Implications for Model Building." *International Journal of Research in Marketing*, 1999, *16*, 177–198.

31. For a model for setting sales-promotions objectives, see D. B. Jones, "Setting Promotional Goals: A Communications Relationship Model," *Journal of Consumer Marketing*, 1994, *11*(1), 38–49.

32. Stern, A. "Measuring the Effectiveness of Package Goods Promotion Strategies." Paper presented to the Association of National Advertisers, Glen Cove, N.Y., Feb. 1978.

33. Dodson, J. A., Tybout, A. M., and Sternthal, B. "Impact of Deals and Deal Retraction on Brand Switching." *Journal of Marketing Research*, Feb. 1978, pp. 72–81.

34. Books on sales promotion include Totten and Block, *Analyzing Sales Promotion: Text and Cases* (Naples, Fla.: Dartnell Corporation, 1994); D. E. Schultz, W. A. Robinson, and L. A. Petrison, *Sales Promotion Essentials*, 2nd ed. Lincolnwood, Ill.: NTC Business Books, 1994; J. Wilmshurst, *Below-the-Line Promotion*. Oxford, England: Butterworth/Heinemann, 1993; R. C. Blattberg and S. A. Neslin, *Sales Promotion: Concepts, Methods, and Strategies*. Upper Saddle River, N.J.: Prentice Hall, 1990. For an expert systems

approach to sales promotion, see J. W. Keon and J. Bayer, "An Expert Approach to Sales Promotion Management," *Journal of Advertising Research*, June–July 1986, pp. 19–26.

35. For an excellent account, see Harris, *The Marketer's Guide to Public Relations*. See also Harris's *Value-Added Public Relations*.

36. Kotler, P., and Keller, K. L. *Marketing Management*, 12th ed. Upper Saddle River, N.J.: Prentice-Hall, 2006, p. 595.

37. "2004 Survey of Planners and Marketers: Summary Results from the Marketing and Planning Leadership Council's On-line Poll." Washington, D.C.: The Advisory Board Company, Fall 2004, p. 7.

38. Goldberg, S. S. "Sponsorship Boot Camp: How Sponsorship Works, What It's Worth, How to Get Results," presented by IEG, LLC, Mar. 3, 2007.

39. Kotler, P. "Atmospherics as a Marketing Tool." *Journal of Retailing*, Winter 1973–1974, pp. 48–64.

40. The Association of National Advertisers has a useful source, *Event Marketing: A Management Guide*, available at http://www.ana.net/publications/cmssearch.

41. Catherwood, D. W., and Van Kirk, R. L. *The Complete Guide to Special Event Management*. New York: Wiley, 1992.

42. Shankin, W. L., and Kuzma, J. "Buying That Sporting Image." *Marketing Management*, Spring 1992, p. 65.

43. Moran, W. T. "Insights from Pricing Research." In E. B. Bailey (ed.), *Pricing Practices and Strategies*, pp. 7–13. New York: The Conference Board, 1978.

44. Shultz, D. E., Tannenbaum, S. I., and Lauterborn, R. F. *Integrated Marketing Communications: Putting It Together and Making It Work*. Lincolnwood, Ill.: NTC Business Books, 1992; Schultz, D. E., and Schultz, H. *IMC, The Next Generation: Five Steps For Delivering Value and Measuring Financial Returns*. New York: McGraw-Hill, 2003.

45. Keller, K. L. *Strategic Brand Management*, 2nd ed. Upper Saddle River, N.J.: Prentice Hall, 2003.

CHAPTER FOURTEEN

1. Mount, I. "Marketing," *Business 2.0*, Aug.–Sept. 2001, p. 84.

2. "An Introduction to Word of Mouth Marketing." Word of Mouth Marketing Association. [http://www.womma.org/wom101/]. May 2007.

3. Ibid.

4. Brown, J. J., and Reingen, P. H. "Social Ties and Word-of-Mouth Referral," *Journal of Consumer Research*, Dec. 1987, *14*, 350–362; E. M. Rogers, *Diffusion of Innovations*, 4th ed. New York: Free Press, 1995; R. Dye, "The Buzz on Buzz," *Harvard Business Review*, Nov.–Dec. 2000, p. 139; S. R. Herriott, "Identifying and Developing Referral Channels," *Management Decision*, 1992, *30*(1), 4–9; P. H. Riengen and J. B. Kernan, "Analysis of Referral Networks in Marketing: Methods and Illustration," *Journal of Marketing Research*, Nov. 1986, pp. 37–78; J. R. Wilson, *Word of Mouth Marketing*. New York: Wiley, 1991; M. E. Cafferky, "Michael E. Cafferky's Free Word-of-Mouth Marketing Tips." [http://www.geocities.com/wallstreet/6246]. May 2007. See also E. Rosen, *The Anatomy of Buzz*. New York: Doubleday, 2000; M. Gladwell, *The Tipping Point: How Little Things Can Make a Big Difference*. Boston: Little, Brown, 2000.

5. Dye, "The Buzz on Buzz," pp. 139–146.

6. Cafferky, M. E. *Let Your Customers Do the Talking*. Chicago: Dearborn Financial Publishing, 1995.

7. Batelle, J. "The Net of Influence." *Business 2.0*, Mar. 2004, p. 70.

8. Meyer, A. "Word-of-Mouth Marketing Speaks Well for Small Business." *Chicago Tribune*, July 28, 2003.

9. Rosen, E. *The Anatomy of Buzz*. New York: Currency, 2000, ch. 12, "Viral Marketing." *Sales & Marketing Automation*, Nov. 1999, pp. 12–14; Silverman, G. *The Secrets of Word-of-Mouth Marketing*. New York: Amacom, 2001.

10. Neff, J. "Spam Research Reveals Disgust With Pop-Up Ads." *Advertising Age*, Aug. 25, 2003, pp. 1, 21.

11. Godin, S. *Permission Marketing: Turning Strangers into Friends and Friends into Customers*. New York: Simon & Schuster, 1999.

12. Dye, R. "The Buzz on Buzz." Harvard Business School Working Knowledge for Business Leaders. [http://hbswk.hbs.edu/archive/1956.html]. Jan. 29, 2001.

13. Gladwell, M. *The Tipping Point: How Little Things Can Make a Big Difference*. Boston: Little, Brown, 2000.

14. "Word of Mouth 101: Positive Word of Mouth Marketing Strategies." Word of Mouth Marketing Association. [http://www.womma.org/wom101/05/]. May 2007.

15. Adapted from R. N. McMurry, "The Mystique of Super-Salesmanship," *Harvard Business Review*, Mar.–Apr. 1961, p. 114. See also W. C. Moncrief III, "Selling Activity and Sales Position Taxonomies for Industrial Salesforces," *Journal of Marketing Research*, Aug. 1986, pp. 261–270.

16. Albers, S. "Salesforce Management—Compensation, Motivation, Selection, and Training." In B. Weitz and R. Wensley (eds.), *Handbook of Marketing*, pp. 248–266. London: Sage Publications, 2002.

17. "The Number of Medical Sales Reps in U.S. to Grow by 24% in 2007." [http://www.przoom.com/news/9962/]. Oct. 26, 2006.

18. Churchill, G. A. Jr., Ford, N. M., and Walker, O. C. Jr. *Sales Force Management: Planning, Implementation and Control*, 4th ed. Homewood, Ill.: Irwin, 1993. See also J. Chowdhury, "The Motivational Impact of Sales Quotas on Effort," *Journal of Marketing Research*, Feb. 1993, pp. 28–41; M. K. Mantrala, P. Sinha, and A. A. Zoltners, "Structuring a Multiproduct Sales Quota-Bonus Plan for a Heterogeneous Sales Force: A Practical Model-Based Approach," *Marketing Science*, 1994, *13*(2), 121–144; W. Chu, E. Gerstner, and J. D. Hess, "Costs and Benefits of Hard-Sell," *Journal of Marketing Research*, Feb. 1995, pp. 97–102; M. Krafft, "In Empirical Investigation of the Antecedents of Sales Force Control Systems," *Journal of Marketing*, July 1999, *63*, 120–134.

19. See P. Kotler, N. Rackham, and S. Krishnaswamy, "Ending the War Between Sales and Marketing," *Harvard Business Review*, July 2006.

20. As a detailed discussion of negotiation principles is beyond the scope of this book, we recommend L. L. Thompson, *The Mind and Heart of the Negotiator*, 3rd ed. Upper Saddle River, N.J.: Pearson Prentice Hall, 2005; and R. Fisher, W. Ury, and B. Patton, *Getting to Yes*. New York: Random House Business Books, 2003.

21. "Sales Force Effectiveness: Getting It Right." [www.eyeforpharma.com]. Dec. 2004.

22. "Revamp, Cut Its Main Sales Force." *Wall Street Journal*, June 20, 2005.

23. Hendrick, B. "Self Diagnosis from TV Drug Ads Can Be Dangerous." *Atlanta Journal Constitution*, Jan. 8, 2007.

24. Kravitz, R. L., and others. "Direct-to-Consumer Advertising May Influence Physicians' Prescribing Decisions." *Journal of the American Medical Association*, 2005, *293*, 1995–2002.

25. Nash, E. L. *Direct Marketing: Strategy, Planning, Execution*, 3rd ed. New York: McGraw-Hill, 1995.

26. Ansari, A., and Mela, C. F. "E-Customization." *Journal of Marketing Research*, May 2003, *40*(2), 131–145.

27. Smith, D. L., and McFee, K. "Media Mix 101: Online Media for Traditional Marketers." [http://advantage.msn.com/articles/MediaMix101_2.asp.]. Sept. 2003.

28. Rayport, J. E., and Jaworski, B. J. *E-Commerce*. New York: McGraw-Hill, 2001, p. 116.

29. Tedeschi, B. "E-Commerce Report." *New York Times*, June 24, 2002, p. C8.

30. "Prime Clicking Time." *Economist*, May 31, 2003, p. 65; Elgin, B. "Search Engines Are Picking Up Steam." *BusinessWeek*, Mar. 24, 2003, pp. 86–87.

31. Desmond, N. "Google's Next Runaway Success." *Business 2.0*, Nov. 2002, p. 73.

32. Godin, *Permission Marketing: Turning Strangers into Friends and Friends into Customers*.

33. Schoenberger, C. R. "Web? What Web?" *Forbes*, June 10, 2002, p. 132.

CHAPTER FIFTEEN

1. Bonoma, T. V. *The Marketing Edge: Making Strategies Work*. New York: The Free Press, 1985. Much of this section is based on Bonoma's work.

2. Goodman, S. R. *Increasing Corporate Profitability*. New York: Ronald Press, 1982, ch. 1. See also B. J. Jaworski, V. Stathakopoulos, and H. S. Krishnan, "Control Combinations in Marketing: Conceptual Framework and Empirical Evidence," *Journal of Marketing*, Jan. 1993, pp. 57–69.

3. For further discussion of this instrument, see P. Kotler, "From Sales Obsession to Marketing Effectiveness," *Harvard Business Review*, Nov.–Dec. 1977, pp. 67–75.

4. Kotler, P., Gregor, W., and Rodgers, W. "The Marketing Audit Comes of Age," *Sloan Management Review*, Winter 1989, pp. 49–62.

INDEX